W9-CIN-113

Second Edition

THE CRITICALLY ILL CHILD

Diagnosis and Management

Edited by

CLEMENT A. SMITH, M.D.

Editor of **Pediatrics**, *1962–1973;*

Professor of Pediatrics, Emeritus,
Boston Hospital for Women, Lying-In Division;
Harvard Medical School,
Boston, Massachusetts

Based on articles appearing in *Pediatrics,*
The Journal of the American Academy of Pediatrics

W. B. SAUNDERS COMPANY
Philadelphia, London, Toronto

W. B. Saunders Company: West Washington Square
                           Philadelphia, PA   19105

                           1 St. Anne's Road
                           Eastbourne, East Sussex BN21 3UN, England

                           1 Goldthorne Avenue
                           Toronto, Ontario M8Z 5T9, Canada

The Critically Ill Child   ISBN   0-7216-8385-1

© 1977 by the W. B. Saunders Company.   Copyright 1972 by W. B. Saunders Company.
Copyright under the International Copyright Union.   All rights reserved.   This book is
protected by copyright.   No part of it may be reproduced, stored in a retrieval system or
transmitted in any form or by any means, electronic, mechanical, photocopying, recording
or otherwise, without written permission from the publisher.   Made in the United States
of America.   Press of W. B. Saunders Company.   Library of Congress catalogue card
number 76-014688.

Last digit is the print number: 9   8   7   6   5   4   3   2

CONTRIBUTORS

MYRON L. BELFER, M.D.

Assistant Professor of Psychiatry, Harvard Medical School. Associate in Psychiatry, Children's Hospital Medical Center, Boston, Massachusetts.
Psychiatric Emergencies

C. WARREN BIERMAN, M.D.

Clinical Professor of Pediatrics, University of Washington Medical School. Chief, Division of Allergy, Children's Orthopedic Hospital and Medical Center, Seattle, Washington.
Status Asthmaticus; Anaphylaxis

LILLIAN R. BLACKMON, M.D.

Assistant Professor of Pediatrics, Assistant Professor of Obstetrics and Gynecology, and Kenan-McBryde Scholar in Neonatology, Duke University Medical Center. Attending Neonatologist, Duke University Medical Center, Duke Hospital, Director of Nurseries, Duke Hospital, Durham, North Carolina.
Respiratory Distress

ALFRED M. BONGIOVANNI, M.D.

Formerly Professor of Pediatrics, University of Pennsylvania. Children's Hospital of Philadelphia, Philadelphia, Pennsylvania. Dean and Professor of Endocrinology, Catholic University of Puerto Rico, Ponce, Puerto Rico.
Acute Adrenal Insufficiency

GEORGE W. BRUMLEY, M.D.

Associate Professor of Pediatrics, Assistant Professor of Obstetrics and Gynecology, and Co-Director, Division of Perinatal Medicine, Duke University Medical Center. Attending Neonatologist,

Duke University Medical Center, Duke Hospital, Durham, North Carolina.
Respiratory Distress

GEORGE R. BUCHANAN, M.D.

Instructor, Harvard Medical School. Assistant in Medicine (Hematology-Oncology), Children's Hospital Medical Center, Boston, Massachusetts.
Bleeding in the Newborn

SIDNEY CARTER, M.D.

Professor of Neurology and Pediatrics, College of Physicians and Surgeons, Columbia University. Attending Neurologist, Presbyterian Hospital, New York, New York.
Status Epilepticus

ROBERT O. CHRISTIANSEN, M.D.

Professor of Pediatrics, Charles R. Drew Postgraduate Medical School. Director, Inpatient Services, Martin Luther King Jr. General Hospital, Los Angeles, California.
Hypoglycemia

ARNOLD G. CORAN, M.D.

Professor of Surgery, University of Michigan School of Medicine. Head of the Section of Pediatric Surgery, University of Michigan Medical Center, Ann Arbor, Michigan.
Intravenous Alimentation

JOHN D. CRAWFORD, M.D.

Associate Professor of Pediatrics, Harvard Medical School. Chief Pediatrician, Shriners Burns Institute, and Chief, Endocrine-Metabolic Unit, Children's Service, Massachusetts General Hospital, Boston, Massachusetts.
Burns

DEAN CROCKER, M.D.

Assistant Professor, Harvard University Medical School. Director of Respiratory Therapy and Associate in Anesthesia, Children's Hospital Medical Center, Boston, Massachusetts. Director of Anesthesia, Massachusetts Hospital School, Canton, Massachusetts.
Tracheostomy

JOHN B. DAS, M.D.

Principal Associate in Surgery, Harvard Medical School. Research Associate in Surgery, Children's Hospital Medical Center, Boston, Massachusetts.
Intravenous Alimentation

DARRYL C. DEVIVO, M.D.

Associate Professor, Departments of Pediatrics and Neurology, Washington University School of Medicine, St. Louis, Missouri. Associate Pediatrician, Division of Neurology, St. Louis Children's Hospital, and Associate Neurologist, Barnes and Allied Hospitals, St. Louis, Missouri.
Head Injury

LOUIS K. DIAMOND, M.D.

Adjunct Professor of Pediatrics, University of California, San Francisco Medical Center. Emeritus Professor of Pediatrics, Harvard Medical School. Pediatric Hematologist, Moffitt Hospital, San Francisco, California.
Sickle Cell Disease

PHILIP R. DODGE, M.D.

Professor of Pediatrics and Neurology, The Edward Mallinckrodt Department of Pediatrics, Washington University School of Medicine, St. Louis, Missouri. Medical Director, St. Louis Children's Hospital, St. Louis, Missouri.
Head Injury

ROBERT M. FILLER, M.D.

Associate Professor of Surgery at Children's Hospital Medical Center, Harvard Medical School. Chief of Clinical Surgery, Children's Hospital Medical Center, Boston, Massachusetts.
Intravenous Alimentation

LAURENCE FINBERG, M.D.

Professor of Pediatrics, Albert Einstein College of Medicine, Bronx, New York. Chairman, Department of Pediatrics, Montefiore Hospital and Medical Center, Bronx, New York.
Dehydration Secondary to Diarrhea

BERTIL E. GLADER, M.D., Ph.D.

Associate Professor of Pediatrics, Stanford University School of Medicine, Stanford, California.
Bleeding in the Newborn

ARNOLD P. GOLD, M.D.

Professor of Clinical Neurology and Pediatrics, College of Physicians and Surgeons, Columbia University. Attending Neurologist and Pediatrician, Presbyterian Hospital, Columbia-Presbyterian Medical Center, New York, New York.
Status Epilepticus

DAVID GOLDRING, M.D.

Professor of Pediatrics, Washington University School of Medicine. Director of Pediatric Cardiology, St. Louis Children's Hospital, St. Louis, Missouri.
Cardiac Failure

STEPHEN I. GOODMAN, M.D., C.M.

Associate Professor of Pediatrics, University of Colorado Medical Center, Denver, Colorado.
Acute Metabolic Disease

ROBERT E. GREENBERG, M.D.

Professor and Chairman, Department of Pediatrics, University of New Mexico School of Medicine, Albuquerque, New Mexico.
Hypoglycemia

ALEXIS F. HARTMANN, JR., M.D.

Professor of Pediatrics, Washington University School of Medicine. Staff Cardiologist, St. Louis Children's Hospital, St. Louis, Missouri.
Cardiac Failure

WILLIAM E. HATHAWAY, M.D.

Professor of Pediatrics, University of Colorado School of Medicine. Attending Pediatric Hematologist, University of Colorado Medical Center, Denver, Colorado.
Disseminated Intravascular Coagulation

ANTONIO HERNANDEZ, M.D.

Assistant Professor of Pediatrics, Washington University School of Medicine. Staff Cardiologist, St. Louis Children's Hospital, St. Louis, Missouri.
Cardiac Failure

JOHN T. HERRIN, M.B.B.S.

Assistant Professor of Pediatrics, Harvard Medical School. Chief, Pediatric Nephrology Unit, Massachusetts General Hospital, Associate Pediatrician, Massachusetts General Hospital, and Assistant Pediatrician, Shriners Burns Institute, Boston, Massachusetts.
Burns

HORACE L. HODES, M.D.

Herbert Lehman Professor and Chairman, Department of Pediatrics, Mount Sinai School of Medicine of the City University of

New York. Pediatrician-in-Chief, Mount Sinai Hospital, New York, New York.
Endotoxin Shock

MALCOLM A. HOLLIDAY, M.D.

Professor of Pediatrics, University of California, San Francisco. Chief, Renal Electrolyte Division, University of California Hospital, San Francisco, and San Francisco General Hospital, San Francisco, California.
Acute Renal Failure

JOHN M. LEEDOM, M.D.

Hastings Professor of Medicine, University of Southern California, School of Medicine. Head, Infectious Diseases Division, Department of Medicine, Los Angeles County–University of Southern California Medical Center, Los Angeles, California.
Acute Bacterial Meningitis

ALLEN W. MATHIES, JR., M.D., Ph.D.

Professor of Pediatrics and Dean, University of Southern California, School of Medicine. Pediatric Staff, Los Angeles County–University of Southern California Medical Center and Children's Hospital of Los Angeles, Los Angeles, California.
Acute Bacterial Meningitis

DONOUGH O'BRIEN, M.D.

Professor of Pediatrics, University of Colorado Medical Center, Denver, Colorado.
Acute Metabolic Disease

SHELDON ORLOFF, M.D.

Clinical Associate, Section on Biochemical and Developmental Genetics, Infant and Perinatal Branch, National Institute of Health, Bethesda, Maryland.
Acute Renal Failure

HOWARD A. PEARSON, M.D.

Professor and Chairman, Department of Pediatrics, Yale University School of Medicine. Chief of Pediatrics and Attending Physician, Yale–New Haven Hospital, New Haven, Connecticut.
Sickle Cell Disease

WILLIAM E. PIERSON, M.D.

Associate Clinical Professor of Pediatrics and Associate Director,

Pulmonary Center, Children's Orthopedic Hospital and Medical Center, Seattle, Washington.
Status Asthmaticus

DONALD E. POTTER, M.D.

Assistant Professor of Pediatrics, University of California, San Francisco.
Acute Renal Failure

ROBERT L. REPLOGLE, M.D.

Professor, The University of Chicago–Pritzker School of Medicine. Attending Surgeon and Head, Section of Cardiac Surgery, The University of Chicago Hospitals and Clinics, Chicago, Illinois.
Trauma and Shock

HERNAN M. REYES, M.D.

Associate Professor of Surgery, The University of Chicago–Pritzker School of Medicine. Attending Surgeon, University of Chicago Hospitals and Clinics, Chicago, Illinois.
Trauma and Shock

ROBERT SCHWARTZ, M.D.

Professor of Pediatrics, Brown University Program in Medicine. Director of Pediatric Metabolism and Nutrition, Rhode Island Hospital, Providence, Rhode Island.
Diabetic Ketoacidosis and Coma

WILLIAM E. SEGAR, M.D.

Professor and Chairman, University of Wisconsin School of Medicine. Chairman of Pediatrics, University of Wisconsin Hospitals, Madison, Wisconsin.
Salicylate Intoxication

GAIL G. SHAPIRO, M.D.

Clinical Assistant Professor of Pediatrics, University of Washington. Attending Physician, University Hospital and Children's Orthopedic Hospital and Medical Center, Seattle, Washington.
Status Asthmaticus

F. ESTELLE SIMONS, M.D.

Assistant Professor of Pediatrics, University of Manitoba, Winnipeg. Head, Section of Allergy and Clinical Immunology, Department of Pediatrics, University of Manitoba, Winnipeg, Manitoba.
Status Asthmaticus

ROBERT M. SMITH, M.D., F.F.A.R.C.S.I.(Hon.)

Chief of Anesthesiology, Children's Hospital Medical Center, Boston, Massachusetts.
Respiratory Arrest

CHARLES TREY, M.B., Ch.B., M.D.

Associate Clinical Professor, Harvard Medical School. Chief, Section Gastroenterology, New England Deaconess Hospital, and Consultant, Children's Hospital Medical Center, Boston, Massachusetts.
Acute Hepatic Failure

PAUL F. WEHRLE, M.D.

Hastings Professor of Pediatrics, University of Southern California, School of Medicine. Director of Professional Services, Pediatric Pavilion, Los Angeles County–University of Southern California Medical Center, Los Angeles, California.
Acute Bacterial Meningitis

PREFACE
TO THE SECOND EDITION

The suggestion of the publisher that a new and revised edition be prepared came surprisingly soon after the first edition was in print. Yet knowledge useful in the treatment of acute illness should perhaps find its way into general circulation more rapidly than knowledge concerning chronic disease is either originated or disseminated. Valuable information may at first be known only to a few, and moreover, the physician may be tempted to adopt potentially dangerous misinformation, as yet untested, in a sufficiently urgent situation. Early revision therefore seems justified. That the publisher is right is confirmed by the amount of new material and the number of recent references received from many of the authors. Some chapters have been completely rewritten. Three new ones have been added, on critical problems not previously covered: bleeding in the newborn infant, status asthmaticus, and certain emotional disturbances of children that may confront the pediatric generalist with particular urgency. Gratitude is therefore expressed to a growing list of contributors.

CLEMENT A. SMITH, M.D.

PREFACE TO THE FIRST EDITION

Life is Short and the Art Long
The Occasion Instant
Experiment Perilous
Decision Difficult

Carved in stone on the wall of at least one medical school, the familiar words have given generations of medical students an unforgettable explanation of purpose. Many may have found such instant occasions less common than they expected in subsequent professional life. Some may wish their educations had given them wisdom and fortitude for the chronic situation rather than resourcefulness for the instant occasion. Nevertheless, all of us, if worth our salt, carry through life the hope of responding quickly and correctly to the critical problems that come our way.

Hence, when Dr. Morris Green, whose own writings have illuminated the area of less acute but often more trying disease, suggested to PEDIATRICS these articles on The Critically Ill Child, response was enthusiastic. Few of those asked to contribute did not rise to the challenge. Subscribers welcomed the monthly appearance of at least one article they could call "practical," because useful in the kind of pediatrics they hoped to practice. Now, through the interest of the W. B. Saunders Company, and with the particular assistance of Mr. Robert B. Rowan, these papers are here made available in one volume. May it help to reduce the peril of experiment and the difficulty of decision.

CLEMENT A. SMITH, M.D.
Editor, PEDIATRICS

CONTENTS

Chapter One

MANAGEMENT OF TRAUMA AND SHOCK IN THE PEDIATRIC PATIENT

ROBERT L. REPLOGLE, M.D.,

HERNAN M. REYES, M.D.

INTRODUCTION

Trauma has long been known to be the leading single killer of children, but the magnitude of its impact is not generally appreciated. Motor vehicle accidents caused the death of 8500 children under the age of 14 years in 1966, and nontransport accidents were responsible for the death of 9000 more, a total of 17,500 deaths from trauma. Contrast this to asthma, which was responsible for 150 deaths in the same age group that year, and pneumonia (7600 deaths), the anemias (360 deaths), malignant neoplasms of all kinds (4200 deaths), heart disease (900 deaths), and congenital malformations of all kinds, which were the cause of 14,000 deaths.[1] With the increasing popularity of the motorcycle and the snowmobile, these figures probably will become even more impressive.[2] The economics of accidental injury are of secondary importance, but it has been estimated that the cost of death and disability from trauma amounts to $17 billion for the 50 million Americans injured each year.[3]

When the severely injured patient is brought into the emergency room, it is desirable that extensive resources be available immediately. Since 50 per cent of traffic accidents occur between 1:00 P.M. on Friday

From the Section of Pediatric Surgery and the Department of Surgery, Pritzker School of Medicine of the University of Chicago, Chicago, Illinois.

and 9:00 A.M. on Monday, it is essential that emergency medical coverage be available 7 days a week, 24 hours a day.[4] The need for methods of transporting trauma victims expeditiously to facilities which have the capability for comprehensive management is emphasized by the study of Waller,[5] who found that the death rate from motor vehicle accidents was substantially higher in rural areas (47 per 100,000 population) than in urban areas (17 per 100,000), even though the extent of the injuries that led to death in the rural accidents was of the same severity as the urban accidents, or even less.

While it is unrealistic to overgeneralize on this kind of study, the implication is that the rural patients remained at the scene of the accident for a longer period, and then, perhaps, were taken to a hospital of limited resources. However, rapid and effective ambulance service is not entirely the answer, as is illustrated by the Philadelphia study,[4] which noted that in 794 traffic fatalities 50 per cent died at the scene of the accident and 72 per cent died either at the scene, in transit, or during the first 10 minutes of hospitalization. It seems apparent that efforts at salvage must begin before hospitalization. Well-designed transport vans engineered specifically for children have been described, and experience has demonstrated the value of such a system.[6] The experience with helicopter evacuation in Vietnam has been very favorable, and several centers are experimenting with the use of this method for civilian injuries.

A basic requirement for emergency care is to provide trained ambulance crews to transport the injured to the designated hospital. These people should be trained in pulmonary resuscitation, techniques of stopping hemorrhage, splinting of extremities, and so on. At least one hospital in a community should be identified as an emergency receiving facility so that its emergency room can be fully prepared and equipped. The widespread custom of transporting patients to the nearest medical facility is not an efficient system, since it means either that every hospital must provide equal resources at the expense of duplication, or that some of them have inadequate facilities. The nurses in the emergency room and the house staff in a teaching institution must be instructed in the treatment of shock and trauma; if the number of real emergencies is not adequate to keep the team smoothly coordinated, nursing in-service education and the staff physicians must regularly be concerned with continuing education. Ideally, coverage by pediatricians, surgeons, orthopedic surgeons, anesthesiologists, neurosurgeons, urologists, and vascular surgeons makes the professional care comprehensive. If a small but strategically located hospital cannot support this large complement of specialists, it is not only possible but necessary to obtain prompt consultation using modern communication devices, provided that the organizational groundwork has been completed previously.

EMERGENCY FACILITIES

As in all areas of medical practice, elegant facilities and equipment are no substitute for well-trained, thoughtful professionals, doctors and nurses. The preparedness and competence of the emergency room staff should be continuously under surveillance.

In each emergency area, all the equipment and supplies necessary for resuscitation in trauma must be maintained, and checked each shift for completeness. The make-up of this resuscitation equipment may vary according to local requirements, but it must always be ready. For a guide, the emergency equipment in our unit is as follows:

General Equipment

1. Direct current defibrillator, with a range from 20 to 400 watt-seconds.
2. Infant (3 cm), pediatric (5 cm), and adult (10 cm) external defibrillator paddles.
3. Electrocardiogram (EKG) machine.
4. Two venous cutdown trays.
5. One tracheostomy tray.
6. One small general surgical tray with abdominal and thoracic retractors.
7. Sphygmomanometer and arm cuffs of various sizes.
8. Blood pressure measuring device, ultrasonic (see further on).

Respiratory Equipment

1. Tracheostomy tubes, sizes 000, 00, 0, 1, 2, 3 and 4 — two each, plastic.
2. Oropharyngeal airways, sizes 0, 1, 2, 3 and 4 — two each.
3. Endotracheal tubes, with connectors, sizes 10 to 26 French, sterile — two each.
4. Laryngoscope, standard handle, extra batteries and bulbs.
5. Laryngeal blades, small straight for infant, Foregger or Flagg for child, and MacIntosh for adult.
6. Hope or Ambu ventilating bag.
7. Various sized face masks for infant or adult.
8. Standard portable suction machine.
9. Oxygen tanks or wall oxygen outlet.
10. Metal tonsil type suction tube. Sterile plastic suction catheters, sizes 5, 8, 10, and 14 French.

Supplies

1. Sterile needles and syringes, including intracardiac needles (22 gauge, 6 cm in length).
2. Plastic intravenous catheters (some at least 40 cm in length), 14, 16, 18, and 20 gauge.
3. Scalp vein needles.
4. Tongue blades.
5. Gauze sponges, alcohol sponges.
6. Antibiotic ointment.
7. Intravenous connection tubing, with and without blood filter.
8. Blood scale and pressure infusor for blood. Calibrated burettes.
9. Three-way stopcocks.
10. Chest tubes, sizes 12, 16, 20, and 24 French (preferably the type with a disposable trocar in the tube).
11. Small tubing for arterial cutdown (size 50 PE — polyethylene — and 90 PE).
12. Needle stub adaptors — 12, 18, 20, and 22 gauge.
13. Knife blades — sizes 10 and 15.
14. Suture material, synthetic and catgut — some with various sized swaged-on needles.

Drugs

1. Sodium bicarbonate — several vials 1 mEq/ml (usual initial dose 2 to 4 mEq/kg repeated each 10 minutes until arterial pH is measured).
2. Epinephrine — several vials, 1:10,000 conc., 0.1 mg/ml (usual dose 0.1 ml/kg by push).
3. Isoproterenol — 0.2 to 0.4 mg/100 ml (usual initial dose 1 to 2 ml, then continuous slow infusion).
4. Dopamine — 200-mg vial (usual dose 10 mcg/kg/min).
5. Calcium chloride — 10 per cent conc., 100 mg/ml (usual dose 0.2 ml/kg).
6. Solutions — 5 per cent serum albumin, 6 per cent dextran (70,000 mol wt), 10 per cent dextran (40,000 mol wt), lactated Ringer's solution, normal saline, dextrose, and water.

MONITORING TECHNIQUE AND INITIAL TREATMENT

Shock in the child is nearly always the result of blood (or fluid) loss, or infection, and frequently the patient has multiple injuries or more than one likely cause for circulatory or respiratory embarrassment. The first objective of the physician is to sort out the various problems quickly so that priorities for treatment can be established. Usually in the severely injured child, several resuscitative measures may be needed simultaneously, and even the most experienced physician should call for help as soon as he or she recognizes the seriousness of the situation.

If the patient is brought in without heartbeat and is making no resuscitative efforts, an instant decision must be made as to whether to attempt resuscitation at all. Unfortunately, there are no infallible signs of brain death that are instantly applicable, and this decision has to be based on "clinical judgment," perhaps by taking a quick history from the parents or ambulance attendants who brought the patient to the hospital. They may be able, for instance, to tell the physician when the child stopped breathing spontaneously, or when the pulse ceased. The stethoscope is a more reliable guide to the presence of a heartbeat in the child than in the adult, but nevertheless an electrocardiographic signal is of utmost importance. If the patient has airway obstruction and still maintains a heartbeat, then either endotracheal intubation or positive pressure ventilation with a mask and oxygen is of primary importance. (It is unwise for the inexperienced physician to spend much time trying to insert an endotracheal tube, since the child nearly always can be well ventilated with the mask and bag.) After respiration has been reestablished, massive hemorrhage should be controlled by the application of manual pressure and unstable fractures splinted.

At the first chance, one nurse should be designated to start a chart on the patient, recording at frequent intervals the vital signs, pupil size and reaction, and the fluids and drugs given. A "systems-oriented" chart which delineates the time and type of treatment for each specific injury in a patient with multiple injuries is of great help in avoiding the confusion that may follow in the aftermath of the initial resuscitation, particularly when more than one patient is received at a time.[7] A second nurse should be assigned the task of connecting a monitor or EKG machine to the patient and preparing the drugs that may be required for cardiac resuscitation, *labeling* each syringe. (The coordination of this team effort is vital, and the most experienced member of the team should assume charge, since without direction the whole scene may degenerate into an unbelievable shambles.) In most instances, the rapid infusion of blood, fluids, or drugs will be essential, and the physician should quickly establish one or more routes for venous infusion. In the child this is best accomplished by cutdown of the greater saphenous vein at the ankle and insertion of a large bore catheter.[8] (Efforts at introducing a needle or catheter percutaneously into a collapsed peripheral vein in a child usually will be very difficult, and unless it is obvious that success is likely, little time should be wasted making multiple attempts.)

One should remember that direct injection of drugs into the heart is a very useful maneuver when time is critical. A 22-gauge 6-cm needle introduced parasternally at the left fifth intercostal space, with the tip of the needle directed toward the posterior right axilla, will enter the right ventricle most of the time. This has been done here on many occasions with no cause found, as yet, for discontinuing this technique. If the patient is injured severely, a catheter should be introduced into the bladder and a central venous pressure line inserted. If the catheter does not pass easily into the bladder, or if there is a pelvic injury, or both, the possibility of a urethral injury must be considered and possibly investigated further.

One needs as much information about the hemodynamic and respiratory status of the patient as it is possible to obtain if a sound evaluation of the effectiveness of treatment is to be made. However, enthusiasm for collecting physiological and biochemical data must be tempered with concern for the clinical progress of the patient, and relatively few measurements are really of practical importance. It is essential to know the arterial blood pressure, but an accurate blood pressure may be difficult to obtain by auscultatory methods in the hypotensive patient. Cohn found that the blood pressure obtained by arm cuff in 39 hypotensive patients averaged 33 mm Hg less than the blood pressure obtained directly by intra-arterial needle puncture, and ranged from 164 mm Hg less to 20 mm Hg more than directly measured pressure.[9] Since it frequently is desirable to have samples of arterial blood for pH, Po_2 and Pco_2 measurements, as well as accurate blood pressure measurements, in most severely injured patients an arterial catheter should be introduced into the radial artery by direct cutdown (Fig. 1). In the infant a #50 PE tube is the proper size for the radial artery, and in the child over 1 year of age, a #90 PE catheter will fit. Continuous infusion of 2 to 3 ml of heparinized lactated Ringer's solution (1000 units heparin per 500 ml solution) per hour can be achieved conveniently using a critical orifice infusion device* or by a constant infusion pump and patency can be maintained for prolonged periods even in the smallest infant. We have performed a great many radial artery catheterizations without a single serious complication. In the newborn an umbilical artery catheter may be used for blood gas monitoring as well as for arterial pressure measurements. If the child is more than 1 day old, a cutdown can be made using an infraumbilical semicircular incision, and either umbilical artery can be dissected free and cannulated without difficulty. A 3.5 to 5 French umbilical artery catheter is introduced into the umbilical artery and directed toward the aorta, and the tip placed just below the level of the diaphragm. The po-

---

*CFS Intraflow, Sorenson Research Co., 4387 Atherton Drive, Salt Lake City, Utah, 84115.

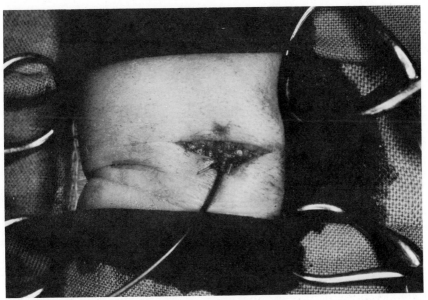

Figure 1. A radial artery catheter can be inserted in even the smallest infant and will provide really meaningful information on arterial Po_2, Pco_2, pH, and blood pressure.

tential complications of this technique must be recognized,[10] and their severity tends to make us prefer peripheral arterial sites. In the older infant, if the radial artery fails, an excellent substitute would be either of the superficial temporal arteries, which can be cannulated with a size #90 PE catheter. A satisfactory substitute for direct intra-arterial blood pressure measurement is provided either by measuring the beginning of blood flow following cuff occlusion, using the transcutaneous Doppler ultrasonic flowmeter,[11] or by Doppler ultrasonic detection of arterial wall motion.[12] Both these techniques give reliable measurements in hypotensive patients of all ages. (It may be redundant to point out that the average systolic pressure during the first week of life is 80 mm Hg, and a systolic pressure of 60 mm Hg during this period may be perfectly normal.[13]) Incidentally, the Doppler flowmeter is extremely valuable in the injured child in whom there is a question of vascular integrity as, for example, in the patient with a fracture-dislocation of the elbow in whom a radial pulse cannot be palpated. We have saved ourselves considerable distress and effort by transcutaneous use of the ultrasonic flowmeter to detect the presence of pulsatile blood flow accurately in distal arteries, even those as small as the digital artery.

Measurement of cardiac output in children has been facilitated greatly by the development of an automated thermodilution device*

---

*Kimray Corp., Oklahoma City, Okla. 73118.

which permits simple, accurate, repeated measurements of cardiac output by the injection of 2 ml to 5 ml of room temperature saline. The balloon-tipped thermistor catheter can be guided into the pulmonary artery and saline injected into the central venous pressure (CVP) catheter. We have found this technique to be very helpful in the management of complex trauma patients[14] (Table 1).

Perhaps the most important advance in the management of the injured patient in the past decade has been the appreciation of the usefulness of the central venous pressure as a method of evaluating the adequacy of blood volume replacement and, indirectly, of cardiac function.[15] The blood reservoir function of the venous system is well known, and is characterized by the relatively slow increase in venous pressure as the intravascular volume is increased, as compared to the arterial side of the system. When the venous reservoir is filled to capacity, the pressure:volume ratio increases very rapidly, indicating that the vascular system is full (Fig. 2).

When the diastolic filling pressure of the ventricles is increased by means of raising the central venous pressure or left atrial pressure by volume infusion, a substantial increase in myocardial contractility is achieved through the Frank-Starling effect, and this results in increased cardiac output (Fig. 3). In the child or young adult in whom coronary artery insufficiency and myocardial dysfunction are of little practical importance, the central venous or right atrial pressure accurately

TABLE 1   Postoperative Studies Following Correction of Fallot's Tetralogy. Cardiac Output During Dopamine Infusion

Patient: F.S.
Age: 23 mos
Wt.:   10.5 kg

Time	Systemic BP	Heart Rate	Right Atrial Pressure	Thermodilution Cardiac Output	Dopamine Infusion	Clinical Status
(hrs)	(mm Hg)	(beats/min)	(cm H_2O)	(L/min $\pm$ SD)	(mcg/kg/min)	
18:42	76/30	147	22.3	0.94 $\pm$ 0.09	0	feet: cool, pale
19:07	68/40	136	23.0	0.89 $\pm$ 0.18	0	cap. filling: 1+
19:55	85/50	160	22.0	1.70 $\pm$ 0.15 ×	10	d. pedis pulse: 0
08:45	93/58	119	13.6	1.58 $\pm$ 0.12 ×	12	
10:00	80/49	119	12.8	1.47 $\pm$ 0.07 ×	12	
11:31	70/45	120	12.8	1.31 $\pm$ 0.12 ×	8	
12:21	75/45	122	12.8	1.63 $\pm$ 0.06 ×	10	feet: warm, pink
17:45	74/45	130	15.2	1.32 $\pm$ 0.11 ×	10	cap. filling: 3+
18:30	74/44	132	16.5	1.31 $\pm$ 0.11 ×	10	d. pedis pulse: 2+
11:25	85/45	136	17.8	1.69 $\pm$ 0.25 ×	10	
13:20	61/39	121	22.6	1.03 $\pm$ 0.07 #	7	
14:10	82/43	144	22.0	1.14 $\pm$ 0.17 #	8	
14:18	87/50	145	20.0	1.34 $\pm$ 0.10 ×	10	

× = Significant change from control (0 mcg/kg/min); $p = <0.001$
= Significant change from control (0 mcg/kg/min); $p = <0.05$

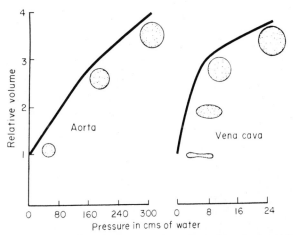

Figure 2. The venous system is more compliant than the arterial circulation, and this is shown in the relatively slow changes in venous pressures, induced by increasing the venous blood volume, until the system is filled. At this point there is a marked increase in venous pressure as volume is further increased.

reflects the left atrial pressure (which, to be precise, determines the left ventricular end-diastolic volume and thus the magnitude of the Frank-Starling effect on systemic output). Figure 4 illustrates this point in a group of normal dogs subjected to hemorrhage followed by replacement of the volume deficit with a variety of colloidal or non-colloidal substances. It is quite apparent that left and right atrial pressures vary closely. If ventricular function is compromised, as illustrated, for example, by the dashed lines in Figure 3, then a higher ventricular filling

Figure 3. Under normal circumstances ventricular stroke volume and contractility are increased as the diastolic filling pressure is increased, by the Frank-Starling mechanism. When intrinsic myocardial contractility is decreased, a greater filling pressure (right atrial pressure) is required to achieve any given value for stroke volume.

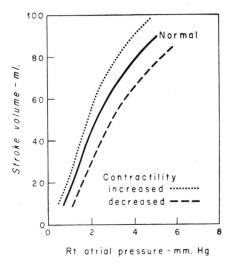

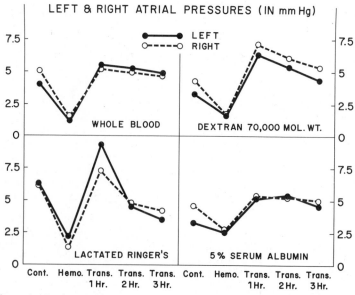

Figure 4. In dogs subjected to hemorrhagic shock and then transfused with blood, colloid, or crystalloid fluids, the right atrial and left atrial pressures were virtually identical throughout. (From R. L. Replogle: Bull. Soc. Int. Chir., 5:370, 1972.)

pressure is required to maintain cardiac output. In patients with coronary heart disease, left ventricular function may be compromised more severely than right ventricular function. In such circumstances, the right atrial pressure may be normal at a time when the left atrial pressure is elevated; continuing to infuse solutions into these patients may precipitate pulmonary edema.[16] In the patient with compromised right ventricular function (as in a postoperative Fallot's tetralogy), or in pulmonary vascular obstructive disease (as in an asthmatic child), the right atrial pressure may be considerably greater than left atrial pressure and again may confuse the issue. The ultimate usefulness of any physiological measurement depends upon the care with which the data are obtained. The central venous catheter should be positioned at the entrance to the great veins into the right atrium or, preferably, in the right atrium.[17] The routine use of radiopaque tubing will make it easier to delineate the location of the catheter tip. If the saphenous vein at the groin is used in infants, it is particularly important to advance the catheter into the thorax, since an artifactually high intra-abdominal pressure may give a falsely high central venous pressure reading. In the newborn use of the umbilical veins is convenient, but may be accompanied by some problems. The catheter must be advanced into the inferior vena cava or right atrium, since the pressure on the portal sinus and ductus venosus may be considerably higher than the central venous pressures[19] (Fig. 5). There is also a possibility that portal vein

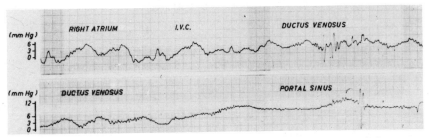

Figure 5. The tracings show the pressures obtained in a newborn infant as an umbilical catheter is pulled back from the right atrium into the inferior vena cava, ductus venosus, and portal sinus. The increased pressure in the portal sinus, easily seen, indicates that this is not a good location for monitoring the central venous pressure. (Courtesy of Dr. R. A. Arcilla.)

thrombosis may develop, which may lead to portal hypertension later in life. A safer means of monitoring central venous pressure is a direct cutdown in the internal jugular vein and a catheter introduced into the superior vena cava or right atrium after tunneling it through the scalp behind the ear. This insures stability and, more important, minimizes infection from the catheter. The complications associated with central venous pressure monitoring are largely preventable but can be mortal, and the physician and nursing service should be familiar with the possibilities.[20, 21] Because any cutdown is susceptible to infection and subsequent septicemia, frequent local application of antibiotic ointment should be routine, since this technique has proved useful.[22]

The predominant, recurring theme in any discussion of the treatment of shock and trauma in the child should be *volume replacement.* As has been mentioned, following the level of the central venous pressure will provide an excellent guide to fluid replacement in the child, since one can nearly always depend on good myocardial function. Blalock first pointed out that the type of fluid used to replace blood loss is of less importance than giving adequate volume.[23] These observations have been confirmed by many investigators.[24, 25, 26, 27] If asanguineous fluids are used, the reduction in red cell concentration and oxygen-carrying capacity of the blood is compensated by the increased cardiac output or more effective oxygen extraction, so that the oxygen consumption remains constant.[28] This is illustrated in Figure 6, which describes the effects on cardiac output in an animal study in which hemorrhage was followed by volume replacement with a variety of fluids. Oxygen consumption measurements showed no statistically significant differences between any of the groups, even though the hematocrit fell as low as 19 per cent (Fig. 7). If non-colloidal fluids are used for volume replacement, the rather rapid loss of solution from the intravascular space into the the extravascular space means one must constantly watch for the signs of hypovolemia, as is illustrated in Figure 8. The choice of fluid for volume replacement in the treatment of shock

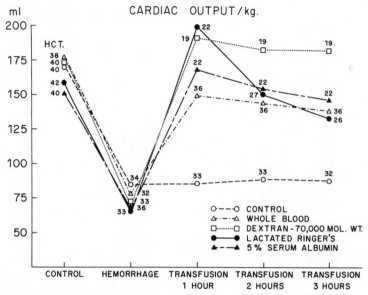

Figure 6. The chart shows changes in cardiac output and hematocrit in dogs subjected to hemorrhagic shock followed by transfusion. The reduced cardiac output associated with hypovolemia was restored by all the fluids, more so with the asanguineous ones than with whole blood. The reduced hematocrit resulted in reduction in systemic vascular resistance as a consequence of reduced blood viscosity. (From R. L. Replogle: Bull. Soc. Int. Chir., 5:370, 1972.)

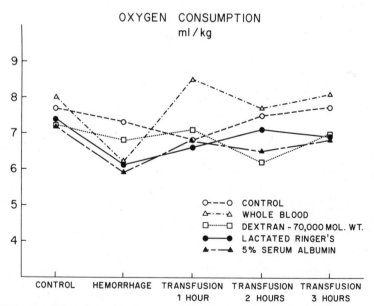

Figure 7. Although the hematocrit fell as low as 19 per cent in animals transfused with asanguineous fluids, there were no significant differences in oxygen consumption between any of the groups. The reduced oxygen-carrying capacity was compensated by increased cardiac output and more efficient oxygen extraction. (From R. L. Replogle: Bull. Soc. Int. Chir., 5:370, 1972.)

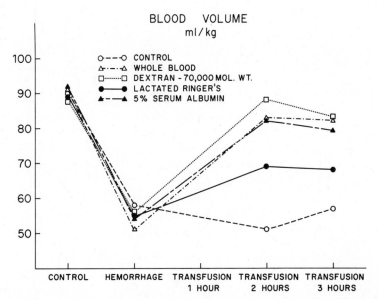

Figure 8.   Whole blood and colloid plasma expanders are more effective and longer-lasting agents in maintaining blood volume after infusion than crystalloid solutions such as lactated Ringer's solution. As illustrated here, despite the fact that the volume of lactated Ringer's solution infused was three times that of the colloid fluids, at the end of 3 hours following transfusion the relative blood volume was 20 per cent less in the lactated Ringer's group. (From R. L. Replogle: Bull. Soc. Int. Chir., 5:370, 1972.)

is, to some extent, a matter of personal preference and experience. We believe that colloidal agents are preferable, since it is possible to predict the degree of expansion from the amount of fluid infused. There are certain disadvantages to the others which make us regard 5 per cent human serum albumin as the first choice. However, there is considerable debate about the use of colloidal agents for the treatment of the patient in shock. Shires and his co-workers[29] emphasize that correction of interstitial fluid volume deficit in a person with hemorrhagic shock is achieved more effectively with the use of electrolyte solutions that quickly equilibrate with the interstitial space, than with colloid-containing solutions that do not diffuse rapidly into the interstitial space. Rowe[30] recommends that protein solutions should be used in a patient in shock only if the oncotic pressure is low and not due to dilution, and it has even been suggested that loss of albumin into the alveolar space during hemorrhagic shock may actively contribute to the development of pulmonary edema.[31] The suggestion has been made that for correction of low oncotic pressure, a 5 per cent albumin solution (10 ml per kg) or 25 per cent albumin solution (4 ml per kg) be given. To maintain normal oncotic pressure, a continuous infusion of 2.5 per cent albumin solution is recommended. Despite the widespread enthusiasm for low molecular weight dextran, there is little solid evidence that its usefulness extends beyond a volume replacement effect; since this material of lower weight leaves the vascular space rapidly, as much as 50 per cent may be lost extravascularly within 2 hours.[32, 33] The higher weight dextran (70,000 mol wt) is a more effective plasma expander than the lower molecular weight material, but if it is given in large quantities (over 1000 ml in an adult), it may have a deleterious effect on blood coagulation.[34]

While there is increasing evidence that moderate hemodilution may have a beneficial effect on perfusion during shock,[35] at the present time it is recommended that blood should be given as soon as it is available unless there is evidence of hemoconcentration (hematocrit higher than 40 per cent), in which case a nonsanguineous fluid is preferable. Under no circumstances should the physician wait for blood to be typed and cross-matched before beginning volume replacement, regardless of the hematocrit value, since immediate volume expansion with whatever material is available is much preferable to any kind of delay for whole blood. There is still some controversy about the emergency use of low titer (less than 1:200 anti-A and anti-B saline isoagglutinins) group O Rho (D) positive universal donor blood. The following evidence leads us to believe that it is best not to use universal donor blood: (1) the fact that even a severely diminished hematocrit does not seem to have deleterious effects, (2) the relative scarcity of this type of blood, (3) the cost of maintaining a supply, and (4) the fact that when blood of the patient's hereditary type is administered later, a hemolytic response may be initiated by the reaction between the incompatible isoagglutinins from the transfused O blood and the red cell antigens in donor blood of the patient's type. If one does give more than the equivalent of 3 units of universal donor blood to an adult, and the patient needs more blood within 2 weeks, it is best to continue giving universal donor blood and not to switch to transfusions with the patient's hereditary blood type.[36]

There has long existed a "clinical impression" that the massive infusion of stored whole blood occasionally is associated with clinical deterioration even in the absence of transfusion reactions. Efforts at relating this impression to hypocalcemia (as a result of the chelation of serum calcium by the citrate solution) or acidosis (from the acidity of the bank blood) have not demonstrated a good correlation. Howland,[37] in a large series, observed that the mortality from ventricular fibrillation following the infusion of calcium during massive transfusion was greater than the risk of hypocalcemia in patients not receiving calcium, even when 5 liters of blood and more were transfused. Miller[38] found no correlation between the amount of stored acid-citrate-dextrose blood administered and the magnitude of acidosis in patients given multiple blood transfusions, and recommended that bicarbonate therapy be reserved for patients with severe metabolic acidosis, established by measurement of arterial pH and Pco_2. However, it has been established recently that red cell concentrations of the organic phosphate, 2,3-diphosphoglycerate, fall rapidly during blood storage, and with the loss of this material the affinity of hemoglobin for oxygen increases markedly. As this affinity increases, the position of the oxyhemoglobin dissociation curve shifts to the left and the delivery of oxygen to the tissues may be compromised. When it becomes necessary to transfuse massively, a substantial amount of blood less than 5 days old should be used, since 75 per cent of the 2,3-diphosphoglycerate is lost after 5 days of storage.[39] Addition of inosine and a small amount of adenine to banked blood will extend the period of normal erythrocytic concentration of 2,3-diphosphoglycerate to from 3 to 5 weeks.[40]

Blood storage is associated with the development of particulate matter, largely platelet aggregates, within the blood over a period of time. Removal of these microaggregates by filtration is indicated if stored blood in large quantities is infused.[41]

It is particularly important to remember that the rapid infusion of cold blood into infants and children frequently results in ventricular fibrillation or standstill. Blood should be *warmed* before it is given rapidly, and there are several convenient methods for doing this.[42, 43]

EVALUATION OF THE TRAUMA PATIENT

The physician should categorize trauma patients rather quickly into those who require *immediate* surgery for massive internal hemorrhage or airway obstruction, those in whom early surgery is probably indicated, and those patients with less obvious major injury.[44] When immediate surgery is required, nothing should be done that will delay the beginning of the operation. The patient should be taken to the operating room at once, and, if possible, intravenous transfusion should be initiated during transportation. The second group of patients consists of those with multiple injuries in whom it would appear that the shock situation can be stabilized and maintained for some time, allowing an interval for certain diagnostic studies. Depending upon the efficiency and experience of the emergency facility and the operating room team, one might spend a few minutes for treatment in the emergency room rather than risk being caught between floors in an elevator with a patient who has suddenly had a cardiac arrest on the way to the operating room. Finally, there are those patients who have sustained injuries which may not be serious, or the seriousness of which may not be readily apparent. In children, this would mean chiefly splenic injury with delayed rupture.

Blood should always be sent for type and cross-match at once, and the wise physician asks for at least one more unit than he or she thinks may be needed. In any serious injury an arterial catheter should be inserted and blood sent for Po_2, pH, and Pco_2 measurements, and a hematocrit. The Foley catheter and the central venous pressure line complete the basic requirements for monitoring. In the young patient who has sustained trauma, hypotension with a low central venous pressure means hypovolemia, and regardless of one's assessment of the adequacy of volume replacement, transfusion should continue until the blood pressure and signs of improved peripheral perfusion return toward normal, or until the venous pressure begins to climb. The level to which the central venous pressure can be pushed without risk of pulmonary edema varies individually, but certainly in the child or young adult there is little danger until the venous pressure goes above 20 cm H_2O.

If major intra-abdominal bleeding is suspected, confirmation can be obtained quickly with about 80 per cent confidence by aspirating the four abdominal quadrants through an 18-gauge needle.[45] The incidence of false negatives can be reduced still further if a plastic catheter is introduced into the abdominal cavity in the infraumbilical region, and 500 to 1000 ml of saline are infused and then aspirated. In most instances a very small quantity of intra-abdominal bleeding can be detected with this technique. The child who is admitted through the emergency room, who has a history of blunt trauma to the abdomen, is in shock, and has an increasingly distending abdomen, is presumed to have serious liver or spleen injury with hemoperitoneum unless proved otherwise. A single aspiration of the peritoneal cavity with the use of an 18-gauge needle is usually diagnostic.

Hemorrhage into the chest is rarely a critical problem unless there is a laceration of the heart or great vessels. If there is doubt about a patient with diminished breath sounds, a chest tube can be inserted (fifth or sixth intercostal space in the anterior axillary line, well away from the liver and spleen), but ordinarily a chest roentgenogram should be obtained to confirm a suspicion of hemothorax. In most instances bleeding from the lung will cease without the need for thoracotomy and the pneumothorax and hemothorax can be treated with the chest tube alone.[46] When there is damage to the heart or great vessels, extremely fast and well-organized teamwork is required for urgent thoracotomy.

It is unfortunate that the changes in social behavior of our times have provided us with greater experience with stab wounds of the various areas of the body. With this newly acquired information have come some suggestions for modifying the traditional approach to treatment. In the past, stab wounds of the abdomen, because they are penetrating, have been considered to be surgical emergencies, and this attitude has been shown to result in unnecessary laparotomy in over 50 per cent of patients.[47] Currently, many experienced clinicians believe that a more selective approach to exploration reduces the number of unnecessary explorations, at little risk to the patient.[48, 49, 50] The decision regarding exploration is based on the usual clinical and laboratory criteria (free intra-abdominal air, hematuria, severe hemorrhage, peritonitis, and so on), as well as radiocontrast injection of the sinus tract to delineate the depth of the wound. With a catheter sewn into the wound, 50 to 75 ml of contrast medium are injected and the patient is x-rayed in several positions to identify contrast in the peritoneal cavity or the bowel. If the radiographic study is negative, the patient is observed clinically for 48 hours and if no signs of peritonitis develop, he or she may be discharged. This protocol has merit and has been very useful and safe.

Stab wounds of the neck are quite different from wounds of the abdomen, since there is a plethora of vital structures close beneath the skin. Major injuries to the airway, blood vessels, or esophagus may result from rather innocent-looking wounds, and routine surgical exploration of penetrating neck wounds is the safest course of action.[51]

The patient suffering blunt trauma to the abdomen may be a diagnostic problem. In the absence of intra-abdominal blood from the peritoneal aspiration, and with no evidence of free air in the abdomen, no fractures, and clear urine, the possibility of subcapsular hematoma of the spleen or liver with delayed hemorrhage still gives cause for concern.[52] The abdomen is usually tender from the trauma and difficult to examine. In certain instances liver or splenic radioisotope scans or selective angiography may be very useful in the evaluation of the extent of injury.[53] Even without signs of major intra-abdominal injury after blunt trauma, it is still wise to maintain the child by intravenous rather than oral food and fluids for 24 hours, since the incidence of paralytic ileus (often from a mesenteric hematoma) is high, and vomiting and distention frequently will follow attempts at early oral feeding.

While the discussion of head injury is the subject of another chapter, it is important to emphasize the fact that, except for the neonate, patients with head injury rarely present in shock.[54] If a child with a head injury is seen with hypotension and shock, *look elsewhere* for hemorrhagic blood loss.

SUPPORTIVE TREATMENT OF SHOCK

In the overwhelming majority of cases, rapid restoration of blood volume is all that is necessary for the resuscitation of the child in shock. On occasion, temporary pharmacological support may be necessary to increase myocardial contractility, reverse metabolic or respiratory acidosis, or simply to maintain arterial pressure until the lost blood can be replaced.

Metabolic acidosis long has been known to accompany reduced tissue perfusion and anaerobic metabolism. Acidosis *per se* has been reported to reduce myocardial contractility, possibly by inhibiting the beta-adrenergic effects of catecholamines on the heart.[55] More recent evidence suggests that this widely held concept may not be entirely correct if it is applied to the patient in shock, since acidosis increases secretion of epinephrine by the adrenal gland, thus enhancing adrenergic activity.[56] Other experimental studies do not support the theory that acidosis, either respiratory or metabolic, has a depressive effect on myocardial function until the pH falls below 6.9.[57] In newborn puppies subjected to hemorrhagic shock, the improvement in cardiovascular function that followed correction of metabolic acidosis with sodium bicarbonate was equally good when other hyperosmotic solutions, such as 3 per cent sodium chloride or 25 per cent mannitol, were given, even though the solutions did nothing to correct the acidosis.[58] Nevertheless, one should not conclude from these comments that metabolic acidosis should not be corrected, since, for one thing, the susceptibility of the heart to ventricular fibrillation does appear to be increased by metabolic acidosis.[59] It should be remembered, however, that metabolic acidosis is a "symptom" of the underlying disease, and every effort must be oriented toward treatment of the basic problem.

Occasionally, it will be necessary to use sympathomimetic drugs, either on a temporary basis while volume losses are being made up, or for more long-term support in the patient with some underlying disorder, such as congenital heart disease or chronic lung disease. Calcium chloride given slowly intravenously, or by intracardiac injection, is extremely useful for improving myocardial function. Isoproterenol also has proved to be of great merit, although some patients have an extreme chronotrophic response, and the tachycardia that develops may be disabling. In the past year we have begun to use dopamine with increasing frequency. This drug does not have the chronotropic effects of isoproterenol,[60] and, in addition, has a direct renal vasodilating mechanism which has been shown to increase renal blood flow.[61] We have evidence from clinical hemodynamic studies that dopamine (10 mcg/kg/min) increases cardiac output in infants and children in low flow situations (Table 1). Higher doses, while raising blood pressure, do not appear to improve cardiac output. In some critical circumstances, glucagon[62] (100 mcg per kg every 30 min) in combination with isoproterenol or dopamine has seemed to be useful clinically, but this is merely an "impression." Nevertheless, if there are no other options, you might want to consider it. Children respond very quickly to volume replacement and, over the long term, catecholamines usually are not required. The physician needs a practical working knowledge of these drugs, and should develop his or her personal protocol.[63, 64, 65]

The use of pharmacological doses of corticosteroids has been advocated in the treatment of shock, some studies indicating a vasodilator effect,[66] others a positive inotropic effect,[67] while still other experimental studies have failed to demonstrate any hemodynamic effects.[68] The role of lysosomal disruption as a consequence of shock, and the apparent stabilizing effect of corticosteroids on the lysosome membrane, may well be of considerable importance.[69] At the present time, although the evidence that large doses of corticosteroids are beneficial in the treatment of shock is not solid, we do have enough experience to know that the very short-term use of this drug is not harmful. Consequently, we frequently use methylprednisolone (25 mg per kg) as an adjunct in the treatment of shock, usually as a single infusion.

The adequacy of urine output remains a very valuable sign of satisfactory circulatory dynamics. The presence of oliguria may simply indicate inadequate volume replacement, or may herald the onset of acute renal failure. (See Chapter 10.) The ratio $\frac{\text{urinary urea nitrogen}}{\text{blood urea nitrogen}}$ is a most valuable aid in establishing the severity of renal dysfunction in the presence of oliguria.[70] Those patients with a $\frac{\text{UUN}}{\text{BUN}}$ below 12 are suspect, and those with a ratio below 5 have severely impaired renal function. While it has been suggested that a urinary (Na^+) of less than 40 mEq/L indicates adequate renal function, this is frequently not the case and may be misleading. When the BUN reaches 30 mg per 100 ml, and the urine output goes below 2 ml/kg/hr, we immediately check the fluid balance and urinary specific gravity. If increasing the fluid load reverses the process, everyone is pleased. If it does not, and the cardiac output seems adequate, we send blood and urine samples for $\frac{\text{UUN}}{\text{BUN}}$ and give furosemide 1 mg per kg in an initial dose, increasing to as much as 20 mg per kg every 6 hours for 24 hours. Stone and Stahl[71] found that furosemide increased renal blood flow during the hypovolemic state. Several reports indicate that furosemide does not affect the intra-renal distribution of blood flow,[72, 73] and since current thinking suggests that a reduction in renal cortical blood flow is a factor in the pathogenesis of acute renal failure,[74] the apparent favorable effect of furosemide may not be on renal blood flow. Furosemide did not reverse *established* renal shutdown in any of our patients or in a reported series,[73] but our experience suggests that impending renal failure can be alleviated if furosemide is used early, and in high doses.[75] If this treatment does not prove effective quickly, high doses of the drug should not be continued, since permanent deafness can occur as a result of eighth cranial nerve damage.[76]

In our experience, once *anuria* has become established, no amount of furosemide has been effective.

One must watch the serum calcium levels closely during treatment with furosemide. We observed remarkably low Ca^+ levels before we became aware that furosemide causes an increase in the urinary excretion of calcium as a result of the inhibition of tubular sodium resorption.[77]

While hypovolemia in the older child may be approached in a manner analogous to its treatment in the adult, a few special aspects pertinent to the treatment of shock in the newborn require mention. First is the relationship of body temperature to the response to shock. It is well known that the index of surface area to body weight is greater in the infant, and that an environmental temperature of 34°C reduces to the lowest level the metabolic activity required to maintain body temperature in the neonate.[78] In the infant with an intact thermoregulatory mechanism, exposure to a cold environment may result in considerable energy expenditure simply to maintain body temperature, and this caloric loss may be detrimental for survival in shock.[79] Therefore, efforts should be made to keep the shocked infant in a warm environment. The most convenient way to maintain a neutral thermal environment is to provide a servomechanism between the infant's skin temperature and a radiant heating device. Maintaining the abdominal skin temperature at 36.5°C minimizes oxygen consumption; at an abdominal skin temperature of 35.9°C, oxygen consumption is increased by 10 per cent.[80] This technique does have the disadvantage of removing one excellent clinical sign (progressive hypothermia) of infant sepsis and intracranial hemorrhage, but, on balance, it is a useful adjunct. While the neuroendocrine response of the infant to hemorrhage is the same as in the adult, the degree of hypotension and the reduction in cardiac output that accompany moderate (15 per cent of blood volume) blood loss are relatively greater in the infant, and replacement of even apparently moderate amounts of blood lost may be important.[81, 82] The sudden infusion of hypertonic solutions, e.g., 20 per cent mannitol (1400 mOsm/kg), or 7.5 per cent sodium bicarbonate (1465 mOsm/kg), may result in a sudden shift of water out of the central nervous system, and this may cause intracranial hemorrhage in the infant. These solutions should be administered slowly.[83] As a matter of fact, anything given intravenously should be given slowly, since an inordinate number of cardiac arrests immediately follow the central intravenous administration of drugs.[84]

If the physician remembers that volume replacement is the name of the game, and that warm feet mean strong heart,[85] he or she will be well rewarded by the rapid, complete, and gratifying recovery of the child in shock.

REFERENCES

1. Vital Statistics of the United States, 1966. Department of Health, Education and Welfare, U.S. Public Health Service, National Center for Health Statistics, Washington, D.C., Government Printing Office, 1968.
2. Withington, R. L., and Hall, L. W.: Snowmobile accidents: A review of injuries sustained in the use of snowmobiles in northern New England during the 1968–69 season. J. Trauma, *10*:760, 1970.
3. Schleuter, C. F.: Some economic dimensions of traumatic injuries. J. Trauma, *10*:915, 1970.
4. Spelman, J. W., Bordner, K. R., and Howard, J. M.: Traffic fatalities in Philadelphia. J. Trauma, *10*:885, 1970.
5. Waller, J. A.: Control of accidents in rural areas. J.A.M.A., *201*:176, 1967.
6. Baker, G. L.: Design and operation of a van for the transport of sick infants. Am. J. Dis. Child., *118*:743, 1968.
7. Katy, N. M., and Ottinger, L. W.: System-structured management of acutely ill surgical patients. Arch. Surg., *111*:239, 1976.
8. Randolph, J. G.: Technique for insertion of a plastic catheter into the saphenous vein. Pediatrics, *24*:631, 1959.
9. Cohn, J. H.: Blood pressure measurement in shock. Mechanism of inaccuracy in auscultatory and palpatory methods. J.A.M.A., *199*:118, 1967.
10. Williams, A. J., Jarvis, C. W., Neal, W. A., and Reynolds, J. W.: Vascular thromboembolism complicating umbilical artery catheterization. Am. J. Roentgenol., *116*:475, 1972.
11. Kazamias, T. M., Gander, M. P., Franklin, D. L., and Ross, J., Jr.: Blood pressure measurement with Doppler ultrasonic flowmeter. J. Appl. Physiol., *30*:585, 1971.
12. Kemmerer, W. T., Ware, R. W., Stegall, H. F., Morgan, J. L., and Kirby, R.: Blood pressure measurement by Doppler ultrasonic detection of arterial wall motion. Surg. Gynecol. Obstet., *131*:1141, 1970.
13. Contis, G., and Lind, J.: Study of systolic blood pressure, heart rates, and body temperature of normal newborn infants through the first week of life. Acta Paediatr. Suppl., *146*:41, 1963.
14. Beyer, J., Lamberti, J. J., and Replogle, R. L.: Validity of thermodilution cardiac output determination: Studies with and without pulmonary insufficiency. J. Surg. Res., 1976 (in press).
15. Wilson, J. N., Grow, J. B., Demong, C. V., Prevedel, A. E., and Owens, J. C.: Central venous pressure in optimal blood volume maintenance. Arch. Surg., *85*:563, 1962.
16. Forrester, J. S., Diamond, G., McHugh, T. J., and Swan, H. J. C.: Filling pressures in the right and left sides of the heart in acute myocardial infarction. A reappraisal of central-venous-pressure monitoring. N. Engl. J. Med., *285*:190, 1971.

17. Liebert, P. S.: Central venous catheters in children—their placement and care. Clin. Pediatr., *10*:218, 1971.
18. Talbert, J. L., and Haller, J. A., Jr.: The optimal site for central venous pressure measurements in newborn infants. J. Surg. Res., *6*:168, 1966.
19. Arcilla, R. A., Oh, W., Lind, J., and Blankenship, W.: Portal and atrial pressures in the newborn period. Acta Paediatr. Scand., *55*:615, 1966.
20. Henzel, J. H., and DeWeese, M. S.: Morbid and mortal complications associated with prolonged central venous cannulation. Awareness, recognition and prevention. Am. J. Surg., *121*:600, 1971.
21. Fitts, C. T., Barnett, L. T., Webb, C. M., Sexton, J., and Yarbrough, D. R., III: Perforating wounds of the heart caused by central venous catheters. J. Trauma, *10*:764, 1970.
22. Moran, J. M., Atwood, R. P., and Rowe, M. I.: A clinical and bacteriologic study of infections associated with venous cutdowns. N. Engl. J. Med., *272*:554, 1965.
23. Blalock, A.: Principles of Surgical Care, Shock and Other Problems. St. Louis, C. V. Mosby Co., 1940, p. 158.
24. Moss, G. S., Proctor, H. J., Homer, L. D., Herman, C. M., and Litt, B. D.: A comparison of asanguineous fluids and whole blood in the treatment of hemorrhagic shock. Surg. Gynecol. Obstet., *129*:1247, 1969.
25. Rush, B., and Eiseman, B.: Limits of non-colloid solution replacement in experimental hemorrhagic shock. Ann. Surg., *165*:977, 1967.
26. Replogle, R. L., and Merrill, E. W.: Hemodilution: Rheologic hemodynamic and metabolic consequences in shock. Surg. Forum, *18*:157, 1967.
27. Takaori, M., and Safar, P.: Treatment of massive hemorrhage with colloid and crystalloid solutions. Studies in dogs. J.A.M.A., *199*:297, 1967.
28. Lako, H., Pilon, R. N., Anderson, W., MacCallum, J. R., and O'Connor, N. E.: Intraoperative prebleeding in man: Effect of colloid hemodilution on blood volume, lung water, hemodynamics and oxygen transport. Surgery, *78*:130, 1975.
29. Shires, G. T., Carrico, C. J., and Canizaro, P. C.: Shock. Philadelphia, W. B. Saunders Co., 1973, pp. 15–41.
30. Rowe, M. I., and Arango, A.: The choice of intravenous fluid in shock resuscitation. Pediatr. Clin. North Am., *22*:269, 1975.
31. Holcroft, J. W., and Trunkey, D. D.: Pulmonary extravasation of albumin during and after hemorrhagic shock in baboons. J. Surg. Res., *18*:91, 1975.
32. Replogle, R. L., Kundler, H., and Gross, R. E.: Studies on the hemodynamic importance of blood viscosity. J. Thorac. Cardiovasc. Surg., *50*:658, 1965.
33. Replogle, R. L., Meiselman, H. J., and Merrill, E. W.: Clinical implications of blood rheology studies. Circulation, *36*:148, 1967.
34. Jacobeus, U.: Studies on the effect of dextran on the coagulation of the blood. Acta Med. Scand., *157* (Suppl. 322): 1957.
35. Replogle, R. L.: Hemodynamic compensation of acute changes of the hemoglobin concentration. *In* Messmer, K., and Schmid-Schonbein, H., eds.: Hemodilution: Theoretical Basis and Clinical Application. Basel, S. Karger, 1972.
36. Barnes, A., Jr., and Allen, T. E.: Transfusions subsequent to administration of universal donor blood in Vietnam. J.A.M.A., *204*:147, 1968.
37. Howland, W. S., Schweizer, O., and Boyan, C. P.: Massive blood replacement without calcium administration. Surg. Gynecol. Obstet., *118*:814, 1964.
38. Miller, R. D., Tong, M. J., and Robbins, T. O.: Effects of massive transfusion of blood on acid-base balance. J.A.M.A., *216*:1762, 1971.
39. Sugerman, J. J., Davidson, D. T., Vibul, S., Delivoria-Papadopoulos, M., Miller, L. D., and Oski, F. A.: The basis of defective oxygen delivery from stored blood. Surg. Gynecol. Obstet., *131*:733, 1970.
40. Dawson, R. B., Edinger, M. C., Ellis, T. J.: Hemoglobin function in stored blood. IV. Red cell adenosine triphosphate and 2,3-diphosphoglycerate in acid-citrate dextrose and citrate-phosphate-dextrose with adenine and inosine. J. Lab. Clin. Med., *77*:46, 1971.
41. McNamara, J. J.: Effective filtration of banked blood. Surgery, *71*:594, 1972.
42. Boyan, C. P., and Howland, W. S.: Cardiac arrest and temperature of bank blood. J.A.M.A., *183*:58, 1963.
43. Schroeder, H. G., and Forbes, A. R.: Massive blood replacement in neonates and children. Br. J. Anaesth., *41*:953, 1969.

44. Shires, G. T., and Jones, R. C.: Initial management of the severely injured patient. J.A.M.A., *213*:1872, 1970.

45. Yurko, A. A., and Williams, R. D.: Needle paracentesis in blunt abdominal trauma: A critical analysis. J. Trauma, *6*:194, 1966.

46. Virgilio, R. W.: Intrathoracic wounds in battle casualties. Surg. Gynecol. Obstet., *130*:609, 1970.

47. Haddad, G. H., Pizzi, W. F., Fleischmann, E. P., and Moynahan, J. M.: Abdominal signs and sinograms as dependable criteria for the selective management of the abdomen. Ann. Surg., *172*:61, 1970.

48. Nance, F. C., and Cohn, I.: Surgical judgment in the management of stab wounds of the abdomen: A retrospective and prospective analysis based on a study of 600 stabbed patients. Ann. Surg., *170*:569, 1969.

49. Wilder, J. R., Haberman, E. T., and Schachner, S. J.: Selective surgical intervention for stab wounds of the abdomen. Surgery, *61*:231, 1967.

50. Steichen, F. M., Efron, G., Pearlman, D. M., and Weil, P. H.: Radiographic diagnosis versus selective management in penetrating wounds of the abdomen. Ann. Surg., *170*:978, 1969.

51. Fitchett, V. H., Pomerantz, M., Butsch, D. W., Simon, R., and Eiseman, B.: Penetrating wounds of the neck. A military and civilian experience. Arch. Surg., *99*:307, 1969.

52. Slate, R. W., Getzen, L. C., and Laning, R. C.: One hundred cases of traumatic rupture of the spleen. Arch. Surg., *99*:498, 1969.

53. Redman, H. C., Reuter, S. R., and Bookstein, J. J.: Angiography in abdominal trauma. Ann. Surg., *169*:57, 1969.

54. Hendrick, E. B., Harwood-Hash, D. C. F., and Hudson, A. R.: Head injuries in children: A survey of 4465 consecutive cases at the Hospital for Sick Children, Toronto, Canada. Clin. Neurosurg., *11*:46, 1964.

55. Darby, T. D., Aldinger, E. E., Gradsden, R. H., and Thrower, W. B.: Effects of metabolic acidosis on ventricular isometric systolic tension and the response to epinephrine and levarterenol. Circ. Res., *8*:1242, 1960.

56. Darby, T. D., and Watts, D. T.: Acidosis and blood epinephrine levels in hemorrhagic hypotension. Am. J. Physiol., *206*:1281, 1964.

57. Andersen, M. N., Border, J. R., and Mouritzen, C. V.: Acidosis, catecholamines and cardiovascular dynamics: When does acidosis require correction? Ann. Surg., *166*:344, 1967.

58. Rowe, M. I., and Arango, A.: The role of buffering, osmolality and sodium in neonatal hemorrhagic shock. Surg. Forum, *21*:34, 1970.

59. Gerst, P. H., Fleming, W. H., and Malm, J. R.: Increased susceptibility of the heart to ventricular fibrillation during metabolic acidosis. Circ. Res., *19*:63, 1966.

60. Holloway, E. L., Stinson, E. B., Derby, G. C., and Harrison, D. C.: Action of drugs in patients early after cardiac surgery. 1. Comparison of isoproterenol and dopamine. Am. J. Cardiol., *35*:656, 1975.

61. Goldberg, L.: Cardiovascular and renal activity of dopamine: Potential clinical application. Pharmacol. Rev., *24*:1, 1972.

62. Polumbo, R. A., Leighton, R. F., and Weissler, A. M.: Efficacy of isoproterenol–glucagon infusion in patients with heart disease. Circulation, *43*:786, 1971.

63. Moran, N. C.: Evaluation of the pharmacologic basis for the therapy of circulatory shock. Am. J. Cardiol., *26*:570, 1970.

64. MacCannell, K. L., McNay, J. L., Meyer, M. B., and Goldberg, L. I.: Dopamine in the treatment of hypotension and shock. N. Engl. J. Med., *275*:1389, 1966.

65. Udhoji, V. N., and Weil, M. H.: Circulatory effects of angiotensin, levarterenol and metaraminol in the treatment of shock. N. Engl. J. Med., *270*:501, 1964.

66. Lillehei, R. C.: Longerbeam, J. K., Bloch, J. H., and Manax, W. G.: Nature of irreversible shock: Experimental and clinical observations. Ann. Surg., *160*:682, 1964.

67. Sambhi, M. P., Weil, M. H., and Udhoji, V. N.: Acute pharmacological effects of glucocorticoids. Circulation, *31*:523, 1965.

68. Replogle, R. L., Kundler, H., Schottenfeld, M., and Spear, S.: Hemodynamic effects of dexamethasone in experimental hemorrhagic shock – negative results. Ann. Surg., *174*:126, 1971.

69. Janoff, A.: Alterations in lysosomes (intracellular enzymes) during shock: Effects of

preconditioning (tolerance) and protective drugs. *In* Hershey, S. G., ed.: Shock. Boston, Little Brown and Co., 1964, p. 93.

70. Porter, G. A., and Starr, A.: Management of post-operative renal failure following cardiovascular surgery. Surgery, *65*:390, 1969.

71. Stone, A. M., and Stahl, W. M.: Effect of ethacrynic acid and furosemide on renal function and intrarenal hemodynamics in acute renal failure. Am. J. Med., *58*:510, 1975.

72. Carriere, S., Dosrosiers, M., Friborg, J., and Brunette, M. G.: The effect of furosemide on intrarenal blood flow distribution in the dog. Can. J. Physiol. Pharmacol., *50*:774, 1972.

73. Epstein, M., Schneider, N. S., and Befeler, B.: Effect of intrarenal furosemide on renal function and intrarenal hemodynamics in acute renal failure. Am. J. Med., *58*:510, 1975.

74. Flamenbaum, W.: Pathophysiology of acute renal failure. Arch. Intern. Med., *131*:911, 1973.

75. Cantarovich, F., Locatelli, A., Fernandez, J. C., Perez, J. L., and Cristhot, J.: Furosemide in high doses in the treatment of acute renal failure. Postgrad. Med. J. (April Suppl.), 13, 1971.

76. Pillay, V. K. G., Schwartz, F. D., Aimi, K., and Kark, R. M.: Transient and permanent deafness following treatment with ethacrynic acid in renal failure. Lancet, *1*:77, 1969.

77. Walser, M.: Calcium clearance as a function of sodium clearance in the dog. Am. J. Physiol., *200*:1099, 1961.

78. Brücke, K.: Temperature regulation in the newborn infant. Biol. Neonate, *3*:65, 1961.

79. Rowe, M. I., and Arcilla, R. A.: Body temperature and the neonatal response to hemorrhage. Ann. Surg., *172*:76, 1970.

80. Buetow, K., and Klein, S.: Effect of maintenance of "normal" skin temperature on survival of infants of low birth weight. Pediatrics, *34*:163, 1964.

81. Wallgren, G., Barr, M., and Rudhe, U.: Hemodynamic studies of induced hypo- and hypervolemia in the newborn infant. Acta Paediatr., *53*:1, 1964.

82. Rowe, M. I., and Arcilla, R. A.: Hemodynamic adaptation of the newborn to hemorrhage. J. Pediatr. Surg., *3*:278, 1968.

83. Kravath, R. E., Aharan, A. S., Abal, G., and Finberg, L.: Clinically significant physiologic changes from rapidly administered hypertonic solutions: Acute osmol poisoning. Pediatrics, *40*:267, 1970.

84. Camarata, S. J., Weil, M. H., Hanashiro, P. K., and Shubin, H.: Cardiac arrest in the critically ill. 1. A study of predisposing causes in 132 patients. Circulation, *44*:688, 1971.

85. Joly, H. R., and Weil, M. H.: Temperature of the toe as an indication of the severity of shock. Circulation, *39*:131, 1969.

Chapter Two

ENDOTOXIN SHOCK

HORACE L. HODES, M.D.

For practical purposes, we may consider that endotoxins of gram-negative bacteria are the cause of endotoxic shock. In general, endotoxins are produced by bacteria which form smooth colonies. However, it should be mentioned that small quantities of endotoxin have been found in colonially rough, gram-negative rods and in some gram-positive bacteria.

Endotoxins are found in the outer layers of the bacterial cell wall. They are so closely associated with other constituents of this structure that their isolation requires strong chemical treatment.[1] Endotoxins are macromolecules which readily form complexes with each other and with other macromolecules. The two major constituents of endotoxins are lipids and polysaccharides. Endotoxins also contain a small percentage of peptides, so we may consider that endotoxins are lipid-polysaccharide-peptide macromolecules. All endotoxins contain phosphorus also. The polysaccharide moiety is composed of a number of different carbohydrates, such as glucose, galactose, and mannose, as well as pentoses, heptoses, and hexosamines.[2] Also present are di-deoxy hexoses, which are found only in endotoxins.

The lipid moiety contains even-numbered saturated and unsaturated fatty acids. The chemical constituents of endotoxins are arranged in three major zones in the macromolecule: the polysaccharide, the lipid-rich, and the amino acid-rich moieties. The backbone of the molecule is polysaccharide, to which are attached amino acids. The fatty acids also are attached to the carbohydrate backbone; these are ester bound to OH groups or amide bound to NH_2 groups of the carbohydrate, probably through such compounds as glucosamine.[2] The endotoxin molecule is unique in its fatty acid–carbohydrate linkages, which

From the Department of Pediatrics, The Mount Sinai School of Medicine of the City University of New York, New York.

have not been found in any other natural substance.[3] Phosphoric acid is found in both the lipid and carbohydrate moieties.

Endotoxins elicit, directly or indirectly, a large number of reactions affecting many organ systems of the host. It seems very likely that most of these toxic reactions are caused by the presence of the lipid moiety, particularly the long-chain fatty acids. Rough mutant, gram-negative bacteria (which contain no polysaccharide moiety) have been shown to contain endotoxins which have full endotoxic action. The polysaccharide moiety probably corresponds to the O antigen of the gram-negative bacilli. This portion of the macromolecule determines the serological specificity of the organism. The peptide moiety appears to have little, if any, endotoxic activity, since removal of this portion of the molecule does not decrease its endotoxic potency.

Although endotoxins have a basic general structure, it should be noted that there is no single type of endotoxin molecule. Several fully active, chemically different molecular complexes may be found in endotoxins prepared from one bacterial culture.[4] Whether or not these different molecules act in exactly the same manner is not known. The greater the heterogeneity of the endotoxin preparation, the greater is its toxicity. It is probable that a number of organs and more than one kind of organelle may be targets for endotoxin. Different endotoxin molecules may injure different cells or different subcellular elements simultaneously, or they may act in sequence. If the latter is the case, a chain reaction might result.[3]

Endotoxin is found soon after its injection into animals in the cells of the reticuloendothelial system. About 90 per cent of the endotoxin appears in the liver and spleen, but endotoxin also accumulates in the endothelium of blood vessels and in the alveoli of the lungs.[5] Endotoxin is adsorbed to the surface of polymorphonuclear leukocytes (or it is actually present in the cytoplasm of these cells) within 10 minutes after it has been injected intravenously.[6] Endotoxin quickly becomes adsorbed to platelets but not to erythrocytes.

BIOLOGIC EFFECTS OF ENDOTOXINS

Endotoxins elicit many of the reactions which we sum up in the term inflammation. These include local vasodilatation, increased vascular permeability which permits plasma and leukocytes to leave the capillaries, enhanced phagocytosis, and stimulation of host resistance. However, many of the reactions caused by endotoxins are not related to inflammation. These include the following:

1. Mobilization of interferon by endotoxin.
2. Induction of local and generalized Shwartzman reactions.
3. Endotoxin, by a number of mechanisms, causes alterations in

the systemic blood pressure which may lead to fatal shock. These actions include the release of kallikreins from leukocytes with the consequent production of kinins, the alteration of the action of epinephrine and norepinephrine on blood vessels, and the release of histamine from mast cells.

4. Endotoxin causes a biphasic febrile reaction; the second peak is probably due to release of an "endogenous pyrogen" from leukocytes.

5. Endotoxin induces leukopenia followed by leukocytosis.

6. Endotoxin causes a fall in number of circulating platelets.

7. Endotoxin causes injury to endothelium of blood vessels.

8. Endotoxin may cause widespread intravascular clotting, with fibrin formation. In this condition there occurs a decrease in circulating platelets, prothrombin, fibrinogen, and intrinsic clotting factors V and VIII. Intravascular clotting may be initiated by activation of Hageman factor (XII) by endotoxin injury of endothelium of blood vessels.

9. Endotoxin causes deleterious changes in carbohydrate and protein metabolism.

10. Endotoxin causes hemorrhagic necrosis in tumors, probably by injury to blood vessels.

11. Mice are protected from a lethal dose of radiation by a prior injection of endotoxin.

It is clear from the very extensive literature on the subject that endotoxins are directly responsible for the shock that occurs during the course of infection with gram-negative bacteria. Changes in the cardiovascular system due in part at least to altered response of the blood vessels to vasoactive substances play an important part in the fatalities that occur in such infections. In addition, extensive intravascular clotting is obvious in some instances, and it is quite possible that some degree of intravascular clotting occurs in all instances. It is also certain that deleterious changes in metabolism occur in many cases, and there is evidence that these alterations are accompanied by cell and organelle injury.

EFFECTS OF ENDOTOXIN ON THE CARDIOVASCULAR SYSTEM

We shall consider first the circulatory changes that are induced by endotoxin. Some confusion has resulted from the fact that endotoxin affects the circulatory system somewhat differently in different animal species. For example, endotoxin brings about the pooling of a large volume of blood in the portal system of the dog, but this does not occur in the monkey.[7] Another factor which has produced conflicting data is the use of anesthesia in some experiments and not in others. This variance may be due to the fact that anesthetics alter the normal circulatory reflexes and may alter the effects of endotoxin. Also, the sequence of the events observed is dependent on the dose of endotoxin used. Finally, the circulatory changes that occur early in the course of endotoxic poisoning may be different from those that are observed later.

It is clear from experiments conducted on unanesthetized rhesus monkeys that the initial response to endotoxin is a decrease in systemic blood pressure which is due to a decrease in peripheral arterial resistance. The decrease in arterial resistance is accompanied by an increase in venous tone. Arterial resistance is decreased in all organs except the spleen, indicating that the microcirculation in the monkey does not undergo selective constriction on exposure to endotoxin. This suggests that the entire microcirculation is involved in potential pooling of blood in the early phase of shock.[8]

Coincident with the peripheral vascular changes, an increase in heart rate and a decrease in cardiac output occur. The decrease in cardiac output reverts to normal in 2 to 3 hours, or rises to above normal values.

Wilson and his colleagues have presented evidence which suggests that the early phase of shock in patients with bacteremia caused by gram-negative organisms is very similar to that seen in endotoxin shock in the rhesus monkey.[9]

Presence of Kinins

It has been shown that in the early phase cardiovascular changes induced by endotoxin in monkeys are accompanied or slightly preceded by the appearance of kinins in the plasma.[10] Recent findings support the belief that kinins may have an essential role in the early phase of endotoxin shock. These include the observation that infusion of kinins in man is followed by all the changes seen in the early phase of endotoxin shock.[11] The fall in blood pressure observed in the early phase of endotoxin shock is due almost entirely to a decrease in peripheral vascular resistance. Kinins are the most potent endogenous vasodilating agents known. The concentration of kinins in the plasma of monkeys injected with endotoxin is sufficient to cause the vasodilation and fall in blood pressure observed in them.

Nies and his co-workers[10] made serial measurements of plasma kinin concentration in the early phase of endotoxin shock in the unanesthetized monkey. Kinin concentration rose from the normal state, in which no kinin is detectable, to concentrations which were as high as 29 ng per ml. The kinins appeared in less than 15 minutes after intravenous infusion of endotoxin was begun (the infusion was conducted over a period of 40 minutes). The appearance of kinins in the plasma preceded or coincided with the beginning of the fall in blood pressure and the decreased peripheral resistance which were observed. The peak concentration of plasma kinin was reached in 1 to 2 hours, and it returned to undetectable levels in the monkeys that survived the dose of endotoxin. Plasma kinin concentration remained slightly elevated for 24 hours in the monkeys that did not survive. As might be expected, plasma concentration of kininogen (the globulin precursor of kinin) fell as the kinin level rose, and returned toward normal values as kinin disappeared from the plasma. Kinins have a short survival time in plasma; they have a half-life of about 30 seconds. They are destroyed by a kininase (carboxypeptidase-*N*). In the experiments of Nies and co-workers[10] described here, kininase remained elevated for at least 24 hours in the monkeys killed by the endotoxin, but very little rise was seen in animals that survived.

In the later (second) phase of endotoxin shock in the unanesthetized monkey, peripheral resistance is elevated rather than greatly reduced, as it is in the first phase.

Also, unlike the earlier phase, cardiac output is decreased in the second phase of shock. Kinin concentration is not elevated in the second phase. Therefore, other vasoactive substances must be involved in the later stages of endotoxin shock. It is probable that epinephrine and norepinephrine are involved in the later stages of shock, while it is clear that kinins and possibly histamine play a key role in the cardiovascular changes in the early phase.[12] Kinins have been shown to have a number of interesting interrelationships with epinephrine, norepinephrine, and histamine, which we shall describe later in this discussion. It is possible that the effect of kinins in the first phase of endotoxin shock determines the occurrence and severity of the later stages of shock.[10] For this reason, a brief discussion of kinins may be useful.

Characteristics of Kinins

Kinins are linear polypeptides, having from 9 to 11 amino acids and a molecular weight of a little over 1000. The two best studied kinins are bradykinin, which is made up of nine peptides, and kallidin, which has the same nine amino acids in the same order as bradykinin, as well as a tenth amino acid—lysine. The structure of these two kinins is shown in Figure 1.

The precursors of kinins are kininogens, which are alpha-2-globulins present in plasma. Kinins are split from kininogens by the ac-

```
                Arg-Pro-Pro-Gly-Phe-Ser-Pro-Phe-Arg              Bradykinin
(N-terminal)                                      (C-terminal)
```

```
                Lys-Arg-Pro-Gly-Phe-Ser-Pro-Phe-Arg              Kallidin
```
Figure 1.

tion of enzymes called kallikreins, which are present in an inactive form (kallikreinogens) in the plasma, in urine, and in the exocrine glands. Kallikrein, or an activator of kallikreinogen, is present in granulocytes also. One of the biochemical pathways which has been proposed for the *in vivo* generation of kinin is the sequence of interdependent reactions, with the product of each one activating the subsequent reaction,[12] shown in Figure 2.

Hageman factor may be activated as a consequence of injury to vascular endothelium. The sequence of reactions outlined here may be set off by the injury endotoxin causes to endothelial cells of blood vessels. Furthermore, there is no doubt that kinins are produced by the action of endotoxin on granulocytes.[10, 13] This probably is brought about by the release of kallikrein (or a kallikrein activator), which is present in granulocytes.

Kinins in nanogram quantities cause vasodilatation of the arterioles of the systemic circulation, including cerebral and coronary vessels. They very probably, at least in part, cause the systemic vascular dilatation and the fall in blood pressure which occurs in the early phase of endotoxin shock. However, kinins are not found in the plasma for more than a few hours. They are not detectable in the plasma in the later stages of shock when there is an increase in peripheral resistance, decreased venous return to the heart, and greatly decreased cardiac output.

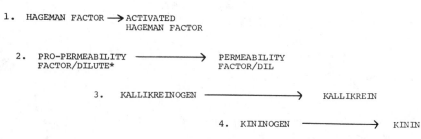

```
1.  HAGEMAN FACTOR ──→ ACTIVATED
                       HAGEMAN FACTOR

   2.  PRO-PERMEABILITY    ──────────→   PERMEABILITY
       FACTOR/DILUTE*                    FACTOR/DIL

        3.  KALLIKREINOGEN  ─────────────→   KALLIKREIN

           4.  KININOGEN   ──────────→   KININ
```

* Permeability factor/dilute is a protein found in serum which causes increased vascular permeability at site of injection into the skin.

Figure 2.

Vasoactive Agents: Epinephrine, Norepinephrine, and Histamine

Kinins may play an indirect part in the later phases of shock by setting in motion chemical changes which lead to the formation of other potent vasoactive agents. These include epinephrine, norepinephrine, and histamine. It is very probable that the first two compounds play a very important role in the vascular changes of endotoxin shock; the importance of histamine is not clear. Large doses of kinins release catecholamines by direct action on the medulla of the adrenal.

A reciprocal relationship between catecholamines and kinins is suggested by the fact that norepinephrine and epinephrine have been shown to cause the formation of kallikrein from tissues. Norepinephrine causes the excretion of kallikrein from salivary glands, and epinephrine infusion of carcinoid tumors also brings about the production of kallikrein. Conversely, epinephrine enhances the action of kininase, thus increasing the destruction of kinin. It is possible that this is one mechanism which serves to control the plasma kinin production.[12, 14, 15]

It is of interest also that kinins cause the release of histamine from mast cells. It has been shown by Hinshaw, Jordan, and Vick [14] that histamine rises in the blood of monkeys given endotoxin. This rise accompanies the fall of blood pressure in the early stage of shock, beginning within 30 minutes after the injection of the endotoxin. In fatally poisoned monkeys, histamine remains in higher than normal concentration in the plasma for at least 10 hours. There is no direct proof that the serum histamine rise is brought about by the action of kinins, but this possibility cannot be excluded. That interactions exist between kinins and the vasoactive amines (histamine, epinephrine, norepinephrine, serotonin) has been well established by experiments on man and laboratory animals. These relationships are shown in Figure 3, which is modified from a paper by Melmon and Cline.[15]

It is probable that all these compounds play a part in the circulatory changes which are induced by endotoxin. Present knowledge indicates that kinins, epinephrine, and norepinephrine may be of more importance than histamine or serotonin.

It was shown by Thomas[16] in 1956 that epinephrine caused hemorrhagic necrosis of the skin in rabbits which previously had been given an intravenous injection of endotoxin. Mixtures of epinephrine and endotoxin injected into the skin caused similar lesions. These observations led to the examination of the possibility that some of the harmful effects of endotoxin might be because it altered the reaction of peripheral blood vessels to epinephrine and norepinephrine. Zweifach, Nagler, and Thomas[17] demonstrated that endotoxin does change the normal vasoconstricting action of epinephrine on blood vessels. Small

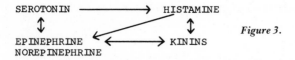

Figure 3.

doses of endotoxin cause epinephrine to exert a greatly increased degree of vasoconstriction. In the presence of endotoxin, prolonged and intense vasoconstriction is caused by a quantity of epinephrine which normally has no effect on blood vessels. A high dose of endotoxin produces a reversal of this effect. With high doses of endotoxin, blood vessels fail to constrict, or actually dilate when they are exposed to epinephrine. Similar results were obtained with norepinephrine.

Zweifach and his co-workers[17] showed that, in the rat, application of threshold doses of epinephrine (0.2 to 0.4 ng per ml) induced transient constriction of terminal arterioles and capillaries, with brief stoppage of capillary blood flow. After 10 to 20 seconds the blood vessels resumed their normal caliber, and blood flow became normal. When endotoxin was given intravenously in small sublethal doses, the application of the same threshold dose of epinephrine caused intense, widespread constriction of arteries, arterioles, venules, and small veins, and complete ischemia of the capillary bed. The venules and veins proved to be more reactive to the combination of endotoxin and epinephrine than were the terminal arterioles. The venous outflow from the capillary bed was stopped completely by quantities of epinephrine which had no effect on the arterioles.

When larger (lethal) doses of endotoxin were given, terminal arterioles and venules became totally unresponsive to epinephrine and norepinephrine, while the arteries and veins continued to be hyperreactive to these amines and remained greatly constricted. As a result, blood became pooled in all the distended capillaries and venules, while the arteries and veins were contracted to threadlike diameter. The distention of the capillaries and venules was followed by the appearance of petechiae.

We shall now consider in more detail the hemodynamic effects which the vasoactive compounds bring about. The changes which are observed probably depend upon which of these compounds (or which combination of them) is acting on the circulatory system at a given time. The amount of time that has elapsed after the beginning of exposure to endotoxin is also of great importance. The dose of endotoxin given, the species of animal studied, and the use of anesthesia all have an influence on the data obtained. When these factors are taken into account, we find that there is general agreement regarding many of the changes which have been observed following administration of endotoxin.

There is a high degree of consensus among investigators concerning the alterations which occur soon after endotoxin is given to the experimental animal. In the anesthetized dog and the anesthetized and unanesthetized monkey, the injection of endotoxin is followed very quickly by a fall in blood pressure. In the dog this is accompanied by a decrease in responsiveness of the precapillary vessels to vasoconstricting substances and an increase in responsiveness of the postcapillary vessels, which become greatly constricted. There is a marked rise in the total peripheral resistance. Blood becomes pooled in the mesenteric and portal venous sytems, and venous return to the heart decreases. Cardiac output decreases, and blood pressure falls. This pooling phenomenon is always observed in dogs.[7]

In the unanesthetized monkey, injection of endotoxin also is followed by a prompt fall in blood pressure. Heart rate increases and cardiac output falls, but these return to normal or even to above normal values within 3 hours.[10] In sharp contrast to the dog, the monkey experiences a fall in total peripheral resistance. This decline is roughly parallel to the decrease in blood pressure. No pooling of blood in portal, splanchnic, or other large areas is found in the unanesthetized monkey.

The decrease in venous return, which probably accounts for the lowering of cardiac output, is believed by some authors[18] to be caused by a net increase in the volume of blood in the small veins throughout the circulatory system. This would amount to a uniform pooling of blood, in contrast to the hepatosplanchnic pooling seen in the dog.

As shock progresses in the dog, dilatation of the arterioles and capillaries progresses while constriction of the veins continues. Blood enters the capillary beds in increasing amounts but is unable to leave them because of the venous constriction. Hydrostatic pressure is increased in the capillary beds, forcing fluid and blood cells out of the circulatory system and into the tissues. Circulating blood volume is decreased, and perfusion of the organs is diminished. Hemorrhagic necrosis of the viscera occurs, with the intestinal mucosa suffering the most severe damage. Venous return to the heart falls further, causing more marked decrease of cardiac output and blood pressure.[19, 20]

Late in the course of endotoxic shock in the unanesthetized monkey, circulatory changes occur which are different from those encountered soon after endotoxin has been injected. In this second phase, which may begin a short time before death, the total peripheral resistance is somewhat increased and cardiac output is decreased. Even at this point, however, no localized pooling of blood is found in the monkey.[10]

Cardiovascular Effects in Man

In man, endotoxin induces circulatory changes which in many ways resemble those it causes in the unanesthetized monkey. The effects on the human circulation are quite different from those suffered by the dog.

It is apparent that endotoxin causes a decrease in the total peripheral resistance (TPR)* in the septic patient. Wilson and colleagues[9] studied the TPR in 12 patients with septic shock uncomplicated by hypovolemia due to massive blood or fluid loss (hypovolemic shock) or by myocardial infarction (cardiac shock). Eleven of these patients with "pure" septic shock had a TPR which was lower than the normal value of 1000 to 1300 dyne-sec/cm[5], one patient had a normal value, and none had an elevated TPR. Similar results are reported by others.[21]

The patients with endotoxic shock studied by Wilson and coworkers[9] had central venous pressure recordings in the normal range. This is in very sharp contrast to the findings in dogs.

Cardiac output has been described as showing a steady decline in patients with endotoxic shock.[21] However, Wilson and colleagues[9] reported that this is not a uniform finding. Three of their patients had a normal cardiac output together with decreased TPR, five had an increased cardiac output, and four had a decreased cardiac output. The cardiac output appeared to be related to survival. Only a small percentage of patients with a cardiac index of 2.0 L/minute/square meter survived. The cardiac index is the cardiac output per square meter of body surface; the normal cardiac index is 2.5 to 3.75 L/minute/square meter.

Wilson and colleagues[9] showed that endotoxic shock differed from the shock caused by hemorrhage or other large-volume fluid loss (hypovolemic shock) and from the cardiac shock of myocardial infarction. This is summarized in Table 1.

TABLE 1   Distinctions Among Types of Shock

Findings	Endotoxic Shock	Hypovolemic Shock	Cardiac Shock
Total peripheral resistance	Low	High	High
Cardiac output	Low, normal, high	Low	Low
Central venous pressure	Normal range	Low	High

Every physician knows that the distinctions among the three types of shock made here often are not very sharp. In a significant number of patients, shock is caused by combinations of endotoxemia, blood and fluid loss, and cardiac disease. Such patients present clinical findings of

---

*TPR is calculated from mean arterial blood pressure (MBP), central venous pressure (CVP), and cardiac output (CO) by the following formula:

$$\text{TPR (dyne-sec/cm}^5\text{)} = \frac{\text{MBP (mm Hg)} - \text{CVP (mm Hg)}}{\text{CO (liters/min)}} \times 80.$$

great complexity. For example, when hypovolemic and endotoxic factors coexist, TPR either may be elevated (as it is in hypovolemic shock), decreased (as it is in endotoxic shock), or normal. Similarly, when myocardial infarction complicates endotoxemia, TPR may be elevated, cardiac output may be decreased, and central venous pressure may be high.

INTRAVASCULAR COAGULATION

Thrombi have been found in the blood vessels of many organs in animals which have been injected with endotoxin. There are also many well-documented examples of widespread intravascular clotting in patients with sepsis caused by gram-negative bacteria, other bacteria, viruses, and rickettsial infections. Perhaps the bacterial infection which most often causes extensive intravascular coagulation is meningococcemia.

It has been demonstrated that endotoxin acts to disturb the intravascular clotting mechanism in a number of ways. We shall consider some of these effects. It has been shown by McGrath and Stewart[22] that endotoxin injures the vascular endothelium of rabbits. Within 1 hour after these animals are given one dose of endotoxin intracardially, histological changes are seen in the endothelium of systemic arteries. The normally elliptical nuclei of the endothelial cells become spindle-shaped and stain irregularly. In some areas the endothelial cell nuclei show vacuolization, and a few red and white blood cells are stuck to the cell surface. Twenty-four hours later the damage is more severe; some of the nuclei are almost unrecognizable. In some parts of the arteries, all cellular structure is destroyed. Clumps of red cells and platelets are adherent to the surface of the injured endothelial cells.

The clear-cut evidence of almost immediate injury of the vascular endothelium is of interest in several ways. First, it is of importance in that it is probable that some injury to the endothelium is necessary for the formation of fibrin clots. Second, it is believed that injury to the endothelium may bring about activation of Hageman factor (coagulation factor XII), which begins the chain of reactions that culminates in the action of thrombin on fibrinogen to form fibrin.

After injection of endotoxin in animals, platelets decrease, probably owing to formation of platelet thrombi. According to Hardaway,[23] intravenous injection of endotoxin into the dog brings about the same widespread intravascular coagulation as does the injection of thrombin. However, thrombin causes clotting by direct action on fibrinogen, while endotoxin does not affect fibrinogen directly. Thrombin removes negatively charged peptides from fibrinogen, and the removal of these repelling charges permits the fibrinogen molecules to aggregate and form a fibrin network. Endotoxin probably starts coagulation by activating Hageman factor. Both agents bring about widespread coagulation in the microcirculation, which causes severe obstruction to blood flow. Hardaway has shown that, within 5 minutes after intavenous injection of endotoxin, the plasma of the dog has undergone a severe decrease in fibrinogen, prothrombin, and coagulation factors V, VII, VIII, IX, X, XI, and XII.

A similar decrease in the components of the intravascular clotting mechanism occurs in man in endotoxemic conditions. Decreases in circulating platelets, coagulation factors V and VIII, prothrombin, and fibrinogen have been demonstrated. Blockage of the circulation may be widespread, causing necrosis of large areas of the skin. Occlusion of vessels large enough to require amputation of extremities may occur.

As soon as fibrin is formed, fibrinolysis begins. This is carried out by a proteolytic enzyme system—the plasminogen-plasmin system. Plasminogen is present in all body fluids, but the highest concentration is in the plasma. Plasminogen is always incorporated into fibrin deposits as they form. Plasminogen activators, which are also present in many body fluids, convert plasminogen to plasmin. Plasmin hydrolyzes fibrin into two large components that are antigenically distinct.

In many instances, soon after intravascular coagulation occurs, plasma fibrinogen is restored to normal or to higher than normal levels, and the platelets in the blood reach or exceed their precoagulation number. However, in some instances fibrinogen and platelets are not restored in proper quantity while fibrinolysis continues, and compounds are formed which interfere with the polymerization of fibrin. In this situation intravascular coagulation may be followed by severe bleeding into the skin, mucous membranes, and internal organs.

EFFECT OF ENDOTOXIN ON METABOLISM

Endotoxin has an adverse effect on carbohydrate and protein metabolism. In addition, animals and patients with endotoxemia are usually in metabolic acidosis. These effects probably are in part the result of cell injury which is secondary to interference with the microcirculation. However, there is reason to believe that endotoxin causes direct injury to cells and cellular organelles. For example, the plasma concentration of the lysosomal enzyme alpha glucosidase rises within 2 hours after the unanesthetized monkey is given an injection of endotoxin.[10] This indicates that the membrane of the lysosome has been injured sufficiently to allow the escape of an enzyme when changes in the microcirculation of the animal are not yet profound.

There is convincing evidence from animal experiments that endotoxin causes derangement of carbohydrate metabolism. It was shown by Berry and co-workers[24] that mice given a large dose of endotoxin suffer severe depletion of blood glucose, liver glycogen and total body carbohydrate. Endotoxin prevents the conversion of injected glucose into liver glycogen, but no effect on muscle glycogen is produced.

It has been shown that endotoxin interferes directly or indirectly with essential molecular reactions in carbohydrate metabolism. For example, endotoxin inhibits the oxidative decarboxylation of pyruvate. This was demonstrated in animals given salmonella or meningococcus endotoxins.[25] Pyruvic acid ($CH_3 \cdot CO \cdot COOH$) normally is converted to acetaldehyde by the enzyme carboxylase and the coenzyme cocarboxylase (thiamine pyrophosphate, or TPP). Then, by a series of reactions involving lipoic acid, flavin adenine dinucleotide (FAD), nicotinamide-adenine dinucleotide (NAD), and coenzyme A (CoA·SH), it is converted to acetyl-coenzyme A. In this form ("active" acetate) it enters the citric acid cycle (Krebs cycle). The conversion of pyruvic acid to acetyl-coenzyme A may be summarized as shown in Figure 4. Endotoxin blocks this reaction. As a result, no pyruvate enters the Krebs cycle in the form of acetyl-coenzyme A, and further carbohydrate metabolism is diminished greatly. Since pyruvate cannot enter the Krebs cycle to be metabolized to ketoglutarate, it is metabolized to lactic acid to a greater extent than is normal. Lactic acid thus becomes the end product of the glycolytic glucose cycle. Accumulation of lactic acid may contribute to the acidemia seen in endotoxin shock. Furthermore, because of the decreased function of the Krebs cycle, fewer energy molecules pass through the cycle, and production of adenosine triphosphate (ATP) is reduced. Endotoxin may interfere with the pyruvate–acetyl-coenzyme A reaction indirectly—by its effect on the microcirculation, an effect which might injure cell mitochondria. If this is the case, the reaction may be blocked by the breakdown of the cytochrome enzyme system, which normally accomplishes the final step in the removal of the hydrogen produced. Or, endotoxin may interfere with enzymes by directly injuring mitochondria.

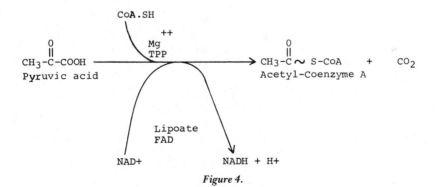

Figure 4.

There is in fact evidence that endotoxin does damage liver mitochondria. Endotoxin causes a decrease in the oxygen uptake of rat liver mitochondria, and it uncouples oxidative phosphorylation in these organelles.[26]

Endotoxin also has been shown to have effects on protein metabolism. It inhibits the induction of the enzyme tryptophan pyrrolase in liver cells. This enzyme, which is an oxygenase, catalyzes the first step in the metabolism of tryptophan.[27]

There is also evidence that endotoxin interferes with the energy production which is required for cell metabolism. Adenosine triphosphate (ATP) production appears to be decreased in cells of animals poisoned by endotoxin. This effect also would result from injury to mitochondria. Takeda and co-workers[28] reported that mice could be completely protected from the effects of a lethal quantity of salmonella endotoxin by intravenous injection of ATP if a dose of 1 mg per 20 gm of body weight was used.

Schumer and Sperling[29] have proposed that we should consider shock as a disorder of the molecules of cells. They believe that the defects in the microcirculation which occur in shock cause damage to cellular function. They imply that the block at the pyruvate–coenzyme A step is due to alteration of cell metabolism, which is caused by the anoxic effect of the decreased microcirculation. Because of this block, lactic acid accumulates. The anaerobic glucose pathway is reversed, with the reaction proceeding from pyruvate to glyceraldehyde to dihydroxyacetone to glucose-6-phosphate. Glucose (which cannot be made into glycogen since endotoxin prevents this process) leaves the cell. Amino acids, which normally enter the glycolytic pathway at the step which produces pyruvate, now leave the cell as the pathway is reversed. A similar course is taken by fatty acids which normally enter the glycolytic cycle at the pyruvate–coenzyme A step. Because of injury to the mitochondria and the decreased activity of the Krebs cycle, less energy and less than the normal amount of ATP is formed. This causes the accumulation of phosphates. Thus, the blockage in anaerobic glucose metabolism leads to the accumulation of lactic acid, phosphates, fatty acids, and amino acids in the plasma, and produces acidemia. With increasing injury to the cell (caused directly by endotoxin or by the microcirculatory deficiency), lysosomal membranes rupture, and phosphatases and hydrolases escape into the plasma.

LABORATORY DIAGNOSIS OF ENDOTOXEMIA

It would be of great assistance to the clinician if a laboratory method for the detection of endotoxin in the blood was available. A number of such methods have been published, but until recently none has been clinically useful. In 1964, and in subsequent reports, Levin and Bang[30] described a method which is of clinical value in some cases. It can be performed in any laboratory and quite often gives a positive result within 3 or 4 hours. The method is extremely sensitive; it detects as little as 0.1 to 1.0 ng of endotoxin per ml of serum. As will be shown further on, even this method has limitations. The method is based on the discovery that a water-clear lysate which gels in the presence of very minute quantities of endotoxin can be obtained from the amebocytes of the horseshoe crab *(Limulus polyphemus)*. In brief, the method of Levin and Bang is carried out in the following manner.

Blood from patients is collected in endotoxin-free glassware containing 5000 units of heparin. The plasma is separated by centrifugation and 0.1 ml of it is added to 0.1 ml of the amebocyte lysate. The mixtures are kept at 37°C for 1 hour and then read for gel formation. The degree of gelation is compared to that which is produced by known quantities of endotoxin.

There is a globulin substance in serum which binds endotoxin. If all the endotoxin in a serum is bound by this globulin, the result of the test described here will be negative. Treatment with chloroform releases the endotoxin from the globulin, enabling one to determine the presence of bound endotoxin also. Specimens of plasma which are negative when tested directly with limulus lysate may be shown to be positive when the chloroform extract is tested. For this reason, the limulus test should be carried out with a chloroform extract of plasma.

In 1970, Levin and co-workers[31] performed the limulus test on the plasma of 98 patients suspected of having bacteremia caused by gram-negative bacteria. Seventeen of these patients had endotoxemia as determined by the limulus test. Twelve of these patients had gram-negative rod bacteremia. In contrast, 77 normal controls and 27 patients with pneumococcal pneumonia or with pneumococcal, streptococcal, or staphylococcal bacteremia all had a negative test for endotoxemia. Levin's results indicate that the limulus test is not invariably positive in gram-negative bacterial infections. Three of his patients who had enterobacter bacteremia gave a negative test result.

A very recent report on the value of the limulus test was published in 1975 by Elin and co-workers.[32] These authors showed that preparations of limulus amebocyte extracts varied greatly in their efficacy. Lyophilized extracts in particular gave a low percentage of positive results, while unlyophilized and unfrozen extracts made by Elin and by Levin[31] yielded a high percentage of positive results. Elin studied a total of 237 samples of 111 patients. Forty-eight plasma samples were positive (all but one was positive with Levin's extract). The Yates modification of the chi-square test showed a statistically significant correlation between a positive limulus test and a positive blood culture ($p = <0.0005$), a positive blood culture for gram-negative organisms

($p = < 0.005$), and an elevated absolute neutrophil count ($p = < 0.0001$). On the other hand, Elin points out that a positive limulus test is not correlated with severity of disease, and that it has no prognostic value. For these reasons, despite the excellent statistical correlation of a positive limulus test with other laboratory indications of endotoxemia, Elin and co-workers conclude that "the test in its present form is not clinically useful in the diagnosis of endotoxemia or gram-negative septicemia." However, we believe that this conclusion is too negative. It is clear that the limulus test does have limitations, but when these are taken into account, a positive result does furnish very useful clinical data often enough to warrant its continued use.

The relatively frequent occurrence of a negative result of the limulus test in patients with gram-negative bacteremia has been taken as an indication that the test is unreliable. This is not the case, however, because it has been shown that most patients with bacteremia have fewer than 100 bacteria per ml of blood, while 1000 bacteria per ml are required to give a positive limulus test. Hence, in most cases the bacteria in the blood would not give a positive result unless endotoxin from some other source has entered the blood. This would occur in peritonitis, for example.

We have stated previously that there is a globulin in normal human plasma which binds endotoxin. This binding is probably the first step in the degradation and detoxification of endotoxin. In studying this globulin, Eugene Ainbender in our laboratory has found that the blood of the newborn infant contains only one tenth of the concentration of the endotoxin-binding globulin that is present in the blood of the mother.

TREATMENT OF ENDOTOXIN SHOCK

There is little doubt that, if endotoxin shock is permitted to go untreated for a long period, its effects may become irreversible. The best time for successful treatment is at the onset of shock. It is of the utmost importance that careful and continuous observation be afforded the patient who is suffering from an infection that may induce endotoxin shock. Such infections include meningococcemia and neonatal sepsis, which is very often caused by gram-negative enteric bacilli. Children with leukemia, lymphoma, and other malignant diseases who are suffering from any bacterial infection are liable to go into shock. Such patients also require special attention.

At the onset of endotoxin shock, there may be changes in the patient's mental state. There may be a loss of alertness or even brief lapses into a torpid or semistuporous state. Often, with the onset of shock, pulse and respiratory rates rise abruptly. The blood pressure should be recorded at regular intervals, since it may drop precipitously. A fall in diastolic pressures may precede a systolic drop. It is our practice to record the blood pressure every hour during the first 8 hours after beginning treatment of patients with meningococcic meningitis; after this period blood pressure is taken every 3 hours for the next 24 hours.

Endotoxin shock is a multiple system disease which exerts a harmful effect on the circulation, on many organs, and on a number of metabolic processes of the patient. These deleterious effects vary with the amount of endotoxemia and with duration of the exposure to the toxin. Furthermore, patients with septic shock often are suffering from other conditions, such as coronary artery disease, malignancy, and surgical trauma. These conditions often complicate or obscure the symptoms caused by endotoxic poisoning. It is not surprising, therefore, that no single drug and no prearranged protocol will be useful for the treatment of all patients with endotoxic shock. Every patient must be treated individually, with careful consideration of all the clinical findings and of all the available laboratory data. In many instances, decisions about treatment must be made almost entirely on clinical grounds. The patient may be too sick to undergo laboratory studies, or his or her condition may be too grave to permit the physician to wait for the results of laboratory studies before beginning therapy. Therapy should be altered promptly if laboratory data provide information that shows that such a change is needed.

With these reservations, we may outline certain principles of treatment which we believe may be useful.

1. Start treatment as soon as the diagnosis of endotoxic shock is made. To delay is to jeopardize the patient's life. In the neonate with gram-negative bacterial sepsis or the patient with meningococcemia, the appearance of any of the clinical symptoms of shock described here warrants institution of anti-shock therapy.

2. Restore blood volume. In many instances, there is no doubt that hypovolemia is present. This is the case in septic infants with diarrhea and vomiting. Children who have undergone surgery and show signs of infection with gram-negative bacteria are often hypovolemic. Glucose and electrolyte solutions may be given as initial therapy, but blood or plasma usually are required to maintain blood volume.

3. Treat with antibiotics the bacterial infection which is the source of endotoxin.

4. Give intravenously a "pharmacological" dose of hydrocortisone. Thirty-five to 50 mg per kg of body weight are recommended. This may be given over a 10-minute period. It may be repeated at 30- to 60-minute intervals for four doses if necessary. Cortisone is recommended because, in the doses recommended here, it exerts many anti-shock effects, which include actions on blood vessels and on molecular reactions. Cortisone acts as an adrenergic blocking agent, relieving the

vascular spasm caused by the abnormal action which epinephrine and norepinephrine exert in the presence of endotoxin. Cortisone exerts a favorable action on carbohydrate metabolism. It counteracts the depletion of glycogen which endotoxin causes. It decreases lactic acid formation by stimulating the pathways that lead to the eventual conversion of lactic acid into glycogen. Cortisone induces the entrance of amino acids into the pyruvate cycle and the entrance of fat into the Krebs cycle; both these actions favor production of ATP.[29] Cortisone has a protective action on lysosomes, preventing their rupture. Cortisone prevents kallikrein from forming kinin from kininogen. It should be noted that the concentration of corticosteroids in the plasma is not decreased in patients with endotoxemia. In fact, in some instances, the corticosteroid level is somewhat elevated. The effects of cortisone described here are obtained only with very high, "pharmacological" doses of cortisone, which raise the plasma level far above that normally found.

It should be noted that the published data indicate that there is no need for "replacement" therapy with adrenal corticosteroids. The concentration of these steroids in the blood may be normal, high, or low in patients with endotoxin shock. Furthermore, several controlled series in which corticosteroids have been used in "physiological" dosage have given negative results.

There is no controlled series which proves the value of "pharmacological" doses of corticosteroids in endotoxin shock. However, the results of animal experiments, and the proved favorable effects of high doses of cortisone in reversing some of the effects of endotoxin, warrant its clinical use. A controlled, large-scale study of this problem is urgently needed.

Many authors have advised against the use of cortisone in the presence of endotoxin-producing bacteria. This recommendation is based on the fear that a generalized Shwartzman reaction might occur if cortisone is used in these circumstances. In fact, in 1952 Thomas and Good[33] reported that a single injection of endotoxin in cortisone-treated rabbits produced a generalized Shwartzman reaction. However, more recently (in 1967), Corrigan and co-workers[34] were unable to produce a Shwartzman reaction with endotoxin in cortisone-treated rabbits, even when they used extremely high doses of cortisone and endotoxin. We do not believe there is convincing evidence that a generalized Shwartzman reaction has been evoked in endotoxemic patients treated with cortisone. We have never observed such a reaction, although we have used cortisone in the treatment of endotoxic shock since 1952.[35]

5. Vasodilators such as isoproterenol and phenoxybenzamine are recommended by some authors. Their value in endotoxin shock is not clearly established. Lillehei[20] was unable to increase the survival of dogs in endotoxin shock by treating them with phenoxybenzamine. Hydro-

cortisone was much more effective. We believe that the vasodilating effect which can be obtained with phenoxybenzamine and isoproterenol may be more effectively obtained with "pharmacological" doses of cortisone.

6. Correct the metabolic acidemia if it is present. Many patients in endotoxic shock are in severe acidemia. This should be corrected by administration of bicarbonate.

7. Intravascular coagulation, when it is extensive, should be treated at once with heparin. Heparin also should be used when the clotting threatens the loss of a limb or of toes or fingers. When there is evidence of less severe intravascular clotting—such as scattered petechiae—it seems best at this time to look for laboratory evidence of coagulopathy before using anticoagulation therapy. If such evidence is found in the presence of symptoms of endotoxic shock or impending shock, heparin therapy should be started. For example, if a low platelet count is found, heparin should be administered; the same is true if there is a decreased concentration of plasma fibrinogen. Abildgaard[36] recommends the use of rapidly obtained screening tests, including observation of the whole blood clot, platelet count, fibrinogen concentration by the semiquantitative heat precipitation method, thrombin time, and partial thromboplastin time.

If a decreased value is obtained by these methods, we may assume that intravascular coagulation has occurred. However, the finding of normal values does not exclude the existence of intravascular coagulation, because, after coagulation has occurred, the clotting factors may be restored rapidly. Thus, we often must make a decision which is based on clinical judgment alone. (See also Chapter 22.)

When heparin is used, it is given intravenously in a dose of 1 mg per kg of body weight every 4 hours. The whole blood clotting time should be kept at 20 to 30 minutes prior to each succeeding dose of heparin.[36] The laboratory screening tests referred to here should be carried out at regular intervals, and, if possible, several more time-consuming laboratory measurements should be made. These include assay of factors V and VIII. Heparin treatment should be continued until coagulation values have returned to normal or until the patient has recovered from the infection which has caused shock.

On occasion, patients under heparin treatment for intravascular clotting may have a hemorrhage from mucous membranes. When this occurs, the action of heparin may be counteracted rapidly by injection of protamine sulfate.

REFERENCES

1. Carey, W. F., and Baron, L. S.: Comparative immunologic studies of cell structure isolated from *Salmonella typhosa*. J. Immunol., *83*:17, 1959.
2. Nowotny, A. M.: Molecular aspects of endotoxic reactions. Bacteriol. Rev., *33*:72, 1969.

3. Nowotny, A. M.: Chemical structure of a phosphomucolipid and its occurrence in some strains of *Salmonella*. J. Am. Chem. Soc., *83*:501, 1961.

4. Nowotny, A. M.: Heterogeneity of endotoxic bacterial lipopolysaccharides revealed by ion-exchange column chromatography. Nature, *210*:278, 1966.

5. Levy, E., Path, F. C., and Ruebner, B. H.: Hepatic changes produced by a single dose of endotoxin in the mouse. Am. J. Pathol., *51*:269, 1967.

6. Rubenstein, H. S., Fine, J., and Coons, A. H.: Localization of endotoxin in the walls of the peripheral vascular system during lethal endotoxemia. Proc. Soc. Exp. Biol. Med., *3*:458, 1962.

7. Hinshaw, L. B.: *In* Overwhelming Bacterial Infections in Childhood. Report of the Fifty-fifth Ross Conference on Pediatric Research. Columbus, Ohio, Ross Laboratories, 1966, pp. 53–57.

8. Forsyth, R., Nies, A. S., Wyler, F., Neutze, J., and Melmon, K. L.: Endotoxin-induced microcirculatory changes in the unanesthetized primate. Clin. Res., *16*:107, 1968.

9. Wilson, R. F., Thal, A. P., Kindling, P. H., Grifka, T., and Ackerman, E.: Hemodynamic measurements in septic shock. Arch. Surg., *91*:121, 1965.

10. Nies, A. S., Forsyth, R. P., Williams, E. H., and Melmon, K. L.: Contribution of kinins to endotoxin shock in unanesthetized rhesus monkeys. Circ. Res., *22*:155, 1968.

11. Mason, D. T., and Melmon, K. L.: Abnormal forearm vascular responses in the carcinoid syndrome: The role of kinins and kinin-generating system. J. Clin. Invest., *45*:1685, 1966.

12. Kellermeyer, R. W., and Graham, R. C., Jr.: Kinins — possible physiologic and pathologic roles in man. N. Engl. J. Med., *279*:754, 1968.

13. Melmon, K. L., and Cline, M. J.: Interaction of plasma kinins and granulocytes. Nature, *213*:90, 1967.

14. Hinshaw, L. B., Jordan, M. M., and Vick, J. A.: Histamine release and endotoxin shock in the primate. J. Clin. Invest., *40*:1631, 1961.

15. Melmon, K. L., and Cline, M. J.: Kinins. Am. J. Med., *43*:153, 1967.

16. Thomas, L.: The role of epinephrine in the reactions produced by the endotoxins of gram-negative bacteria. J. Exp. Med., *104*:865, 1956.

17. Zweifach, B. W., Nagler, A. L., and Thomas, L.: The role of endotoxin in the reactions produced by the endotoxins of gram-negative bacteria. J. Exp. Med., *104*:881, 1956.

18. Hinshaw, L. B., Emerson, E. T., Jr., and Reins, D. A.: Cardiovascular responses of the primate in endotoxin shock. Am. J. Physiol., *210*:335, 1966.

19. Lillehei, R. C., Longerbeam, J. K., Bloch, J. H., and Mannax, W. G.: The nature of irreversible shock. Ann. Surg., *160*:682, 1964.

20. Lillehei, R. C.: *In* Overwhelming Bacterial Infections in Childhood. Report of the Fifty-fifth Ross Conference on Pediatric Research, Columbus, Ohio, Ross Laboratories, 1966, pp. 58–63.

21. Gilbert, R. P.: Mechanisms of the hemodynamic effects of endotoxin. Physiol. Rev., *40*:245, 1960.

22. McGrath, J. M., and Stewart, G. J.: The effects of endotoxin on vascular endothelium. J. Exp. Med., *129*:833, 1969.

23. Hardaway, R. M.: *In* Overwhelming Bacterial Infections in Childhood. Report of the Fifty-fifth Ross Conference on Pediatric Research. Columbus Ohio, Ross Laboratories, 1966, pp. 34–35.

24. Berry, L. J., Smythe, D. S., and Young, L. G.: Effects of bacterial endotoxin on metabolism. I. J. Exp. Med., *110*:389, 1959.

25. Kun, E., and Abood, L. G.: Mechanism of inhibition of glycogen synthesis by endotoxins of *Salmonella aertrycke* and type 1 meningococcus. Proc. Soc. Exp. Biol. Med., *71*:362, 1949.

26. Mager, J., and Theodor, E.: Inhibition of mitochondrial respiration and uncoupling of oxidative phosphorylation by fractions of the *Shigella paradysenteriae* type III somatic antigen. Arch. Biochem., *67*:169, 1957.

27. Berry, L. J., and Smythe, D. S.: Effects of bacterial endotoxin on metabolism, VII. J. Exp. Med., *120*:721, 1964.

28. Takeda, Y., Miura, Y., Sazaki, H., and Kasai, N.: The elimination of metabolic disturbances produced by the injection of *S. typhi*, *S. paratyphi B*, *S. flexneri* and the

prevention of animals from death through the application of adenosine triphosphate. Jap. J. Exp. Med., *25*:133, 1955.

29. Schumer, W., and Sperling, R.: Shock and its effect on the cell. J.A.M.A., *205*:215, 1968.

30. Levin, J., and Bang, F. B.: The role of endotoxin in the extracellular coagulation of *Limulus* blood. Bull. Johns Hopkins Hosp., *115*:265, 1964.

31. Levin, J., Poore, T. E., Zauber, N. P., and Oser, R. S.: Detection of endotoxin in the blood of patients with sepsis due to gram-negative bacteria. N. Engl. J. Med., *283*:1313, 1970.

32. Elin, R. J., Robinson, A. R., Levine, A. S., and Wolff, S. N.: Lack of clinical usefulness of the limulus test in the diagnosis of endotoxemia. N. Engl. J. Med., *293*:521, 1975.

33. Thomas, L., and Good, R. A.: The effect of cortisone on the Shwartzman reaction. J. Exp. Med., *95*:409, 1952.

34. Corrigan, J. J., Abildgaard, C. F., Seeler, R. A., and Schulman, I.: Quantitative aspects of blood coagulation in the generalized Shwartzman reaction. Pediatr. Res., *1*:99, 1967.

35. Hodes, H. L., Moloshok, R. E., and Markowitz, M.: Fulminating meningococcemia treated with cortisone. Pediatrics, *10*:138, 1952.

36. Abildgaard, C. F.: Recognition and treatment of intravascular coagulation. J. Pediatr., *74*:163, 1969.

Chapter Three

ACUTE ADRENAL INSUFFICIENCY

ALFRED M. BONGIOVANNI, M.D.

CAUSES

Acute adrenal insufficiency in infancy and childhood has several causes. It may be due to primary aplasia of the adrenal gland and may be accompanied by other congenital anomalies such as anencephaly. Hypoplasia of the adrenal with a longer period of survival has also been described.

Bilateral adrenal hemorrhage, usually in the newborn, may be the result of a traumatic delivery. The symptoms occur early and resemble those of overwhelming septicemia. Without immediate recognition and vigorous treatment, the condition is fatal. Certainty of such diagnosis in an infant who survives is difficult, although calcification of the adrenal glands may be visible by x-ray in later life.

Temporary hypofunction of the adrenal cortex in early life also has been described and may represent a defect in the biosynthesis of aldosterone. However, the indiscriminate treatment of numerous infants presumed to have this condition, as has been promulgated from time to time, is not endorsed by this writer.

Fulminating infections may be accompanied by acute adrenal insufficiency, as in the Waterhouse-Friderichsen syndrome. The mortality is high and postmortem examinations often reveal damage to the adrenal cortex. Although suitable therapy as described herein may be required for adrenal insufficiency *per se,* there is little to support the notion that empirical employment of large doses of adrenal steroids exerts a beneficial effect in the treatment of a variety of infections.

From the Department of Pediatrics, School of Medicine, University of Pennsylvania, and Children's Hospital of Philadelphia, Pennsylvania.

In about one-fourth of patients with the adrenogenital syndrome (and this incidence varies from clinic to clinic) due to congenital adrenal hyperplasia, the condition is complicated by an electrolyte disturbance attributable to a deficiency of the salt-retaining steroids. Infants affected with this condition fail to thrive and have emesis, dehydration, and shock in the early weeks of life. In contrast to other forms in which steroid levels in blood and urine are low, there is a rise in urinary 17-ketosteroids as well as other "abnormal" adrenal products.

The sudden withdrawal of adrenal steroids administered for purposes other than primary adrenal disease may be followed by acute adrenal failure. Adrenal crisis also may occur after unilateral adrenalectomy for a tumor causing Cushing's syndrome, since the other gland in such cases is usually atrophic. Finally, acute insufficiency may occur in chronic adrenal disease (Addison's disease) and often is precipitated in this condition by superimposed infection or injury.

TREATMENT

With deficiency of adrenocortical steroidal hormones, there is a loss of extracellular water and sodium into the urine, the intracellular compartment, and possibly bone. There is also loss into the sweat. This leads to extracellular dehydration and hypotension. On the other hand, there is potassium retention. Thus, supplementary potassium in the treatment of this condition is contraindicated unless hypokalemia develops later as a consequence of excessive treatment with adrenal steroids.

The keys to therapy of adrenocortical failure thus include fluid and electrolyte replacement as well as appropriate steroid hormone replacement. Approximately 100 to 120 ml of isotonic saline solution per kilogram of body weight should be administered intravenously within the first 24 hours to children weighing up to 20 kg, and 75 ml per kilogram should be administered when body weight is above 20 kg. These recommendations are based on the special situation applicable to the dehydration of adrenal failure in which extracellular fluid loss predominates. When shock is especially severe, 5 ml of plasma per kilogram of body weight may be substituted, volume for volume, as part of the initial replacement fluid. About 20 to 25 per cent of the total may be given carefully during the first 2 hours. After the first day, maintenance may be continued as half isotonic saline solution in 5 per cent glucose, about one-third to one-half the volume stated here.

When liquids may be taken by mouth, ordinary fluids may be administered as tolerated, with additional sodium chloride, 1 gm per each 10 kg of body weight.

Simultaneously, it is necessary to administer those steroid hormones which are believed to be deficient. This writer strongly urges that the "newer" steroids be avoided, and that cortisone or hydrocortisone always be used in the treatment of acute adrenal insufficiency. Initially, one of the soluble hydrocortisone products, either hemisuccinate or phosphate, should be given intravenously, 1.5 to 2.0 mg per kilogram of body weight. Hydrocortisone phosphate has a longer duration of action, but this is of secondary importance since it is well to administer hydrocortisone (or cortisone acetate) intramuscularly, 2 mg per kilogram, as soon as possible, to be repeated daily for several days. The intramuscular dose is absorbed slowly; the plasma level does not reach its peak for several hours and then is maintained for 24 hours or longer, thus obviating the need for further intravenous steroid. It is also necessary to give one of the salt-retaining steroids, and for this purpose desoxycorticosterone acetate is most often employed intramuscularly in a dose of 2 mg on the first day and 1 mg a day thereafter. This compound restores the electrolyte regulation and diminishes the salt requirements.

Often a vasopressor substance is required. About 25 mg of metaraminol bitartrate may be added to 250 ml of 5 per cent glucose and connected via a Y tube to the system delivering the recommended electrolyte solution. The rate of flow which will support the blood pressure is maintained. In severe adrenal cortical insufficiency, vasopressor drugs may be without effect until after the administration of hydrocortisone. After complete restoration, the steroids may be tapered rapidly in the hospital, by 25 per cent diminution per day, over 4 days. The decision to proceed with such a course depends on the patient's reaction. On the other hand, if chronic adrenocortical insufficiency supervenes, maintenance doses of cortisone (about 20 mg per square meter per day by mouth) and, less often, salt-retaining steroids are required.

Some recommendations are necessary in order to avoid the occurence of acute adrenal insufficiency in situations well known for their association with this condition. Such situations include the child about to undergo unilateral (or bilateral) adrenalectomy; the child who has been treated for a long time with large doses of steroids and now requires surgery for one reason or another; and the child previously maintained on suitable treatment for chronic adrenocortical insufficiency (including the adrenogenital syndrome), who is suddenly confronted with the stress of serious illness or injury.

We have advised that some children carry on their person an identification card or tag, which gives, or directs the finder to, instructions in case of sudden need. Under such circumstances adrenal crisis may be averted by the use of cortisone acetate, intramuscularly, 2 mg per kilogram of body weight daily. It is unwise to rely upon continued oral treatment during an emergency and this intramuscular route provides a satisfactory depot for the maintenance of adequate blood levels for 24 hours or longer. In addition 1 mg of desoxycorticosterone acetate in oil may be given daily. Throughout the period of stress the serum electrolytes should be determined daily. Usually within a few days it is possible to return to the previous routine of control.

It is to be recalled that the adrenal steoids exert some of their beneficial influence on the salt-water balance by shifts between the extracellular and intracellular compartments. Thus the sodium requirements must be given careful consideration and excess administration of sodium should be avoided when the adrenal steroids are used, as they should be, concomitantly. Overtreatment may lead to hypertension, edema, cardiac failure, hypernatremia, and hypokalemia with muscle weakness. The child should be observed repeatedly for undue elevation of the blood pressure, pretibial edema, and impending heart failure. The serum electrolytes should be determined daily and frequent electrocardiograms are advisable.

Following the successful management of the acute episode, the commitment of the child with apparent adrenal failure due to unknown causes to indefinite therapy may be unwarranted. As the patient recovers from the crisis, the treatment with steroids should be slowly discontinued and the adrenocortical function carefully evaluated to differentiate between temporary and chronic adrenal deficiency. For example, after unilateral adrenalectomy the contralateral gland, at first atrophic, usually recovers its function and is restored to normal.

SUMMARY

Acute adrenal insufficiency in infancy and childhood must be recognized quickly and treated adequately at once. Both the rapid replacement of fluids and electrolytes and suitable steroid therapy are essential. Because the dehydration is primarily extracellular, isotonic saline is appropriate. Rapid correction is essential and overtreatment must be avoided, particularly when adrenal steroids are employed, since they will counteract the prior loss of sodium and retention of potassium within the extracellular compartment. During recovery the child should be studied carefully in order to determine the rate at which the various therapeutic measures may be withdrawn and in order to distinguish between acute and chronic adrenal insufficiency. The indiscriminate assignment of nonspecific diseases in childhood to the category of acute adrenal insufficiency is decried.

REFERENCES

Bongiovanni, A. M.: Fluid therapy in adrenocortical failure. Pediatr. Clin. North Am., *11*:791, 1964.

Bongiovanni, A. M.: Disorders of steroid biogenesis. *In* Stanbury, J. B., Wyngaarden, J. B., and Fredrickson, D. S., eds.: The Metabolic Basis of Inherited Disease. 3rd ed., New York, McGraw Hill, 1972.

Gardner, L. I.: Review article: Adrenocortical metabolism of the fetus, infant and child. Pediatrics, *17*:897, 1956.

Jaudon, J. C.: Further observations concerning hypofunctioning of the adrenals during early life. J. Pediatr., *32*:641, 1948.

Kock, R., and Carson, M. J.: Meningococcal infections in children. N. Engl. J. Med., *258*:639, 1958.

Liddle, G. W.: Sodium diuresis induced by steroidal antagonists of aldosterone. Science, *126*:1016, 1957.

Migeon, C. J., and Stempfel, R. S., Jr.: Laboratory diagnosis in pediatric endocrinology. Pediatr. Clin. North Am., *4*:959, 1957.

Pakravan, P., Kenny, F. M., Depp, R., and Allen, A. C.: Familial congenital absence of the adrenal glands. J. Pediatr., *84*:74, 1974.

Ulick, S., Vetter, K. K., Gautier, E., Nicolis, G. L., Markello, J. R., and Lowe, C. U.: An aldosterone biosynthetic defect in a salt-losing disorder of infancy (abstract). J. Clin. Invest., *43*:1261, 1964.

Visser, H. K. A.: Hypoadrenocorticism. *In* Gardner, L. I., ed.: Endocrine and Genetic Diseases of Childhood and Adolescence. 3rd ed., Philadelphia, W. B. Saunders Co., 1975, pp. 513–538.

Weiss, L., and Mellinger, R. C.: Congenital adrenal hypoplasia—an X-linked disease. J. Med. Genet., 7:27, 1970.

Chapter Four

THE SERIOUSLY BURNED CHILD

JOHN T. HERRIN, M.B.B.S., F.R.A.C.P.,
JOHN D. CRAWFORD, M.D.

INCIDENCE AND PREVENTION

Burns are the third most important cause of accidental death in childhood, outranked only by automobile casualties and drownings.[1] In the United States 12,000 deaths occur annually, but over the same period 2,000,000 patients seek medical attention for burns. Among these, a very large number of children must undergo prolonged, painful, and restrictive hospitalization, from which they emerge with scars to both body and personality profoundly affecting their social and emotional development.[2]

The tragedy is that the great majority of burn injuries are preventable.[3, 4, 5, 6, 7] Seventy per cent occur in children under 5 years, generally at times when supervision of activities is minimal. The periods of greatest jeopardy are the early morning hours when parents are still in bed and the interval between the end of school and suppertime. Burns in this age group are far more frequent in large than in small families. In the toddler stage the most common accident occurs when the youngster reaches up and pulls on a pot handle at the front of the stove and thereby receives a scald of the extended arm, shoulder, and chest. Another frequent accident at this stage is the mouth burn from chewing on an electric cord.

Burns have a seasonal incidence. House fires are more frequent in cold weather, particularly in rural areas where dwellings are of wooden construction and facilities for heating are apt to be makeshift. These

From the Shriners Hospitals for Crippled Children, Burns Institute, Boston Unit, the Children's Service of the Massachusetts General Hospital, and the Department of Pediatrics, Harvard Medical School, Boston, Massachusetts.

Supported in part by grants from the Shriners Hospitals for Crippled Children and from the National Institute of Child Health and Human Development (5 T1 HD 00033), United States Public Health Service.

51

factors result in increased risks in winter in the South, where demands for home heating are only occasional. With the advent of summer, burns from the outdoor barbecue become epidemic. These flash flame burns of face, hands, arms, and chest, usually in boys, follow explosive ignition of the outdoor fire on which the victim has poured gasoline, kerosene, or other highly flammable starter fluid. The pant-leg burn is prevalent during autumn when the burning of leaves is common. In all seasons one encounters burns of the chest and arms in young girls when loose, frilly night clothes ignite from too close proximity to an open fire, gas range, or candelabrum.

Burns resulting from ignition of clothing carry a significantly higher mortality than those due to scalds or contact with hot solid objects or chemicals. Mandatory treatment of cloth with fire retardants could greatly reduce the incidence of these injuries at a negligible cost.[8] As early as possible children should be taught never to run if their clothing ignites but rather to fall to the ground and smother the fire by rolling. Should they be bystanders, they can help to extinguish the flame rapidly by throwing a coat, a rug, a blanket or a similar item that is immediately available on the victim. Cool water, milk, or virtually any bland, non-flammable, readily available fluid doused on burning or smoldering clothing or clothes wet from scalding water will put out the fire and rapidly remove the injurious thermal energy source.[9]

The frequency of burn injuries, as of other types of childhood accidents, is much increased in families in which there is marital discord. Fire-setting by small boys is often to be interpreted as a signal of distress over the dissolution of the family, and especially the loss of the father. Conversely, many serious injuries, both scalds and flame burns, prove to be a form of child battering. The unwanted child, frequently the product of an extramarital affair, is likely to be the last one rescued from a burning house.

TREATMENT

In dealing with an extensive burn, an established routine is helpful to eliminate the possiblity of error or oversight. Special measures are required to prevent or treat shock, to control infection, to obtain early skin covering, and to restore both physical function and psychological well-being.

First aid treatment should consist of no more than reassurance and wrapping the involved area in clean cotton or linen until the extent and severity of the burn can be rapidly evaluated at the nearest medical facility. In general, there is a tendency to underestimate the seriousness of the local problem, especially in burns due to scalds or alkali, and to overlook respiratory involvement. Inhalation injury is far more frequent when burns have been sustained in enclosed spaces. No child should be transported until any respiratory difficulties are relieved and control of the airway obtained. If it is necessary to transfer the patient elsewhere, intravenous fluid therapy should be commenced, and circulation stabilized. A concise record should accompany the patient giving the time and history of the burn, including notation as to whether it occurred indoors or out, an account of the vital signs and urine formation, and a record of the drugs and fluids administered. Whenever possible, a qualified nurse or medical attendant involved in the initial care should accompany the patient to supervise and record treatment during transit, observe trends in vital signs, and facilitate assumption of responsibility by the team undertaking definitive treatment.

In the makeup of the team assuming ultimate care, there must always be a captain primarily responsible for therapeutic decisions, but all team members, including nurses, physical therapist, social worker, and dietician, should meet the patient as early as possible. Only in this way can changes in the child's condition be recognized promptly and a well-coordinated treatment program be planned and carried through.

The following is an outline of initial evaluation and treatment measures for a patient with an acute, extensive burn, as carried out at the Shriners Burns Institute of Boston. The order of procedure is only approximate and frequently several of the functions can be carried on simultaneously.

1. Check adequacy of airway and provide oxygen, intubation, and/or ventilatory assistance as indicated. Avoid tracheotomy.
2. Sedate patient only if necessary, using the intravenous route.
3. Remove clothing and weigh patient.
4. Establish an intravenous line adequate to deliver fluids at a high rate of flow. A central venous pressure line is desirable in patients with extensive burns.
5. Evaluate extent and depth of burn (Fig. 1.).
6. Consider need for escharotomy and/or fasciotomy for circumferential burns of extremities and chest.
7. Cover flame or contact burns with gauze dressings wet with 0.5 per cent silver nitrate solution. Use mafenide acetate (Sulfamylon) or silver sulfadiazine (Silvadene) cream for facial burns, Silvadene for scald burns.
8. Splint areas of potential contracture.
9. Obtain blood sample for baseline laboratory studies.
10. Calculate fluid requirements and establish fluid regimen.
11. Insert Foley catheter and obtain urine specimens for analysis.
12. Commence "critical care" type of tabular chart of intake, output, vital signs, and chemical values for blood and urine.
13. Initiate low dosage penicillin prophylaxis.
14. Give appropriate protection against tetanus.
15. Obtain detailed history, including circumstances and time of injury.
16. Consider means of achieving temporary and permanent skin cover.
17. Plan nutritional support, treatment of anemia and hypoproteinemia, and rehabilitation, including physiotherapy and emotional support.

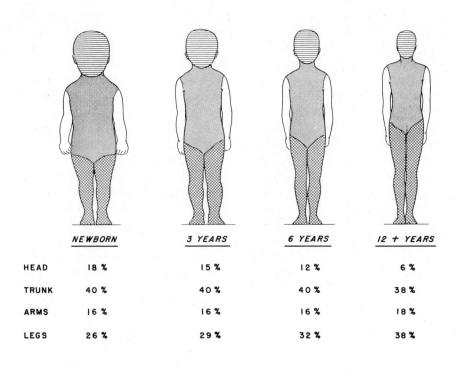

	NEWBORN	3 YEARS	6 YEARS	12 + YEARS
HEAD	18 %	15 %	12 %	6 %
TRUNK	40 %	40 %	40 %	38 %
ARMS	16 %	16 %	16 %	18 %
LEGS	26 %	29 %	32 %	38 %

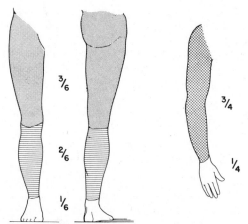

Figure 1.   The percentage figures in the chart refer to front and back. For example, if an individual suffered a burn of the whole anterior chest, this would comprise 10 per cent of his body surface. (From Talbot, N. B., Richie, R. H., and Crawford, J. D.: Metabolic Homeostasis. Cambridge, Harvard University Press, 1959. After Lund, C. C., and Browder, N. C.: The estimation of areas of burns. Surg. Gynecol. Obstet., 79:352, 1944.)

It is imperative immediately after a patient arrives at the treatment center to check the adequacy of the airway and to reappraise this periodically, especially in burns that have occurred indoors, when there is involvement of the face, or when prolonged exposure to smoke has occurred. Attention to color, respiratory rate, character of the voice, appearance of the pharynx, and presence or absence of restlessness will usually tell if there is glottic swelling, respiratory "burn," or significant reduction in oxygen carrying capacity of the blood due to methemoglobinemia. Hemoglobin in serum or urine is another sign of pulmonary inhalation injury and should alert one to the need for respiratory care. A decision to intubate the patient at once or to observe while monitoring the arterial blood gas concentrations should be made at this stage.

In cases of respiratory inadequacy, a nasotracheal tube should be passed. Tracheotomy in children with burns is associated with a prohibitive mortality and should be avoided if at all possible.[10] Nasotracheal intubation allows for the delivery of appropriately humidified air enriched with oxygen, if necessary; it permits use of positive and expiratory pressure, is a beneficial adjunct in the treatment of inhalation injury, and facilitates use of a respirator if the patient requires assistance.

In circumferential burns of the chest with formation of a thick, leathery, inelastic surface, escharotomies may be required to permit adequate respiratory excursions.

Pulmonary complications remain a major problem.[11, 12] Even without a specific inhalation injury, increased minute ventilation is generally present by the third day, increasing to a maximum by 5 days, then gradually declining. This change is reflective of the adaptive increase in metabolic rate and is more marked in large burns. In cases of inhalation injury, airway resistance is elevated but pulmonary shunting is rare.[13] The new fiberoptic bronchoscopes permit direct assessment of airway injury, and in older children the examination can be carried out in the admitting room without anesthesia.

Blood gas changes immediately following a burn resemble those seen in non-thermal injuries. A Po_2 of 80 mm Hg or less is common early and, in the absence of an inhalation injury, returns to normal values by 1 week. Remember that in carbon monoxide poisoning the arterial Po_2 remains normal. The carotid body is not stimulated so that respirations are characteristically shallow; since the affinity of hemoglobin for oxygen is increased, the patient's color remains good despite marked tissue anoxia.[13] The diagnosis of carbon monoxide intoxication should always be considered in children brought to the hospital from burning buildings, and treatment with humidified 100 per cent oxygen inhalation should be given until the possibility of this much underdiagnosed, potentially lethal complication has been eliminated, as by determination of the carboxyhemoglobin blood level or oxyhemoglobin dissociation curve.

Corticosteroids in large doses (dexamethasone, 2 to 10 mg per square meter every 8 hr)* have been recommended to combat pulmonary inflammatory changes secondary to inhalation of irritating products of combustion. Their efficacy has not been fully established.

Electrical burns from contact with high voltage lines (i.e., greater than 1000 volts), a special hazard to the teen-age boy, are among the most mutilating of injuries.[15, 16] Characteristically, there is a burn at the site of entry and another at the point of exit. These can be relatively small and innocent in appearance but between them, beneath normal skin, can be found extensive destruction of muscle bundles, nerves, and blood vessels. Victims require great care in evaluation. Because so many of the injuries occur during climbing, fractures, ruptured viscera, and concussive head injuries are frequent accompaniments.

Sedation should not be considered a routine part of early treatment. Since restlessness is very often a sign of hypoxia, respiratory depressants are contraindicated. Deep third degree burns are seldom painful in the early hours after injury; paradoxically, morphine (6 mg per square meter) or meperidine (25 mg per square meter) are most often indicated to relieve the pain of extensive first and second degree burns. When given in the early stages of a burn injury, these medications should be administered intravenously because absorption of agents given subcutaneously or intramuscularly is erratic. Most children who have suffered severe burns are fully conscious; anxiety is a major component of their distress and requires constant attendance, interpretation, and reassurance.

Once the respiratory status has been evaluated and the immediate needs provided, all clothing should be removed, and the patient weighed. The exact extent and severity of the burn should be mapped and the percentage of the child's total surface area computed by reference to standard charts.

There is little to be gained from an attempt to discriminate deep second from third degree involvement, nor should an inordinate period be spent in meticulous débridement. If blisters are broken they should be totally unroofed. Great care must be taken to evaluate the influence of circumferential burns of the extremities on the vascular supply of distal parts. Prompt escharotomies or fasciotomies may prevent loss of fingers and toes through ischemic gangrene (Fig. 2). If there has been mechanical trauma in association with the burn injury, rapid examination for fractures, ruptured spleen, and similar consequences should be conducted.

With all possible dispatch deeply burned areas should be wrapped without constriction in loose mesh gauze wet with warm 0.5 per cent silver nitrate solution to a thickness of one-half inch. Superficial scald

---

*The estimation of body surface area, a useful parameter for calculation of drug dosage, fluid requirements, and extent of burns, is readily made from weight, or better, height and weight, using tables or nomograms that have been widely reprinted.[14]

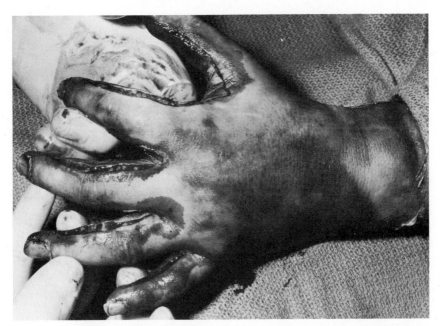

Figure 2. Escharotomies done to prevent ischemic gangrene and loss of digits. A full thickness flame burn involving the wrist circumferentially, the entire dorsum of the hand, portions of the palm, and volar surfaces of the fingers of this 16-year-old girl resulted in swelling under the inelastic eschar. The incisions shown were made approximately 12 hours after injury and resulted in an improved blood supply. Staged excisions of all non-viable skin were carried out at 2 and 5 days after injury, with initial application of allografts, later replaced by autografts. The fingers were maintained in a position of function during healing by the use of Zimmerman pins placed through the distal phalanges. The escharotomies were instrumental in preventing the loss of digits and in the final achievement of a fully functional hand.

burns should be smeared with silver sulfadiazine cream and left open or only lightly covered. Splints or traction should be applied to maintain joints in extension if the burn involves areas such as the antecubital space, popliteal fossa, or axilla. When the hands are burned, the wrist should be maintained slightly cocked and the metacarpophalangeal joints moderately flexed. Burns of the anterior neck require that the child be placed on a half mattress extending up to the shoulder so that when supine the neck is extended. Skeletal traction to maintain joints in a position of function has been used with a high degree of success.[17] Not only are contractures prevented but elevation of burned extremities is more easily obtained, nursing and grafting procedures are facilitated, and the incidence of osteomyelitis and septic complications has been remarkably low.

There has been a recent trend in fluid therapy toward using balanced saline solutions rather than the large amounts of plasma formerly advocated in the early treatment of burns.[18, 19] Crystalloids, in the large amounts adequate to maintain the circulation, give rise to a much greater degree of early edema, but the interstitial fluid is more rapidly reabsorbed because of lesser entrapment of protein in the extravascular spaces once the normal permeability of capillaries is restored, 36 to 48 hours following the accident. During the first 24 hours while the capillary membrane no longer provides a structural barrier, colloid administration is of no unique benefit. Expansion of plasma volume is then dependent on rate of administration rather than fluid type.[20] In the succeeding 24 hours, as capillary integrity is renewed, plasma or albumin replacement becomes more useful to maintain plasma volume. It is our practice to use intravenous fluids in all deep burns involving more than 10 per cent of the body surface, commencing treatment with Ringer's lactate solution and providing 2 to 3 ml/per cent burn/kg plus 1500 ml/square meter per 24 hours for maintenance. Since individual requirements vary, this formula is only a rough guide.[21] It has been suggested that the critical common denominator of successful early resuscitation in the burn patient is sodium administration.[20] Expansion of plasma volume, extracellular fluid volume, and normal cardiac output requires as much as 0.5 to 0.7 mEq sodium/kg/per cent burn. This makes it possible to resuscitate using hypertonic sodium solutions if one can accept a deficit in cardiac output and plasma volume to decrease subsequent edema. This may be important in the presence of preexisting cardiopulmonary disease and pulmonary burn injury.

The adequacy of intake is monitored by means of urinary output plus, in larger burns, measurement of central venous pressure. An increase in the rate of infusion of Ringer's lactate is required if the urine output falls below 30 ml/square meter per hour, or if the hematocrit rises above 50 per cent. If, in the early phase of treatment, difficulty is experienced in maintaining blood pressure, central venous pressure, or urine output at adequate levels despite an increase in rate of infusion of the Ringer's lactate to as much as 300 ml/square meter/hr, rapid delivery of plasma (300 ml per square meter) or an equivalent amount of albumin is recommended. Otherwise, enough plasma or albumin is administered to provide 0.5 to 1.0 gm of protein per kg if the serum protein concentration falls to less than 3.5 gm per 100 ml in the acute phase of therapy.

After diuresis the serum total protein should be maintained above 5.5 gm per 100 ml. Similarly, in the acute phase, blood transfusion should be given if the hematocrit falls below 30 per cent; later, values should be maintained between 35 and 40 per cent. If greater than 50 per cent of the body surface is burned, fluid requirements calculated as for a 50 per cent burn provide the maximum volume tolerated and it is usually necessary to supply colloid in addition to the Ringer's lactate. The rate of fluid administration must be decreased if anesthesia or surgery is necessary because these procedures so commonly lead to antidiuresis.[22, 23] Oliguria also may develop as a consequence of pigment nephropathy (*vide infra*), and this, too, is an indication for slowing the rate of fluid delivery to prevent vascular overload. Our aim through the first 5 to 7 days after injury is to keep urine flow at 40 ml per square meter per hour, the urinary sodium concentration between 20 and 80 mEq/L, the serum sodium between 130 and 140 mEq/L, and the potassium concentration between 3.5 and 5.0 mEq/L.

The requirements for sodium chloride are very much increased by silver nitrate wet dressings. Because of hypotonicity, osmotic forces favor egress of sodium chloride, the principal extracellular electrolyte at areas of injury; additional surface chloride losses are the result of formation of an insoluble complex with silver ion, and excess urinary sodium losses are due to the requirement of the absorbed nitrate ion for companion cation. As a result, needs approximate 3.5 mM per day per 100 sq cm (the area of an adult's palm) of deep second or third degree burns.[24]

In the early phase of therapy, if hemoglobinuria is present (often a sign of inhalation of toxic products of combustion and extensive pulmonary involvement), alkalinization of the urine is advantageous because of the insolubility of hematin in acid solution. Alkalinization of the urine can be accomplished by giving sodium bicarbonate (0.5 mM/kg) and maintaining or establishing good urine flow with mannitol (0.5 gm/kg) or furosemide (1 to 2 mg/kg).

In the first few days oliguria is more commonly the result of inadequate fluid replacement than of acute renal failure. However, isotonic urine in volumes of less than 0.5 ml/kg/hr suggests renal failure and requires examination of the urine for pigment casts and for a combination of high sodium concentration, low osmolality, and low urea concentration (Table 1).[25] Renal failure is uncommon in burns of less than 20 per cent of the body surface; it occurs more frequently after flame burns sustained indoors than after scalds. It is most common with extensive electrical burns in which myoglobinemia often complicates the pigment load to be dealt with by the kidneys. It is ordinarily preventable if oliguria is promptly recognized and appropriately treated. Dialysis is the only resort should anuria supervene.

TABLE 1   DIFFERENTIAL DIAGNOSIS OF OLIGURIA DEVELOPING IN TREATMENT OF PATIENT WITH SEVERE BURNS

Cause	Clinical Findings	Urinary Volume	Urinary Sodium	Urinary Osmolality	Urinary Urea[1]	BUN and Serum Creatinine
Prerenal						
Hypovolemia Dehydration Salt depletion		Low	10–20 <10	Increased >800 mOsm/kg (SG > 1.025)	3000	Both increased (Ratio 40:1)[2]
Parenchymal Acute tubular necrosis	Hypotensive episode	Low	40	Isotonic −300 mOsm/kg (SG 1.010)	300	Both increased (Ratio 15:1 but may show elevation early)
Cortical necrosis	Hypotensive episode	Very low	20	Often increased (SG 1.015)	800–2000	Both increased (Ratio 15:1)

[1]Mg per 100 ml.
[2]The ratio normally is 15:1 but in prerenal oliguria will rise to 40:1 or higher in most cases.

One-half of the estimated first day's fluid requirement should be given in the initial 8 hours after the burn (not 8 hours from commencement of therapy) and one-fourth in each of the second and third 8-hour periods. On the second day the requirement for Ringer's lactate is approximately two-thirds of the volume required on the first day. Since Ringer's lactate does not contain dextrose, the fluid should be enriched with 2.5 to 5 per cent dextrose if measured blood glucose levels fall below 140 mg per 100 ml. Oral fluids are best withheld in the early shock phase but may be begun after 24 to 48 hours. Oral intake should not be relied upon for support of vascular volume, although it is often adequate to meet the needs for maintenance fluid. After 48 to 72 hours, a diuretic phase is entered. At this stage interstitial fluid is being returned rapidly to the vascular bed, and it is important not to overload the patient's circulation with large amounts of fluid given in an endeavor to match urine output.

A skilled, well-coordinated team is necessary for institution of acute therapy. Evaluation of the pulmonary situation and the extent and severity of the burn requires experience and careful judgment. Most children in incipient or full-blown shock will require a venous cut-down, and unless an operator skilled in this procedure or in percutaneous introduction of a large bore intravenous catheter is available, time will be wasted. A centrally placed venous catheter with a suitable manometer attachment may be used both as an intravenous line and as a means to monitor central venous pressure. When appropriate care is taken to avoid dead space dilutional errors, the catheter can also serve for blood sampling.

Experienced nursing help is required for expeditious bandaging and splinting and an additional person should be available to initiate an accurate record of vital signs, medications and fluids administered, urine output, and values for blood Po_2, Pco_2, pH, hematocrit, total protein, and sodium, chloride, and potassium concentrations.

Vital signs and urine output are measured at half-hour intervals initially and hourly thereafter. Rectal temperature is taken at not greater than 2-hour intervals initially, for hypothermia is frequently a complication not only when the patient is uncovered but also as a response to evaporative heat loss when he or she is wrapped in wet dressings.[26] A continuous temperature record using a direct reading probe is advantageous in very severe burns. Urinary sodium content and osmolality, serum electrolyte concentrations and hematocrit, total protein, and blood gases should be monitored and recorded not less often than at intervals of 6 hours in large burns. A skilled technician in a close-at-hand laboratory equipped with modern analytical instruments designed to give rapid answers on small samples can improve chances for survival of the extensively burned child immeasurably.

Because of their susceptibility to rapidly spreading cellulitis from beta-hemolytic streptococci, all patients with serious burns are given relatively low doses of parenteral penicillin (200,000 units every 6 hr) at entry. If previously immunized they also receive a booster dose of tetanus toxoid (0.5 ml). Penicillin is continued for 10 to 14 days or until the serum IgG immunoglobulin levels are restored. The sharp fall in these levels following a burn usually reaches its nadir at 4 to 5 days.

Continuous topical application of 0.5 per cent silver nitrate solution with wet dressings or silver sulfadiazine (Silvadene) or mafenide acetate (Sulfamylon) as creams gives a high level and broad spectrum of surface bacterial control.[27, 28, 29, 30] The effectiveness of these agents depends upon close contact with residual viable tissue. None can adequately penetrate a leathery eschar, but mafenide acetate is the best in this respect; silver sulfadiazine is the agent of choice for scald burns of the thin skin of infants and small children. Irrespective of the choice, the topical agent must be totally removed daily and the burn surface carefully débrided of necrotic tissue easily separable from the granulating bed. Special care must be taken to identify and unroof abscesses forming beneath the leathery eschar resulting from flame or electrical burns. Initial and subsequent daily cultures should be taken from representative areas of the injury to provide constant knowledge of the bacterial flora. If invasive infection supervenes it should be treated early and vigorously with the appropriate systemic antibiotics. Bear in mind that the doses of antibiotics, especially gentamicin and the penicillins, may have to be increased above those employed for other illnesses. In patients with burns, there are unusual losses of the antibiotics in exudates and, with aggressive fluid therapy, extraordinarily high rates of urinary clearance may be seen. Determination of peak and lowest antibiotic levels in plasma is essential to optimal therapy.

Continuous fever, tachycardia, an elevated respiratory rate, and leukocytosis with a "left shift" are invariable sequelae of an extensive burn. These are manifestations of an adaptive state of hypermetabolism and will be intensified by superimposed infection, but they are not, *per se*, indications for a change in the antibacterial regimen. In addition to evidence from cultures and sensitivity tests, a change in systemic antibacterial therapy requires good judgment and perspective. Infection markedly augments surface losses of electrolytes and an appropriate increase in sodium chloride supplementation will be required.[24]

A significant advance in the care of burned patients has been the introduction of the laminar air flow isolation units, one of which is shown in Figure 3. Bacteria-free air is introduced through ceiling panels which distribute it in a uniform "shower" descending over the patient. The air pressure is maintained slightly positive in respect to the external environment to exclude entry of air-borne organisms from outside and the unit is exhausted through floor panels on either side of the bed. Humidity and air temperature are individually controlled. With use of silver nitrate wet dressings humidity is maintained at 80 per cent to reduce evaporation and, for patient comfort, the tempera-

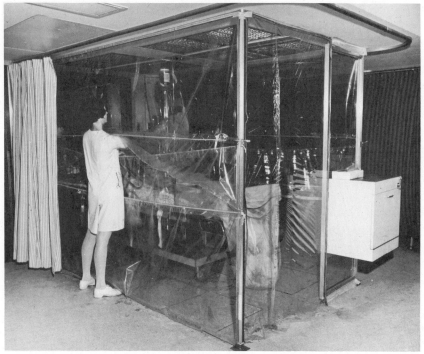

Figure 3. Laminar air flow in a bacteria-free nursing unit. Plastic curtains permit child to maintain contact with nurses, parents, and other children. The need for use of masks and gowns by attendants is obviated. The nurse shown wears thin, plastic gauntlets extending to her shoulders. The white box at the foot of the bed is a pass-through for trays and equipment which subjects all items to ultraviolet sterilization.

ture is set at approximately 84°. In combination with the new topical antiseptics, these units have resulted in a sharp drop in septic complications.

Children with very large, "statistically fatal" burns have been treated recently by early excision and cover with compatible allograft skin using immunosuppression to prolong graft survival. Serial harvesting from the host's limited donor sites has made possible ultimate replacement of all allografts and withdrawal of immunosuppression.[31]

A frequent complication of childhood burn injuries both large and small, is central nervous system dysfunction.[32] The clinical manifestations range from hallucination, personality change, and delirium to seizures and coma. "Burn encephalopathy" has been thought to have an obscure etiology but in our experience the cause usually has been readily discoverable: in about one-third of our patients it has been due to hypoxia, with hypovolemia, hyponatremia, and septicemia each contributing about 15 per cent to the total incidence. Once the cause is determined, treatment is readily provided. It is notable that in spite of prolonged and serious manifestations, full neurological recovery has been the rule.

Hypertension is another complication of serious burn injuries.[33] Its etiology is generally related to a number of factors. Elevated levels of norepinephrine, renin, aldosterone, and cortisol contribute as does aggressive fluid therapy. Hypercalcemia secondary to immobilization is occasionally the pathogenesis. Control of hypertension of clinical significance is readily achieved using the ordinary diuretic and anti-hypertensive drugs.

In the past, encephalopathy,[32] nephropathy,[34] and the so-called Curling's or stress ulcer[35] have been the principal non-infectious complications of the acute stage of severe burns. Their incidence has fallen dramatically over the 8 years since the opening of this Burns Institute. It is our impression that the single most important factor contributing to the decline of each of these entities is early, aggressive, but closely monitored fluid therapy. Nonetheless, use of antacids during periods of fasting, and especially when corticosteroids are in use, is important in the prevention of stress ulcers or hemorrhagic gastroduodenitis. Magnesium and aluminum hydroxides in suspension generally are given by nasogastric tube, affording an opportunity to monitor their effectiveness by measurement of the pH of gastric aspirates.

The amount of scarring and contracture following a major burn depends, in general, upon the rapidity of achievement of skin coverage. Early excision of small but sharply demarcated full thickness burns much reduces the time required for healing. It has become increasingly evident that excision is advantageous in large burns also, especially since the introduction of allografting,[36] xenografting,[37] and use of human amniotic membranes[38] as highly effective methods of hastening preparation of the burned areas for autografting. The development of a method for preservation of cadaver skin by freezing allows flexibility in such therapy and, in the future, tissue matching may increase the survival time of allografts (Fig. 4). Nonetheless, whatever the means employed in dealing with the local injury, the condition of the patient remains precarious until the majority of the burn surface is reepithelialized.

It is during the period preceding reepithelialization, generally beginning within 48 hours of the injury and frequently lasting for many weeks, that nutrition is of paramount importance. A high caloric intake is essential to sustain the adaptive hypermetabolism mentioned earlier, to replace the protein lost by exudation, and to support synthesis of immunoglobulins and structural protein.[39, 40] It is not sufficient simply to write in the order book "high caloric intake." Great ingenuity is required to devise the kind of diet that will appeal to the often anorexic and frequently manipulative child. In the early phase after the burn, a liquid diet is often better tolerated than solids. Enormous patience, understanding and explanation, and a consistent firmness of approach are necessary to insure that the food is taken. Success in use of a nasogastric tube to supplement what the child can take by mouth is

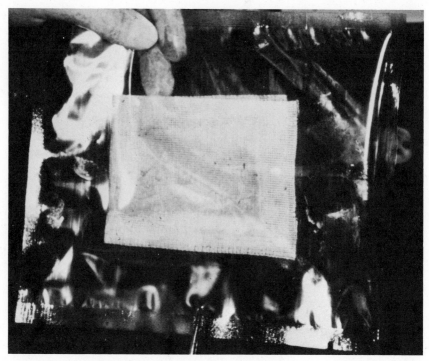

Figure 4. Sealed, plastic envelope of frozen skin for use in allografting. These packets of glycerolized tissue spread on gauze are maintained in liquid nitrogen until used. Supplies of the patient's own skin may be similarly preserved for primary autografting delayed to allow time for better preparation of the graft site or for secondary repair of areas of graft loss. This results in a lesser need for repeated anesthesia because application of such grafts can be accomplished at the bedside.

largely dependent upon the attitude of the staff. In general, an intake of at least 3000 calories per square meter or, differently expressed, 60 calories per kg, plus 30 per 100 square centimeters of burn, is required daily to meet the needs for energy metabolism and healing. This will almost automatically supply sufficient protein (3 to 5 gm/kg/day). Higher protein intakes are apt to be distasteful and it is well to recall that the availability of ingested protein for synthetic processes varies directly with the number of calories provided from fat and carbohydrate.

Figure 5 gives information concerning the realimentation of a 16-year-old boy admitted 2 months after a 26 per cent full thickness burn injury. During the interval between the injury and his transfer to this hospital there had been a failure to recognize and to meet adequately his caloric needs. The result had been no progress in the healing of his original wounds, while his donor sites had been converted to full thickness skin losses. He had lost 55 pounds from his preinjury weight of 116 pounds and was beginning to manifest the symptoms of high intestinal obstruction characteristic of superior mesenteric artery syndrome.[41] This malnutrition syndrome, which can be prevented if

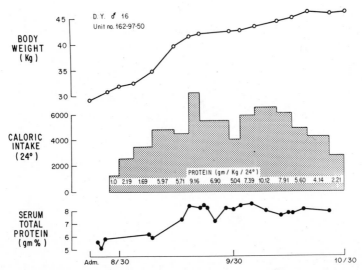

Figure 5. Realimentation in syndrome of postburn malnutrition. The patient had incurred a 55-pound weight loss in the 2 months following an injury originally involving only 26 per cent of the body surface. The restoration of his weight was accomplished by steady advancement of his food intake. A nasogastric tube was used to supplement what he could take by mouth during the first 3 weeks. The average daily caloric intake between weighings (*top*) is shown by the height of the columns in the center portion of the figure. Average daily protein intakes are shown by the numbers in the clear zone of the stippled columns. The serum total protein values are shown at the bottom of the figure.

adequate attention is paid to the principles stated in the foregoing paragraph, has been seen so often as to deserve special attention.

In this instance, the patient was encouraged to sit up and take all he could by mouth. The importance to his healing of a high caloric intake was carefully explained and the use of a nasogastric tube presented as a means to help him achieve the requisite food intake. The constituents of normal, appetizing meals were blended to an appropriate consistency to pass easily through the nasogastric tube using milk or water as a diluent. This practice may have nutritional advantages over use of some of the commercially prepared mixtures and has significant psychological merit. To avoid overloading the bowel and the development of diarrhea, the initial prescription was for 1200 calories daily. As seen in Figure 5, this was advanced stepwise to reach ultimately an intake in excess of 6000 calories per day. Use of the nasogastric tube was discontinued after approximately 3 weeks. The figure shows the response in terms of weight gain and the rise in serum total protein. Equally dramatic was the rapid healing of the original burn injuries and the donor sites.

In very large burns, anorexia, delayed gastric emptying, and diarrhea secondary to high solute tube feedings make it necessary to give at least a portion of the caloric requirement by parenteral routes. A substantial caloric supplement can be delivered by peripheral intravenous infusion utilizing a fat emulsion (Intralipid) with amino acids and low sugar concentrations.[42, 43] Infusion of hypertonic glucose solutions necessitates the placement of central vein catheters.[44] Low insulin[45] high glucagon[46] pseudodiabetes in seriously burned patients may necessitate the concurrent use of insulin. Further problems include technical difficulties in placement of a suitable catheter and the compromise of sterility by débridement and dressing changes, increasing the ever-present threat of sepsis. Even with these techniques, high fluid loads are necessary to provide adequate calories and water retention may require the intermittent use of diuretics to maintain water balance.[47] Nevertheless, impressive results in terms of reduction of body protein losses have been obtained and further advances in the preparation of more suitable fluids and techniques of administration are anticipated. In patients so treated, particular attention needs to be paid to the level of red cell 2,3-diphosphoglycerate.[48] Deficiency of this compound, which plays such an important role in the release of hemoglobin-bound oxygen to the tissues, may develop as a result of a markedly depressed serum inorganic phosphate, massive transfusion of depleted bank blood, or other as yet not fully defined circumstances. The consequence of 2,3-DPG deficiency is tissue hypoxia due to an increase in the affinity of hemoglobin for oxygen, shifting the oxygen saturation curve to the left. The patient exhibits the anxiety and hyperventilation of oxygen starvation despite normal arterial Po_2 values, with a tendency to low Pco_2 tension and elevated arterial pH.

During treatment with silver nitrate, extra sodium chloride (350 mM per square meter of burn per day) must be supplied to counterbalance the losses resulting from silver nitrate treatment. Once the period of mandatory intravenous therapy is passed, the salt supplement can be given by mouth, along with other food to avoid gastrointestinal irritation. Adequacy of salt replacement can be judged conveniently by monitoring urine sodium concentration. The latter should be maintained in the range of 20 to 80 mEq/L; lower values suggest a maximal effort to conserve, and higher levels can indicate substantial salt or vascular volume surfeit, with the attendant risk of hypokalemia. Use of Sulfamylon over significantly large body surface areas (30 per cent) may be associated with an acidosis and hyperventilation which can be confused with respiratory disease.[49] This results from the carbonic anhydrase inhibitory activity of degradation products of Sulfamylon and may require sodium bicarbonate supplementation. Maintenance of a large urine output will help to minimize metabolic effects by insuring adequate clearance of such products.

After the acute phase of edema and diuresis has passed, repeated transfusions of albumin or plasma to keep total serum protein above 5.5 gm per 100 ml and packed erythrocytes to maintain the hematocrit between 35 and 40 per cent are often necessary. Spontaneous reepithelialization and graft acceptance are never optimal unless the granulations are relatively sterile, nonedematous, and richly oxygenated.

Children with severe burns commonly exhibit retrogressive behavior beginning soon after the injury and persisting until skin coverage is all but complete. This behavior is aggravated by the requisite, but nonetheless painful, daily débridement and dressings, the physical therapy to prevent joint contractures, the fixation to restrict motion following grafting, and the increasingly distorted body image conjured up by the children as they view their wounds. This change in personality makes care emotionally traumatic to physicians, nurses, physical therapists, dieticians—indeed, all with whom patients have contact, including their parents.

Changing dressings and other painful procedures should not be scheduled immediately before mealtimes. Analgesics and brief-acting anesthetics have their role but the pain threshhold is principally lowered by apprehension; thus, reassurance, efficient workmanship, and encouragement of participation by the child are often of more value. Members of the team caring for the child must be judicious in their word choice during all "professional" discussions. By and large, these should be carried on away from the child, and conversations at the bedside should be primarily with the child. One must at all times strive to furnish a cheerful environment and encourage visits from parents and relatives. Visitors as well as nurses and other attendants will need to be counseled in techniques to provide diversion and to promote constructive thinking in the child and to reestablish channels of communication between the child and the world, which so many fear to reenter.

In the years intervening between the Coconut Grove tragedy in 1942, that great stimulus to burns research at this hospital, and the present time, enormous advances in lifesaving and rehabilitation have been made. Nonetheless, few illnesses still pose so great a problem as the severe burn. Even with physical survival and accomplishment of full skin coverage, scarring, contractures, and distortion of the self-image (often unwarranted from the objective viewpoint) all too frequently culminate in "social death."[50] Much research is still required on every facet of the care described here, and the efforts of every member of the team—pediatrician, surgeon, anesthesiologist, orthopedist, psychiatrist, pharmacologist, nurse, nutritionist, social worker, biochemist, immunologist, and epidemiologist—are needed.

REFERENCES

1. Berman, W., Jr., Goldman, A. S., Reichelderfer, T., and Mofenson, H. C.: Childhood burn injuries and deaths. Pediatrics, *51*:1069, 1973.
2. Bernstein, N. R.: Emotional Care of the Facially Burned and Disfigured. Boston, Little, Brown & Co., 1976.
3. Smith, E. I.: The epidemiology of burns. The cause and control of burns in children. Pediatrics, *44*:821, 1969.

4. Iskrant, A. P.: Statistics and epidemiology of burns. Bull. N.Y. Acad. Med., *43*:636, 1967.
5. Caudle, P. R. K., and Potter, J.: Characteristics of burned children and the after effects of the injury. Br. J. Plast. Surg., *23*:63, 1970.
6. Borland, B. L.: Prevention of childhood burns: Conditions drawn from an epidemiologic study. Clin. Pediatr., *6*:693, 1967.
7. Biggs, J. S. G., and Clarke, A. M.: Burns in children: A five year survey of a burns unit. Med. J. Aust., *1*:787, 1964.
8. Oglesby, F. B.: The flammable fabrics problem. Pediatrics, *44*:827, 1969.
9. Epstein, M. F., and Crawford, J. D.: Cooling in the emergency treatment of burns. Pediatrics, *52*:430, 1973.
10. Eckauser, F., Billote, J., Burke, J. F., and Quinby, W. C.: Tracheostomy complicating massive burn injury: A plea for conservatism. Am. J. Surg., *127*:418, 1974.
11. Shuck, J. M., and Moncrief, J. A.: The management of burns. Part I. General considerations and the Sulfamylon method. Curr. Prob. Surg., Feb. 1969.
12. Pruitt, B. A., Jr., DiVincenti, F. C., Mason, A. D., Jr., et al.: The occurrence and significance of pneumonia and other pulmonary complications in burned patients: Comparison and topical treatments. J. Trauma, *10*:519, 1970.
13. Mellins, R. B., and Park, S.: Respiratory complications of smoke inhalation in victims of fires. J. Pediatr., *87*:1, 1975.
14. Shirkey, H. C.: The dose of drugs. *In* Nelson, W. E., Vaughan, V. C., III, and McKay, R. J., eds.: Textbook of Pediatrics. 10th ed., Philadelphia, W. B. Saunders Co., 1975, p. 1713.
15. Skoog, T.: Electrical injuries. J. Trauma, *10*:816, 1970.
16. McLoughlin, E., Joseph, M., and Crawford, J. D.: Epidemiology of high-tension electrical injuries in children. J. Pediatr., *89*:62, 1976.
17. Evans, E. B., Larson, D. L., and Yates, S.: Preservation and restoration of joint functions in patients with severe burns. J.A.M.A., *204*:843, 1968.
18. Blocker, T. G., Jr., Lewis, S. R., Lynch, J. B., and Blocker, V.: Early treatment of severe burns. Part IV: Fluid therapy. Trends away from blood and plasma in the early treatment of severe burns. Ann. N.Y. Acad. Sci., *150* (Art 3):912, 1968.
19. Davies, J. W. L., Jackson, D. M., and Cason, J. S.: Early treatment of severe burns. Part IV: Fluid therapy. A comparison of the efficacy of plasma and sodium salts. Ann. N.Y. Acad. Sci., *150* (Art. 3):852, 1968.
20. Pruitt, B. A., Jr., Mason, A. D., Jr., and Moncrief, J. A.: Hemodynamic changes in the early post-burn patient: The influence of fluid administration and of a vasodilator. J. Trauma, *11*:36, 1976.
21. Crawford, J. D., Antoon, A. Y., Baxter, C. R., Boswick, J. A., Jr., Pruitt, B. A., Jr., Moncrief, J. A., and Feller, I.: How to determine the fluid needs of burned patients. Mod. Med., *41*:61, 1973.
22. Aprahamian, H. A., Vanderveen, J. L., Bunker, J. P., Murphy, A. J., and Crawford, J. D.: The influence of general anesthetics on water and solute excretion in man. Ann. Surg., *150*:122, 1959.
23. Moran, W. H., Jr., and Zimmermann, B.: Mechanisms of antidiuretic hormone (ADH) control of importance to the surgical patient. Surgery, *62*:639, 1967.
24. Burke, J. F., Bondoc, C. C., and Morris, P. J.: Early treatment of severe burns. Part II: Metabolism. Metabolic effects of topical silver nitrate therapy in burns covering more than fifteen percent of the body surface. Ann. N.Y. Acad. Sci., *150* (Art. 3):674, 1968.
25. Cameron, J. S.: Disturbances of renal function in burn patients. Proc. R. Soc. Med., *62*:49, 1968.
26. Roe, C. F., Kinney, J. M., and Blair, C.: Water and heat exchange in third degree burns. Surgery, *56*:212, 1964.
27. Monafo, W. W., and Moyer, C. A.: Effectiveness of dilute aqueous silver nitrate in the treatment of major burns. Arch. Surg., *91*:200, 1965.
28. Moncrief, J. A., Linberg, R. B., Switzer, W. E., and Pruitt, B. A.: The use of a topical sulfonamide in the control of burn wound sepsis. J. Trauma, *6*:407, 1966.
29. Altemeier, W. A., and MacMillan, B. G.: Comparative studies of topical silver nitrate, Sulfamylon and gentamicin. Ann. N.Y. Acad. Sci., *150*:966, 1968.
30. Stanford, W., Rappole, B. W., and Fox, C. L., Jr.: Clinical experience with silver sulfadiazine, a new topical agent for control of *Pseudomonas* infections in burns. J. Trauma, *9*:377, 1969.

31. Burke, J. F., Quinby, W. C., Bondoc, C. C., et al.: Immunosuppression and temporary skin transplantation in the treatment of massive third degree burns. Ann. Surg., *182*:183, 1975.

32. Antoon, A. Y., Volpe, J. J., and Crawford, J. D.: Burn encephalopathy in children. Pediatrics, *50*:609, 1972.

33. Lowrey, G. H.: Hypertension in children with burns. J. Trauma, 7:140, 1967.

34. Cameron, J. S., Miller-Jones, C. M. H., and Trounce, J. R.: Renal function and renal failure in severely burned patients. Second Conference on Renal Failure and Replacement of Renal Function (Newcastle upon Tyne, 1965, Vol. 2). Amsterdam, Excerpta Medica, International Congress Series, *103*:27, 1965.

35. Czaja, A. J., McAlhany, J. C., and Pruitt, B. A., Jr.: Acute gastroduodenal disease after thermal injury: An endoscopic evaluation of incidence and natural history. N. Engl. J. Med., *291*:925, 1974.

36. Burke, J. F., Quinby, W. C., and Bondoc, C. C.: Primary excision and prompt grafting as routine therapy for the treatment of thermal burns in children. Surg. Clin., North Am., *56*:477, 1976.

37. Bromberg, B. E., Song, E. C., and Mohn, M. P.: The use of pig skin as a temporary biological dressing. Plast. Reconstr. Surg., *36*:80, 1965.

38. Robson, M., Krizek, T., Koss, N., and Samburg, J.: Amniotic membrane as a temporary wound dressing. Surg. Gynecol Obstet., *136*:904, 1973.

39. Good, R. A.: The relation between nutritional deprivation and immunity. Adv. Exp. Med. Biol., *29*:321, 1973.

40. Kinney, J. M., Duke, J. H., Jr., Long, C. L., et al.: Tissue fuel and weight loss after injury. J. Clin. Pathol., *23*:65, 1970.

41. Law, E. J., MacMillan, B. G., Gelfand, D. W., and Day, S. B.: Prospective upper gastrointestinal series in the evaluation of burned children. Am. J. Surg., *126*:366, 1973.

42. Popp, M. P., Law, E. J., and MacMillan, B. G.: Parenteral nutrition in children with burns: Experience in the Shriners Burns Institute in Cincinnati. *In* Bode, H. H., and Warshaw, J. B., eds.: Parenteral Nutrition in Infancy and Childhood. Adv. Exp. Med. Biol., *46*:240, 1974.

43. Antoon, A., and Bode, H. H.: Parenteral nutrition in children with burns: Experience in the Shriners Burns Institute, Boston. *In* Bode, H. H., and Warshaw, J. B., eds.: Parenteral nutrition in Infancy and Childhood. Adv. Exp. Med. Biol., *46*:247, 1974.

44. Filler, R. M., and Coran, A. G.: Total parenteral nutrition in infants and children: Central and peripheral approaches. Surg. Clin. North Am., *56*:395, 1976.

45. Hinton, P., Littlejohn, S., Allison, S. P., and Lloyd, J.: Insulin and glucose to reduce catabolic response to injury in burned patients. Lancet, *1*:767, 1971.

46. Wilmore, D. W., Lindsey, C. A., Moyland, J. A., et al.: Hyperglucagonaemia after burns. Lancet, *1*:73, 1974.

47. Moncrief, J. A.: Medical Progress—Burns. N. Engl. J. Med., *288*:444, 1973.

48. Benesch, R.: How do small molecules do great things? N. Engl. J. Med., *280*:1179, 1969.

49. White, M. G., and Asch, M.: Acid-base effects of topical mafenide acetate in the burned patient. N. Engl. J. Med., *284*:1281, 1971.

50. MacGregor, F. C.: Facial disfigurement and problems of employment: Some social and cultural considerations. Chap. 10, in Rogers, B. O., ed.: Facial Disfigurement: A Rehabilitation Problem. Proceedings of a Conference of the Institute of Reconstructive Plastic Surgery of the New York University Medical Center, March 21–22, 1963, New York. Washington, D.C., U.S. Government Printing Office, 1966, pp. 123–133.

Chapter Five

DIAGNOSIS AND MANAGEMENT OF HEAD INJURY

DARRYL C. DEVIVO, M.D.,
PHILIP R. DODGE, M.D.

Head injury ranks high among the causes of death and disability in childhood. And it is the rare child who attains adulthood without ever having sustained a significant bump or blow to the head. Although accurate statistics are not available, the majority of children who suffer such injury do not require hospitalization, and probably only a fraction of them are seen by the family doctor or pediatrician. Yet it has been estimated that 200,000 children are hospitalized each year for evaluation and treatment of a head injury and perhaps 5 to 10 per cent of this number exhibit neurological signs. Some indication of the scope of the problem in a pediatric setting is indicated by the fact that during the 21-month period from January 1974, to September 1975, 1522 children were evaluated for head injury in the emergency room of St. Louis Children's Hospital, and that 200 (7.6 per cent) of this group were hospitalized for further observation and treatment. In addition, 224 children were admitted directly to our hospital usually as patient transfers from other hospitals. The total number admitted to St. Louis Children's Hospital for head injuries during this 21-month interval, then, was 424 children. Only 19 (4 per cent) of the children required neurosurgery.

From the Edward Mallinckrodt Department of Pediatrics and the Department of Neurology and Neurosurgery (Neurology), Washington University School of Medicine, and the Division of Neurology, St. Louis Children's Hospital, St. Louis, Missouri.

This work supported in part by the Allen P. and Josephine B. Green Foundation of Mexico, Missouri, and Grant #TO l-NS 5633 from the National Institute of Neurological Diseases and Stroke.

Over the past 30 years many investigators have attempted to quantitate the effects of closed head injury. Denny-Brown and Russell, in developing an experimental model to study concussion, demonstrated that a much greater force is necessary to render an animal unconscious when the skull is held firmly in place than when the skull is free to move after impact.[2] They termed these two circumstances compression concussion and acceleration concussion.

In the majority of human situations, acceleration-deceleration is more descriptive of the circumstances surrounding head injury. Thus, the rate of change in head position after impact and the associated deformation of the skull at the time of impact have become the major factors used in evaluating the effects of experimentally induced head injury. The force transmitted to the intracranial contents which produces acceleration and deformation of the skull gives rise to significant distortion and cavitation of the brain. There is little or no change in the volume of brain substance at the time of injury, but there is substantial change in its shape. This distortion causes bruising or laceration of brain which may occur at the site of injury (coup), or at a distance (contrecoup).

A shearing force may tear small arteries and veins and produce parenchymatous bleeding, or subdural hemorrhages in the case of those bridging vessels which are coursing from the cerebral surface through the meninges to enter the dural sinuses. Less well recognized stretching or shearing effects can be transmitted to ascending and descending fiber tracts as they pass through the brain stem, separating these long processes from their cell bodies.[3] An appreciation of these several effects of a blow to the head leads to an understanding of various clinical syndromes which follow an acute head injury. (See Figure 1.)

CLINICAL SYNDROMES AND PATHOLOGY

Concussion

The term concussion refers to the reversible neuronal dysfunction associated with loss of awareness and responsiveness (unconsciousness) which follows immediately upon a head injury and which persists for a brief period of time, usually measured in terms of minutes or hours. If the patient is observed carefully during this period, the duration of impaired consciousness can be noted precisely; but if one must rely on the history given by the patient at a later date, a false impression as to the duration of unconsciousness will be obtained. The reason for this is that the patient will be amnesic not only for the period of unconsciousness but also for events immediately before and after this. This loss of memory surrounding a concussion, termed post-traumatic amnesia

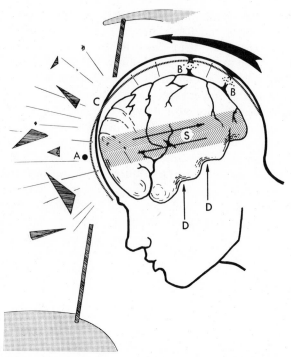

Figure 1.   Diagrammatic representation of the mechanical distortions of the cranium following closed head injury. There is local deformation of the skull at the impact site with *(A)* representing the preinjury contour and *(C)* the immediate postinjury contour. Subdural veins *(B)* are torn as the brain rotates forward and the inferior temporal and frontal lobes *(D)* are traumatized by the restraining floors of the middle and anterior fossae. Shearing forces *(S)* are maximal at the brain surface and extend toward the center of rotation within the brain. (From Grubb, R. L., and Coxe, W. S.: Central nervous system trauma: Cranial. *In* Eliasson, S. G., Prensky, A. L., and Hardin, W. B., Jr., eds. Neurological Pathophysiology. New York, Oxford University Press, 1974.)

(PTA), is considered by many investigators the single most important clinical phenomenon reflecting the extent and severity of injury to the brain following blunt trauma.

Post-traumatic amnesia is composed of two parts: retrograde amnesia, or that period of time before impact for which the patient has no memory; and anterograde amnesia, or the period of memory loss after injury. Both periods tend to shrink with time, but the patient is always left with some permanent amnesia. It is usually said that no significant pathological counterpart of concussion can be found when the brain is examined by light microscopy. It should be mentioned here that concussion and PTA may not occur in injuries caused by sharp objects striking the head at high velocity and penetrating the skull (and even the brain) without producing significant deformities of the skull or acceleration-deceleration of the head. Under these circumstances severe focal damage to cerebral tissue and consequent neurological defects can occur.[4]

Experimentally, concussion in animals is characterized by loss of consciousness, respiration, postural tone, and corneal and pinnal reflexes, associated with a rapid rise in blood pressure, and followed by recovery. These findings relate to autonomic functions in the lower brain stem; and certain investigators believe the primary lesion is damage to the large fibers in the ventral surface of the upper cervical cord from cervical extension and consequent stretching of the cord around the odontoid process.[5, 6] Preliminary physiological and pharmacological studies of experimental concussion have demonstrated interruption in the sensory-evoked responses in the reticular activating system and the liberation of large quantities of free acetylcholine into the cerebrospinal fluid.[7] Although the significance of these observations at present remains unclear, such investigations may lead ultimately to a better understanding of the mechanism underlying concussion.

Contusion and Laceration

If visible injury to the brain exists, the terms contusion and laceration are used to describe the bruising or tearing of cerebral tissue, respectively, frequently accompanied by parenchymatous hemorrhage. The contusion or laceration is characteristically directly beneath the site of impact but, as noted earlier, the lesion may be remote from the site of direct trauma. Often in serious accidents there may be multiple sites of injury. The poles and undersurfaces of frontal and temporal lobes are injured most frequently.

Focal disturbances in strength, sensation, or visual awareness may result from such injury unless the damage involves so-called silent areas. Such disturbances on examination need not, however, always imply this type of cerebral injury. Focal signs also may follow seizures (Todd's paresis), but in these cases are quite transient, usually resolving within 2 or 3 days after the cessation of seizure activity. Rapidly clearing focal findings in the absence of seizure activity may represent localized disturbances in neuronal function, referred to as "local concussion."[4] We have proposed that such a mechanism might underlie the transient loss of vision seen after mild head injury.[8] In some instances, development of such focal signs is delayed, suggesting that local edema and ischemia may be responsible.

Epidural and Subdural Hemorrhages

Hemorrhages developing between the calvarium and cerebral surfaces will compress the underlying brain. If the hemorrhage results from arterial bleeding, the temporal course of the resulting neurological syndromes will be more rapid than if the bleeding is from veins.

Epidural bleeding usually is accompanied by roentgenographic evidence of skull fracture; however, in children a fracture may be absent radiographically and at surgery in more than a quarter of the cases.[1] This fact presumably is attributable to the reactive plasticity of the child's skull and the looseness with which the dura mater is attached to the overlying calvarium. For similar reasons, the hematoma may derive from diploic veins or dural sinuses rather than from an arterial source. Consequently, even in the absence of radiographic evidence of skull fracture, one must be alert to the possibility that an epidural hemorrhage can supervene.

Symptoms and signs of cerebral compression from acute subdural hemorrhage usually evolve within hours or days of injury. Or the hemorrhage may develop more slowly, the clot undergo dissolution, and a chronic subdural effusion result. It is taught that symptoms and signs of epidural or subdural hemorrhage develop after a transient period of normalcy (lucid period) following concussion or other immediate effects of head injury. Clinically, however, this sequence of events is seldom recognized. More often in serious head injury the effects of a developing mass lesion appear before recovery from the immediate effects of the trauma has occurred.

Skull Fracture

Breaks in the calvarium may be associated with any of the aforementioned clinical syndromes. The location and nature of the fracture may suggest additional complications. For example, if the fracture line extends through the squamous portion of the temporal bone, the possibility of an epidural hemorrhage from laceration of the middle meningeal artery is increased.

Fractures extending through the base of the skull may be associated with leakage of cerebrospinal fluid into either the auditory or nasal passages, resulting in otorrhea or rhinorrhea, and presence of either implies a break in the skull bone even though the fracture cannot be demonstrated radiographically. The observation of intracranial air on x-ray films after trauma always means anatomical continuity between nasal or ear cavities and the interior of the skull. This finding may exist even in the absence of obvious otorrhea or rhinorrhea. Rarely, such basal fractures also injure the pituitary stalk and cause transient or, less often, permanent diabetes insipidus. If the fracture line involves the rim of the foramen magnum, acute respiratory failure may occur secondary to direct injury of the lower brain stem or to subsequent compression of this region by a blood clot. Cranial nerve signs also may reflect direct injuries to these nerves captured in the line of fracture as they course through various bony canals.

The likelihood of a complicating intracranial infection is increased when there is a fracture, particularly when it extends through the base of the skull. Nuchal rigidity and peripheral leukocytosis frequently accompany head injury, particularly if there has been bleeding into the subarachnoid space. Even though a low grade fever also may follow severe head injury as a direct consequence of the injury itself, its occurrence always should raise the possibility of a complicating meningitis or parameningeal infection, especially when there is evidence of disruption of the natural anatomical barriers to entrance of bacteria from the outside. In the face of any of these findings, diagnostic lumbar puncture is indicated, although this test should not be performed routinely following every head injury. The potential risk of neurological deterioration developing in the patient with increased intracranial pressure after a lumbar puncture must be remembered; but this perhaps overemphasized potential hazard should not countermand the use of such a test to evaluate the possible existence of an intracranial infection suggested by the clinical circumstances.

Cerebral Edema

Some degree of brain swelling is to be expected following significant craniocerebral trauma. Cerebral edema may coexist with any of the aforementioned clinical syndromes, or it may be the only recognizable tissue alteration causing increased intracranial pressure.[9] Theoretically, cerebral edema may result from direct cellular injury (cytotoxic) or from vascular injury (vasogenic).[10] The fluid accumulation is intracellular in the cytotoxic form and interstitial in the vasogenic form, and plasma proteins leak into the brain when the vascular integrity is impaired. In actual fact, cerebral edema represents a mixture of both the cytotoxic and vasogenic forms in most clinical settings and certainly in relation to head injury.[11]

HISTORY AND EXAMINATION

Even though the diagnosis of head injury seems obvious, a detailed present and past history is essential. That it is important in management to know that the unconscious child also may suffer from drug allergies, hemophilia, diabetes mellitus, or epilepsy is obvious, but it is surprising how frequently historical data germane to the problem are missed on the initial assessment of the patient.

Similarly, a precise knowledge of the details immediately surrounding the injury may help the examiner to interpret the significance of the injury. For example, if the child stumbles while running and strikes his head on the pavement, it is reasonable to assume that the resulting neurological syndrome is the direct result of the injury. On the other hand, if a child crumples to the ground and, in doing so, strikes his head on the pavement, one would have to consider seriously why he fell and search for predisposing factors, which could include a seizure or an intracranial hemorrhage. Similarly, if the injury is minor and the neurological deficit profound, aggravation by the trauma of a preexisting, clinically compensated intracranial disease process, such as a tumor, should be considered. Over the years, numerous examples of each of these several combinations have been witnessed.

Finally, a precise understanding of the circumstances surrounding the accident often will suggest to the physician sites of additional injury which could prove to be important if shock or sepsis develops. It is axiomatic that multiple sites of trauma, as well as the presence of coexisting disease, demand consideration in every seriously injured child. The vigilant pediatrician can serve the vital function of coordinating the efforts of several other specialists, each focusing upon a particular facet of a complex problem. Unfortunately, this rarely obtains. In our experience, the average pediatrician fails to assume this role.

Following a minor head injury, such as might occur in a fall from bed, the child commonly will exhibit a transient period of lethargy usually associated with one or more episodes of vomiting. To the inexperienced parent or physician, this sequence of events may evoke great concern and immediately bring to mind the question of an evolving intracranial catastrophe. In the majority of such cases, however, this concern is unrealistic, particularly when consciousness has been preserved during the acute period. This is best assessed by determining that the baby cried immediately after injury. Nevertheless, careful evaluation of the infant or child is mandatory before one can justifiably return him to the care of his parents, who must continue to observe him until recovery is complete. The vast majority of children who sustain minor trauma with or without a brief period of unconsciousness can be managed with the expectation that they will recover uneventfully.

With severe head injury, as may occur following a fall from a significant height or as associated with a vehicular accident, prompt evaluation and recognition of developing complications and treatment are essential if the outcome is to be favorable. These patients constitute true emergencies, demanding a thorough understanding of the nature of the problem requiring medical or surgical therapy.

Awareness of the rapidity with which complications of acute head injury can evolve may lead to fear and uncertainty and impede the methodical evaluation of the patient by the pediatrician. All too frequently, recently injured patients will be sent for tests such as skull radiographs before an adequate clinical evaluation has been completed. Without accurate baseline clinical information, subsequent examinations of the patient are rendered more difficult and early recognition of developing complications may be delayed. Whenever possible, serial examinations by a single observer are strongly recommended. Only in this way can subtle worsening in the neurological status over time be appreciated. Alterations in mental status, including increased difficulty in arousing the patient and mounting agitation, almost invariably imply an extension of the basic pathological process. Developing focal or lateralizing neurological findings or alarming changes in the vital signs, including those detailed in the succeeding paragraphs, should alert the examiner to the presence of a progressive lesion. It should be noted, however, that careful serial examinations of the child's level of alertness are fatiguing not only for the examiner but also for the patient. A desire to fall asleep under these circumstances is not unreasonable, and should not be confused with depression of consciousness due to progressing cerebral dysfunction.

The child's level of consciousness, heart rate, blood pressure, and breathing should be assessed rapidly, with primary attention to those vital circulatory and ventilatory functions upon which life depends; also, impaired circulation, hypoxia, and hypercapnia, if not life-threatening, will all compromise cerebral functions and tend to elevate intracranial pressure further by increasing cerebral edema and vascular volume. Rising systemic blood pressure associated with slowing of the pulse rate and irregularity of breathing usually implies increasing intracranial pressure. Rapid pulse with marked hypotension and irregularity of respiration must reflect disturbed brain stem function, as occurs with occipital fractures involving the foramen magnum; these alterations may lead to fulminant pulmonary edema. But the same combination of findings in an injured child always should raise the question of occult hemorrhage, ruptured viscus, aspiration, sepsis, or massive fat embolization.

In the young infant, bleeding into the subdural space may be of such magnitude as to lower the hematocrit significantly; in such circumstances the associated increase in intracranial pressure should produce obvious evidence of the probable site of bleeding. The signs of acute subdural hemorrhage may include vomiting, enlarging head size, full fontanelle, squint, and retinal hemorrhage. In older children, the volume of blood lost into the cranial cavity is usually insignificant.

Although the relative fixation of the cranial bones at the suture lines precludes a significant increase in head size, other signs of increased intracranial pressure should be evident. In the absence of significant intracranial hemorrhage, the prompt increase in intracranial pressure which all too frequently follows head trauma in children has been related to rapidly developing cerebral swelling ("flash edema").[9] Careful assessment of responsiveness and of pupillary size can give important additional signs of such an increase in pressure. Surprisingly, perhaps, the significance of pupillary changes, always stressed in the evaluation of raised intracranial pressure, is incompletely understood by physicians. A dilated pupil, poorly reactive or unreactive to light, most often indicates compression of the third nerve on that side by the herniating mesial portion of the temporal lobe through the incisura of the tentorium, caused by increased pressure. While this may be due to cerebral edema as well as to intracranial hematoma, the latter surgically remediable lesion should be kept foremost in mind, and appropriate contrast studies performed to verify its presence. This pupillary finding often is accompanied by paresis of the oculomotor nerve on the same side and contralateral, ipsilateral, or bilateral body weakness or intermittent decerebrate posturing.

It is important to be certain that no one has instilled a mydriatic preparation into the conjunctival sac before concluding that the above circumstances apply. In general, mydriatic drugs should be avoided; but if administered, a sign should be placed on the patient's bed and on his or her chart to make this fact clear to all those involved in his or her care. The dilation of one pupil also may occur during a seizure.[12] Conjugate jerking of the eyes away from the side of the seizure discharge often accompanies the pupillary dilation, which may occur on either the contralateral or ipsilateral side. The intravenous administration of an anticonvulsant, such as diazepam (Valium), may result in prompt equalization of pupillary size, cessation of the ocular jerking, and return to consciousness of the patient. Direct injury to the eye, or to the second or third cranial nerves, also may result in a dilated and poorly reactive pupil.

Bleeding into the subarachnoid or subdural spaces may be suggested by retinal or preretinal hemorrhages. These usually develop in the face of a marked increase in intracranial pressure, and may be coupled with venous distention and early signs of papilledema. Well-developed papilledema usually is not seen during the first hours or days of injury. When it is, associated but unrelated cerebral lesions, e.g., a brain tumor, must be considered. Spontaneous pulsations of the retinal veins usually reflect normal intracranial pressure, particularly if the systemic blood pressure is not elevated, and may be a reassuring finding in the child with head injury.

SPECIAL TESTS

After a thorough clinical evaluation, skull and other roentgenograms usually are indicated, especially if the patient lost consciousness following the injury. If hyperextension or flexion injury to the cervical spine is a consideration, appropriate x-ray films of this region should be obtained. Cervical cord injury is not uncommon following severe, blunt head injury and should be considered even in the absence of recognizable spinal fracture.

In the infant or young child, paracentesis of the subdural spaces through the coronal sutures may establish the presence of an extracerebral clot. Acute epidural or subdural hemorrhages are not associated with increased transillumination; rather, there is usually less of a glow about the rim of the light in such circumstances. Only when the subdural hematoma undergoes dissolution and the fluid becomes less turbid, and eventually xanthochromic, is excessive transillumination found.

Electroencephalography is not particularly helpful as an emergency procedure, but may become so in the acute period after head injury to define a focal destructive lesion or seizure activity, thus confirming or supplementing the clinical impression and assisting in the design of appropriate therapy. Echoencephalography (the recording of an ultrasonic echo from the interface of intracerebral structures normally midline), considered by some to be useful in the management of head injury, has been of limited value in our experience. Isotopic scan techniques similarly have contributed relatively little to diagnosis. Lumbar puncture is inadvisable as a routine procedure following craniocerebral injury, but may be necessary when the diagnosis is obscure, and should be performed if intracranial sepsis, especially meningitis, is a serious diagnostic consideration, as noted earlier. Cerebral angiography may contribute much to diagnosis and management. In particular, extra- or intracerebral hemorrhages may be outlined by this technique or, equally important, their presence rendered unlikely. Also, damage to the extracranial portions of the major blood vessels may be visualized during these studies. It is self-evident that these special tests must be performed by physicians experienced in their use.

Computerized transaxial tomography (CTT scan) has contributed enormously to the accuracy of neurological diagnosis.[13] When it is available, the need for other diagnostic procedures frequently is obviated. The CTT scan is non-invasive and it can be repeated serially to reassess the intracranial relationships, particularly with the patient who remains comatose or who exhibits further neurological deterioration. This technique permits identification of hemorrhage and cerebral edema and clearly outlines the ventricular cavities.

MANAGEMENT

The majority of infants and children who have not lost consciousness following head injury can be cared for by their parents, after a careful examination satisfies the physician that no serious intracranial injury exists. Those patients who have focal or diffuse neurological disturbances and all who have been rendered unconscious for a period of time, with or without an associated skull fracture, should be hospitalized until their condition is stable and the neurological signs abate.

In the obtunded or comatose patient, intravenous fluids may be necessary, particularly if vomiting persists. Maintenance fluids of a balanced electrolyte solution such as 5 per cent dextrose and Isolyte-M should be restricted to 1000 to 1200 cc per square meter of body surface area per day. This solution, although hypotonic after metabolism of the glucose, has proved to be safe if the volume administered is monitored carefully. The primary purpose of restricting fluids is to avoid hypotonicity which will aggravate brain swelling, so common after trauma. Accurate recording of fluid intake and output, daily weights, and serum osmolalities (the serum sodium level in mEq/L $\times$ 2 plus 10 approximates the osmolality) should be followed closely. When non-ionic solutes such as urea, glucose, or mannitol have been administered, the serum sodium does not reflect accurately the osmolality, and the determination of serum osmolalities is essential. These data are absolutely necessary to avoid weight gain from water retention, excessive dehydration, and states of hypotonicity or hypertonicity. Hypertonicity also may occur when injury to the hypothalamus or pituitary stalk has produced diabetes insipidus. As stated earlier, this is usually a transient disorder. Sedatives and hypnotics should be avoided, although persistent vomiting may be treated with an appropriate antiemetic such as trimethobenzamide hydrochloride (Tigan).

Certain problems will require further consideration by the neurosurgeon. With skull fracture, rhinorrhea persists more commonly as a clinical problem than does otorrhea and may require surgical repair of the anatomical defect. Of course, the risk of intracranial infection remains as long as the defect exists. Depressed fractures should be referred to the neurosurgeon for possible elevation. Compound fractures require prompt surgical treatment, with debridement and removal of bone fragments, hair, and other foreign material which predisposes to intracranial infection.

When serial examinations suggest that the intracranial pressure is increasing significantly, various measures to minimize this complication should be employed. Glucocorticoids, hyperosmolar agents, and assisted ventilation may help forestall herniation of cerebral tissue at either the tentorial opening or foramen magnum.

Dexamethasone (Decadron) and methylprednisolone sodium succinate (Solu-Medrol) are the two glucocorticoids most commonly used; Decadron is administered usually in a dose of 10 to 12 mg, and Solu-Medrol in a dose of 40 to 50 mg per square meter of body surface area per day in four divided doses intramuscularly.[14, 15] One half of the first day's dose usually is given in the initial injection. Recent evidence suggests that glucocorticoids act primarily on the normal brain tissue to prevent cellular decompensation and increasing cerebral edema.[16]

Hyperosmolar agents are used to develop a transient osmotic gradient between the blood and the brain which will cause water to move from the brain tissues into the blood. Water moves from other cells as well, and the result is an expanded extracellular (including the vascular) space. Under usual circumstances the solute and water are excreted by the kidneys. Urea, as a smaller molecule, enters cells more rapidly than does mannitol; therefore, if urea is used a higher osmolality must be achieved in the blood to effect comparable shifts of water from the brain. Mannitol, readily available for intravenous infusion as a 20 per cent solution (Osmitrol), contains 1.1 mOsm per ml. To increase the serum osmolality approximately 10 to 20 mOsm per liter, it is given in a dosage of 2 to 3 gm per kilogram of body weight. Urea, stored as a lyophilized crystal, must be reconstituted with a 10 per cent invert sugar solution before it can be administered; also, it is usually necessary to warm the solution to facilitate solubilizing the urea crystals. After reconstitution, urea represents a 30 per cent solution containing 5.8 mOsm per ml, and is infused at a dosage of 1 to 1.5 gm per kilogram of body weight. Intravenous infusion time should be 45 to 60 minutes with mannitol or urea. Too rapid a rate of infusion of these hyperosmolar solutions may produce a sudden increase in the intravascular volume with resulting cardiac decompensation. Also, following infusion of these substances, a brisk diuresis develops and catheterization of the bladder may be necessary to prevent acute urinary retention in the unconscious patient.

The hyperosmolar solutions are most effective when the integrity of cerebral blood vessels has been maintained. Both urea and mannitol normally pass through these vessels into the cerebral tissue to some extent; after clearance of these substances by the kidneys, the resulting increased osmolality of the cerebral tissue draws water back into the brain, transiently increasing the intracranial pressure—the so-called rebound phenomenon. Risk of this is increased in extensive injury to cerebral blood vessels, when hyperosmolar solutions may pass more readily from the intravascular compartment into surrounding brain tissue.

The technique of assisted ventilation also can reduce the intracranial pressure transiently by producing cerebral vasoconstriction, thereby decreasing the size of the vascular compartment. Through this mechanism of action, brain perfusion is reduced, together with the intracranial pressure which could accentuate the injury to brain tissue by enhancing the cerebral ischemia and resulting tissue anoxia.

When the clinical situation dictates emergency treatment—and action cannot be delayed while the precise nature or extent of the intracranial pathology is delineated—it is justified to utilize such temporizing maneuvers, despite the theoretical limitations of each method, until additional studies can be performed to define surgically remediable lesions. Extracerebral and intracerebral hematomas can be evacuated with very gratifying results. Unfortunately, there is no generally accepted surgical treatment for extensive contusion or laceration of brain substance or for cerebral edema.

Continuous monitoring of intracranial pressure has become a valuable technique in managing patients with cerebral edema resulting from head injury.[17] Constant monitoring allows the physician to intercept elevations in intracranial pressure before further neurological deterioration becomes manifest clinically. Uncontrolled elevations in intracranial pressure eventually compromise perfusion of blood through cerebral vessels, which in turn intensifies the edema and the probability of brain herniation. The outcome in any given case is the summation of the "primary" injury at the time of the accident and the delayed or "secondary" injury which occurs in the acute post-traumatic period. Vigorous control of brain edema to minimize ischemia and hypoxia appears crucial in attenuating the magnitude of the "secondary" injury.

Other proposed adjuncts to treatment include the lowering of the body temperature to decrease the metabolic requirements of compromised cerebral tissue, and the use of anticonvulsants. Hypothermia, to be truly effective in this regard, would require lowering of the body core temperature to 90 to 92°F, a level usually resulting in violent shivering and heightened metabolic activity which nullifies the advantage sought in the treatment. Drugs such as promethazine hydrochloride (Phenergan) or chlorpromazine (Thorazine) will eliminate the shivering reflex but frequently will depress the level of consciousness and further accentuate any hypotensive tendency. Furthermore, at these low body temperatures, one can expect increasing cardiac irritability with the possibility of a serious arrhythmia. We therefore strive simply to keep the patient afebrile.

Although anticonvulsants probably do not lessen the liability to post-traumatic epilepsy, we advocate their use in severe head injury in which cerebral contusion or laceration is suspected, because of the impression that such therapy minimizes the occurrence of seizures during the immediate postinjury period. Either phenytoin (Dilantin) at a dosage of 5 mg per kilogram of body weight per day or phenobarbital at 4 mg per kilogram per day is an acceptable drug, although the former is less likely to obtund the patient.

PROGNOSIS

Children as a group demonstrate a remarkable capacity for recovery, even when substantial neurological disturbances follow acute head injury. In general, the total duration of post-traumatic amnesia can be correlated directly with the degree of brain damage, and as Smith[18] has concluded, with the ultimate prognosis. The long-term effects of severe closed head injury and protracted coma have been summarized by Richardson.[19] He evaluated 10 children who were comatose for 7 to 47 days following severe head injury, with post-traumatic amnesia ranging from 25 to 65 days. All were rehabilitated and returned to school in the community despite substantial residual neurological and psychological deficits. Persisting specific defects in rote memory were demonstrated in most of these children on formal psychometric testing. In a larger and less severely injured group, Dencker examined 117 head-injured children, removed on the average by 10 years from the acute injury, and as a control their uninjured twins; he failed to demonstrate any difference in the psychometric scores, range of symptoms, electroencephalograms, or personality integration.[20] This study further substantiates the capacity of the young child to recover after significant closed craniocerebral injury.

This capacity for functional recovery must be remembered when evaluating any program of physical rehabilitation. Many sophisticated programs have been credited with the quality and quantity of recovery in the injured child, and as such, have unjustifiably increased the total financial expense incurred by parents. Yet there is no evidence that elaborate and time-consuming programs of physiotherapy offer any more than do simple passive and active range of motion exercises to minimize joint contractures and maintain muscle tone and strength.

The possibility of post-traumatic epilepsy is largely dependent on the site of injury. Certain areas of the brain, when damaged, give rise to epileptogenic foci more frequently than do others. The most vulnerable areas include the cortex of the medial temporal, posterior frontal, and anterior parietal lobes. In the given case the site of injury appears more important in the etiology of post-traumatic epilepsy than does an underlying genetic predisposition.[21] The incidence of post-traumatic epilepsy following closed head injury is probably less than 10 per cent. Patients with evidence of significant contusions or lacerations are especially prone to this complication. Those suffering from seizures at or shortly after injury may be more likely to develop post-traumatic epilepsy than others who have sustained comparable lesions without fits during the immediate post-traumatic period. Jennett and colleagues[22] have enumerated several determinants of post-traumatic epilepsy which include seizures within the first week after injury, compound depressed skull fractures, tearing of the dura mater, and post-traumatic amnesia exceeding 24 hours. Approximately 50 per cent of the patients destined to suffer post-traumatic epilepsy developed their seizures within the first year after the accident.

Electroencephalography is of little help in anticipating which children ultimately will develop a seizure disorder. Though many EEG recordings are focally or diffusely disordered and may show epileptiform activity during the acute period, serial tracings usually show a gradual return toward a more normal pattern. Occasionally, an abnormal electroencephalogram with some epileptiform activity persists in a clinically asymptomatic patient; conversely, a large percentage of patients with post-traumatic epilepsy demonstrate a relatively normal EEG between seizures.

Chronic subdural effusions represent a major problem because of the lack of any uniformly effective treatment. Diagnostically, such a lesion may be suspected in a child whose head is increasing too rapidly in circumference, particularly if the contour is brachycephalic and transillumination shows a marked increase in the glow of light. The outcome in such cases appears to correlate primarily with the extent of damage sustained by the underlying cerebral substance during the acute head injury.[23] This realization, coupled with the knowledge that the efficacy of all forms of treatment remains unproved, encourages us to be conservative in our approach and to attempt only to discourage disproportionate increases in head size by periodic paracentesis.

Enlarging skull fractures associated with leptomeningeal cysts or erosion of the skull occur in a small minority of children who have suffered acute head injury. Taveras and Ransohoff have suggested that rupture of the dura mater during the acute injury, with herniation of the arachnoid membrane into the fracture line, produces this condition.[24] Aided by the normal pulsations of the brain, this entrapped arachnoidal hernia gradually erodes the edge of the bone and also may compress the underlying cerebral cortex.

In conclusion, it should be pointed out that much of the management of the patient with acute head injury has been arrived at empirically, and many of the clinical regimens suggested, including the choice and dose of various therapeutic agents, are arbitrary. Ritualistic adherence to any particular program will serve only to perpetuate our state of ignorance and preclude further clarification of the problems which attend head injury. As is true of so many areas of medicine, clinical and basic research is sorely needed in relation to common problems associated with head injury.

REFERENCES

1. Mealey, J., Jr.: Pediatric Head Injuries. Springfield, Ill., Charles C Thomas, 1968, Chap. 1.
2. Denny-Brown, D., and Russell, W. R.: Experimental cerebral concussion. Brain, *64*:93, 1941.
3. Strich, S. J.: Shearing of nerve fibers as a cause of brain damage due to head injury. A pathological study of twenty cases. Lancet, 2:443, 1961.
4. Dodge, P. R.: Tangential wounds of scalp and skull. *In* Heaton, L. D., Coates, J. B.,

Jr., and Meirowsky, A. M., eds.: Neurological Surgery of Trauma. Washington, D.C., U.S. Government Printing Office, 1965, pp. 143–159.

5. Friede, R. L.: Experimental acceleration concussion. Arch. Neurol., 4:449, 1961.

6. Friede, R. L.: Specific cord damage at the atlas level as a pathogenic mechanism in cerebral concussion. J. Neuropathol. Exp. Neurol., 29:266, 1960.

7. Ward, A. A., Jr.: The physiology of concussion. In: Caveness, W. F., and Walker, A. E., eds.: Head Injury: Conference Proceedings. Philadelphia, J. B. Lippincott, 1966, pp. 203–208.

8. Griffith, J. F., and Dodge, P. R.: Transient blindness following head injury in children. N. Engl. J. Med., 278:648, 1968.

9. Pickles, W.: Acute focal edema of the brain in children with head injuries. N. Engl. J. Med., 240:92, 1949.

10. Klatzo, I.: Neuropathological aspect of brain edema. J. Neuropathol. Exp. Neurol., 26:1, 1967.

11. Manz, H. J.: The pathology of cerebral edema. Hum. Pathol., 5:291, 1974.

12. Pant, S. S., Benton, J. W., and Dodge, P. R.: Unilateral pupillary dilatation during and immediately following seizures. Neurology, 16:837, 1966.

13. New, P. F. J., and Scott, W. R.: Computed Tomography of the Brain and Orbit (EMI Scanning). Baltimore, Md., Williams & Wilkins, 1975.

14. Sparacio, R. R., Lin, T. H., and Cook, A. W.: Methylprednisolone sodium succinate in acute craniocerebral trauma. Surg. Gynecol. Obstet., 121:513, 1965.

15. Long, D. M., Hartmann, J. F., and French, L. A.: The response of experimental cerebral edema to glucosteroid administration. J. Neurosurg., 24:843, 1966.

16. McLaurin, R. L.: Some metabolic aspects of head injury. In Caveness, W. F., and Walker, A. E., eds.: Head Injury: Conference Proceedings. Philadelphia, J. B. Lippincott, 1966, pp. 142–157.

17. Lundberg, N.: Continuous recording and control of ventricular fluid pressure in neuro-surgical practice. Acta Psychiatr. Neurol. Scand. (Suppl.), 149:1, 1960.

18. Smith, A.: Duration of impaired consciousness as an index of severity in closed head injuries. Dis. Nerv. Syst., 22:69, 1961.

19. Richardson, F.: Some effects of severe head injury. A follow-up study of children and adolescents after protracted coma. Dev. Med. Child Neurol., 5:471, 1963.

20. Dencker, S. J.: Closed head injury in twins. Arch. Gen. Psychiatry, 2:569, 1960.

21. Marshall, C., and Walker, A. E.: The value of electroencephalography in the prognostication and prognosis of post-traumatic epilepsy. Epilepsia, 2:138, 1961.

22. Jennett, B., Teather, D., and Bennie, S.: Epilepsy after head injury. Lancet, 2:652, 1973.

23. Rabe, E. F., Flynn, R. E., and Dodge, P. R.: Subdural collection of fluid in infants and children. Neurology, 18:559, 1968.

24. Taveras, J. M., and Ransohoff, J.: Leptomeningeal cysts of the brain following trauma with erosion of the skull: A study of 7 cases treated by surgery. J. Neurosurg., 10:233, 1953.

Chapter Six

STATUS EPILEPTICUS

SIDNEY CARTER, M.D.,
ARNOLD P. GOLD, M.D.

Status epilepticus is the clinical definition of a state in which the patient has a series of recurrent convulsions without recovering consciousness between episodes.[1] It can occur with any seizure type, but a true medical emergency usually exists only with the generalized or focal motor varieties of status epilepticus. This definition of status epilepticus clearly excludes epilepsia partialis continua, in which there is no alteration of the state of consciousness, and serial epilepsy, in which consciousness is regained between attacks.

Petit mal status epilepticus is characterized by a prolonged blurring of the state of consciousness lasting from minutes to hours, during which time there may be repetitive movements of the mouth and eyelids. The EEG shows continuous discharges of the characteristic 3 per second spike and wave variety. In some epileptic children, status epilepticus may be manifested only by behavioral changes that mimic psychotic or retarded states.

Status epilepticus occurs in 5 to 10 per cent of children with epilepsy, and may result in postepileptic paralysis or psychosis.[2] It requires immediate and continued medical attention, for, if uncontrolled, death or permanent neuronal damage could result. Death occurs in approximately 15 per cent of patients and either may be related directly to status epilepticus or, as emphasized by Lombroso,[3] may result from the untoward effect of intravenous sedatives or hypnotic compounds on the already depressed medullary centers. The immature nervous system is particularly vulnerable to status epilepticus; in one recently reported study, slightly over 50 per cent of the children were 2 years of age or less.[4] Prompt management is mandatory, since both the neuro-

From the Division of Pediatric Neurology, Department of Neurology, Columbia University, College of Physicians and Surgeons, New York, New York.

logical residua from irreversible cerebral damage and the rate of mortality are higher in this young age group.

The true pathophysiology of status epilepticus is poorly understood. However, the condition is more common in children with symptomatic epilepsy of infectious, metabolic, vascular, or structural etiology than in those with the so-called idiopathic variety. Status epilepticus may be the initial manifestation of meningitis or encephalitis, hypertensive encephalopathy, occlusive cerebrovascular disease, uremia, or acute electrolyte disturbances such as hyponatremia. It may follow head trauma and, on rare occasions, be a manifestation of a brain tumor. Intercurrent infections and rapid or sudden withdrawal of anticonvulsants are the common triggering mechanisms. Injudicious withdrawal of drugs, either prior to an electroencephalogram or after a seizure-free state of relatively short duration, and a sudden change in the anticonvulsant regimen are frequent precipitating factors.

MANAGEMENT

Status epilepticus must be considered a life-threatening condition which requires immediate treatment. The four essential steps in management are: (1) suppression of convulsions as rapidly as possible, (2) general supportive measures, (3) initiation of daily maintenance therapy, and (4) concomitant investigation of the condition responsible for the status epilepticus.

Suppressive Therapy

Suppressive therapy is of primary importance and is an indication for the immediate use of intravenous anticonvulsants. Specific compounds always must be given in amounts large enough to arrest all seizure activity. Common errors include the administration of the drug by the intramuscular route and use of small aliquots with resultant toxicity and continued status. A variety of agents have been used in the treatment of grand mal and focal motor status epilepticus. These range from barbiturates, hydantoins, local anesthestic agents, and paraldehyde to hypertonic solutions of mannitol and glycerol. Petit mal status epilepticus has been treated by trimethadione (Tridione) and inhalation of 10 to 20 per cent carbon dioxide. Traditionally, sodium phenobarbital (10 mg/kg) or paraldehyde in a 4 per cent solution has been the drug of choice. Diazepam (Valium) has largely replaced both these agents, and should now be employed as the initial anticonvulsant in the management of all types of status epilepticus.[5-11] It has the capacity to suppress seizure activity within minutes, and the untoward effects, respiratory depression and hypotension, are rare.

Generally, 0.3 mg per kilogram of diazepam, with a maximum dose of 5 mg in children 5 years or less and of 10 mg in older children, is both safe and effective when administered by slow intravenous injection. It should be administered at the rate of 1 mg per minute. Diazepam is dispensed commercially in 10-mg quantities in 2 ml of buffered solution. Seizures may cease before the total anticipated dose is administered. If the first dose is ineffective, the same quantity should be readministered in a similar fashion after a period of 15 minutes. A third dose may be necessary to achieve control of the status. When diazepam is ineffective, sodium phenobarbital or 4 per cent paraldehyde, or both, should be given intravenously in sufficient quantities to control all seizure activity. Respiratory depression and hypotension may occur when parenteral paraldehyde or phenobarbital is administered in addition to Valium.[12] Diazepam, as presently available in its injectible form, is a potent bilirubin-albumin uncoupler. It is of interest that the diazepam itself is not responsible for this uncoupling of bilirubin, but rather the benzoic acid, as found in the stabilizer preservative. This hyperbilirubinemic effect poses a risk above all others to the neonate in status epilepticus.[13]

Intravenous phenytoin (Dilantin) is considered by some to be an effective therapeutic agent in the treatment of status epilepticus. It must be administered slowly at a rate not to exceed 50 mg per minute, during which time both blood pressure and electrocardiographic monitoring must be maintained. Intramuscular phenytoin is absorbed so poorly that its use is contraindicated in the treatment of status. Likewise, intramuscular and rectal paraldehyde have varying rates of absorption, thus limiting their use. When parenteral suppressive measures fail, it may be necessary to use volatile anesthetics.

On occasion, specific therapeutic measures are indicated. Hypertonic sodium chloride is essential in the management of hyponatremic convulsions, calcium solutions in hypocalcemic seizures, and hypertonic glucose in hypoglycemic states.

Supportive Therapy

On arrival at the hospital the child, often in coma with failing vital signs, requires a vigorous program of supportive therapy. Ideally, such children are best managed in a pediatric intensive care unit. General supportive measures include maintaining an adequate airway, administration of oxygen, and intravenous hydration. Close observation is essential, and impending respiratory failure is an indication for tracheostomy and the use of an artificial respirator. Antibiotics are not used prophylactically, but are employed if specific infectious conditions are delineated.

Maintenance Therapy

Concomitant with the acute emergency therapy of status epilepticus, long-acting drugs, preferably phenytoin (Dilantin), 5 mg per kilogram per day, should be initiated by the intravenous route. Once the child is able to swallow, these long-acting compounds should be given orally in divided doses. Ethosuximide (Zarontin) is the drug of choice in the treatment of petit mal. Children 5 to 10 years of age usually require 250 mg two to four times a day.

Investigation of the Etiological Factors

This phase of the management is initiated almost immediately in order to determine those conditions which require specific therapy other than anticonvulsants. Blood samples are drawn for determination of electrolytes, glucose, calcium, and blood urea nitrogen. Children receiving anticonvulsants should have blood level determinations. Inadequate anticonvulsant levels may indicate failure of compliance; adequate levels may indicate the need for another anticonvulsant agent. Cerebrospinal fluid is examined for inflammatory disease. Toxic conditions, above all lead poisoning, should be ruled out by appropriate tests. The other less common causes of status epilepticus usually are investigated when seizure control has been attained.

Electroencephalography is not essential in the acute management of status epilepticus, but may be helpful when petit mal status is suspected. Subsequent investigations are designed to delineate an etiological factor responsible for the convulsive disorder and the associated status epilepticus. These include skull x-rays, electroencephalograms, echoventriculograms, brain scans, and computerized axial tomography, and, on rare occasions, contrast studies such as pneumoencephalograms and cerebral arteriograms.

REFERENCES

1. Schmidt, R. P., and Wilder, B. J.: Epilepsy. Contemporary Neurology Series, vol. 2. Philadelphia, F. A. Davis Company, 1968.
2. Hunter, R. A.: Status epilepticus — history, incidence and problems. Epilepsia, *1*:162, 1959.
3. Lombroso, C. T.: Treatment of status epilepticus with diazepam. Neurology, *16*:629, 1966.

4. Calderon-Gonzales, R., and Mireles-Gonzales, A.: Management of prolonged motor seizure activity in children. J.A.M.A., *204*:544, 1968.
5. Gordon, N. S.: Treatment of status epilepticus with diazepam. Dev. Med. Child Neurol., *8*:668, 1966.
6. Prensky, A. L., Raff, M. C., Moore, M. J., and Schwab, R. S.: Intravenous diazepam in the treatment of prolonged seizure activity. N. Engl. J. Med., *276*:779, 1967.
7. Lalji, D., Hosking, C. S., and Sutherland, J. M.: Diazepam (Valium) in the control of status epilepticus. Med. J. Aust., *1*:542, 1967.
8. Bailey, D. W., and Fenichel, G. M.: Treatment of prolonged seizure activity with intravenous diazepam. J. Pediatr., *73*:923, 1968.
9. Sawyer, G. T., Webster, D. D., and Schut, L. J.: Treatment of uncontrolled seizure activity with diazepam. J.A.M.A., *203*:913, 1968.
10. Brett, E. M.: Diazepam—the new wonder drug. Dev. Med. Child Neurol., *12*:655, 1970.
11. Tutton, J. C.: Status epilepticus treatment with diazepam. N. Y. State J. Med., *70*:2425, 1970.
12. Lombroso, C. T.: The treatment of status epilepticus. Pediatrics, *53*:536, 1974.
13. Schiff, D., Chan, G., and Stern, L.: Fixed drug combinations and the displacement of bilirubin from albumin. Pediatrics, *48*:139, 1971.

Chapter Seven

ACUTE BACTERIAL MENINGITIS

PAUL F. WEHRLE, M.D.,
ALLEN W. MATHIES, JR., M.D., PH.D.,
JOHN M. LEEDOM, M.D.

Although many of the serious and life-threatening infectious diseases of childhood have been controlled, no effective preventive approach is presently available for most forms of bacterial meningitis. Reduction of disability and death caused by this important group of infections is dependent upon early clinical recognition of the disease, accurate and specific laboratory diagnosis, vigorous supportive and antimicrobial therapy, and subsequent attention to rehabilitative measures. Despite improvements in both antimicrobial and supportive treatment, meningitis remains one of the most serious of the infectious diseases, and should be regarded as a true medical emergency.

The most common cause of bacterial meningitis is *Hemophilus influenzae,* type b. This organism, *Neisseria meningitidis,* and *Diplococcus pneumoniae* are responsible for an overwhelming proportion of cases of purulent meningitis in patients older than 2 months of age. These three organisms are the "usual" causes of bacterial meningitis. Occasionally, other bacteria, which might be called "unusual" organisms, are found in patients older than 2 months of age. However, clinical features detectable at the time of admission, such as lesions permitting direct communication with the dura, endocarditis, immunological defects, or other underlying diseases, should alert the clinician to suspect "unusu-

From the Departments of Pediatrics and Medicine, University of Southern California School of Medicine, the Communicable Disease Service, Los Angeles County–University of Southern California Medical Center, and the Hastings Foundation Infectious Disease Laboratory.

al" organisms. In the neonatal period *Escherichia coli,* other enteric bacteria, group B streptococci, and other organisms are found which do not commonly cause meningitis in older patients. The relative frequency of various causes of acute bacterial meningitis by age is shown in Table 1.

CLINICAL RECOGNITION

The clinical symptoms and signs characteristically associated with meningeal irritation, such as nuchal rigidity and positive Kernig and Brudzinski signs, are frequently absent in young infants and in children with fulminant or overwhelming disease. In infants, a high-pitched cry, fretfulness or irritability, frowning, poor feeding, or vomiting, together with fullness of the fontanelle, may be the only signs leading the physician to suspect meningitis. The frequent absence of fever, definite meningeal signs, or definite bulging of the fontanelle presents a particular problem in clinical diagnosis during early infancy.

The clinical symptomatology is more consistent in older infants and children. Fever, headache, and vomiting, together with the customary signs of meningeal irritation, are often the presenting complaints. At times the presence of cranial bruits, a recently described clinical sign,[1] may be helpful in the diagnosis. Fulminant illness, accompanied by convulsions, coma, cutaneous rash, and shock, is seen with greatest frequency in meningococcal infections. These grave signs also are seen occasionally with other types of meningitis, but skin lesions and purpura are characteristically associated with fulminant meningococcal infections. Convulsions, coma, and shock will supervene if recognition and proper therapy of the early stages of any type of bacterial meningitis are delayed.

TABLE 1   Organisms Recovered From Patients With Acute Bacterial Meningitis of Known Etiology*

Age Group	H. influenzae	Meningo- cocci	Pneumo- cocci	E. coli	Klebsiella- Aerobacter	Strepto- cocci	Miscel- laneous	Total†
<2 mo	9	1	6	62	23	22	40	163
2–11 mo	266	67	63	3	–	4	12	415
1–4 yr	359	126	49	3	2	6	3	548
5–14 yr	41	74	39	–	–	–	6	160
15+ yr	19	160	205	12	4	17	25	442
TOTAL	694	428	362	80	29	49	86	1728

*Periods considered: July 1, 1963 to December 31, 1970, for ages 2 months and over; 1961 to 1970 data for <2 months group. Study performed at Los Angeles County-University of Southern California Medical Center.

†Total does not include an additional 302 patients with purulent meningitis from whom no organism was recovered; many were partially treated prior to admission.

An exanthem is seen in two thirds of children with meningococcal disease, and is usually most evident on the lower extremities. Although the skin lesions are typically petechial when fully developed, an evanescent morbilliform rash may appear initially. Rarely, skin lesions resembling erythema nodosum have been observed. Purpuric lesions, ranging in size from a few millimeters to many centimeters in diameter, are seen in fulminant cases of the disease. Petechiae or purpura may appear during the course of the acute meningococcemia, before definite clinical invasion of the meninges has occurred. Bullous lesions are infrequent but do occur. They usually appear after at least 24 hours of illness and are most frequently found adjacent to the larger purpuric areas. It should be noted that petechial skin lesions and purulent meningitis are not diagnostic of meningococcal disease. Meningitis and petechial skin lesions sometimes accompany endocarditis (particularly prominent in the acute staphylococcal variety), and are less common concomitants of severe sepsis due to other organisms.

Joint involvement occurs in about 5 per cent of patients with meningococcal disease. A few patients, particularly those with fulminant disease, present with arthritis of multiple joints due to direct seeding of the synovia with organisms. More characteristic, and presenting a diagnostic and therapeutic dilemma to the uninformed, is arthritis with onset late in the first week of the illness. Pain and sterile effusion, usually involving a single large joint, are characteristic. Fever may persist or return. Neither type of meningococcal arthritis requires special treatment; both subside within 2 weeks, and late sequelae are unknown. Arthritis may occur as a septicemic complication in bacterial meningitis due to other organisms. These arthritides are quite different from those due to the meningococcal infections. They are purulent arthritides. There is active replication of bacteria in the joint space, and prompt drainage (open or closed) is necessary to prevent sequelae.

Presence of Underlying Disease

The evaluation of the patient must include a careful history with special emphasis on evidence of prior trauma, particularly skull fracture, other mechanical defects of the dura, localized infections, and immunological defects. Meningitides in patients with prior skull fractures and two or more attacks of purulent meningitis are most frequently pneumococcal in etiology,[2] as are those associated with mastoiditis and sickle cell disease.[3] The presence of acute endocarditis, particularly with a petechial rash, suggests staphylococcal or streptococcal meningitis. Communicating dermal sinuses and prior neurosurgical procedures, particularly those involving insertion of a foreign body, seem particularly likely to be associated with staphylococcal meningitis, often due to coagulase-negative organisms. Infections in patients with ruptured meningomyeloceles, and in those with immunological defects are likely to be due to "unusual" organisms, often those found in the enteric flora, or associated with the hospital environment. Meningitis occurring 5 days or later after open or penetrating head wounds is often due to staphylococci, enteric bacilli, or anaerobic organisms.[4]

Specific Diagnosis

Blood and cerebrospinal fluid (CSF) cultures should be obtained when the patient is first suspected of having meningitis and before antibiotic therapy has been initiated. Determination of the cell count, type of cells present, glucose and protein content of the CSF, plus gram stain of sedimented CSF, in most instances will indicate the type of infection present (Table 2). Exceptions to the findings listed in Table 2 may occur. Patients with acute meningococcemia may present to the physician prior to invasion of the central nervous system. In overwhelming pneumococcal infections of the newborn and older individuals with impaired resistance, organisms may be present without cellular response or a decrease in glucose.

The direct examination of CSF, using the gram-stain technique on sediment, is particularly important as it provides a presumptive-specific diagnosis in approximately two thirds of patients at the time of admission to the hospital. This examination should be completed, regardless

TABLE 2   Differential Characteristics of Cerebrospinal Fluid in Meningitis of Various Etiologies

CSF Findings	Type of Meningitis		
	Bacterial	AFB* and Fungi	Viral
Total cells	High: 500 to several thousand	Low: usually <500	Low: usually <500
Cell type	Predominantly neutrophils	Predominantly mononuclear	Predominantly mononuclear
Glucose	Low	Low	Normal
Protein	Elevated	Elevated	Elevated
Organisms	Present†	Present†	Absent

*AFB = Acid-fast bacillary.
†Present—usually detectable by microscopic examination of CSF sediments or by cultural techniques.

of cell count, since bacteria may be present without cellular response. The use of fluorescent antibody techniques, while theoretically providing additional accuracy, does not significantly improve the frequency or accuracy of clinical diagnosis in laboratories with experienced personnel,[5] although it may permit a rapid specific diagnosis in individual instances. If *H. influenzae* is suspected after examination of the gram stain, a quellung reaction should be attempted by use of type-specific antiserum to confirm the diagnosis promptly; nearly all invasive strains of *H. influenzae* are of type b.

Gram-stained smears of scrapings from petechial lesions frequently will provide presumptive-specific bacteriological diagnosis upon admission to the hospital.

SUPPORTIVE THERAPY

Blood pressure must be monitored frequently; if instability of the blood pressure is noted, an indwelling central venous catheter should be inserted. Rapid infusion of fluids (saline, albumin, dextran, or blood) frequently will restore an effective arterial circulation.[6, 7] If central venous pressure increases without concomitant improvement in arterial circulation, administration of isoproterenol by intravenous drip may lead to restoration of the arterial blood pressure. Digitalis may be helpful in those patients who do not respond to this approach.

While pharmacological doses of hydrocortisone or other glucocorticoids have been suggested (and data are available indicating their effect in the restoration of arterial circulation), satisfactory data indicating increased survival after their administration are not yet available. Low plasma cortisol levels have been observed in children with adrenal hemorrhage,[8] but clinical benefit from replacement therapy has not been established.

Attention to the maintenance of an adequate airway is essential. Tracheostomy, or assisted ventilation, or both, occasionally are required.

Cerebral edema represents a serious problem and does not respond as well to urea or mannitol therapy as does edema following acute brain trauma. If either of these agents is used, full therapeutic doses are required, and relatively rapid infusion is suggested to insure maximum diuresis. Attention to electrolyte balance is particularly important in patients in whom extensive diuresis has been induced. Dexamethasone also appears to be of no definite value in reducing cerebral edema associated with infection.

Persistent fever may indicate continued sepsis, brain abscess formation, improper therapy, subdural effusion, lateral sinus thrombosis, sinusitis, mastoiditis, or localized tissue necrosis (particularly at the sites of large ecchymotic lesions in meningococcal disease). Persistent fever also may indicate nosocomial infections, such as urinary tract infections (in patients who have been catheterized during their acute illnesses), or pneumonia (most frequently after aspiration and in those patients requiring respiratory assistance). Drug fever, perhaps the most frequently overlooked cause of persistent fever, is readily suspected when fever returns after the fourth day. The patient does not appear to be in a toxic condition, lacks localizing signs, and none of the readily diagnosed causes noted previously are found. The impression may be confirmed by discontinuing or changing therapy, with the prompt return of the temperature to normal levels.

Diffuse intravascular clotting has been described in meningococcal disease.[9, 10, 11] This phenomenon is associated with poor prognosis; and, while the clotting defect may be corrected by the use of heparin, there is a lack of convincing clinical evidence proving that such therapy is beneficial. (See also Chapter 22.)

Obstruction to spinal fluid flow with resultant hydrocephalus occurs occasionally. While enzymes of various types (e.g., plasmin activators such as streptokinase) can produce lysis of fibrin clots, insufficient experimental data are available to justify their intrathecal use, even with grossly purulent CSF.

Hypothermia also has been suggested by some. Insufficient data as to potential benefit are available to justify the real hazard of this procedure when used in an acutely ill child.

SPECIFIC ANTIMICROBIAL THERAPY

In the selection of specific therapy for an individual with meningitis, three patient categories should be considered: (1) infants younger than 2 months of age, (2) "normal" individuals older than 2 months of age who have no underlying diseases, and (3) individuals older than 2 months of age who have underlying or concomitant diseases known to be associated with an increased frequency of "unusual" organisms. The antibiotic regimens suggested for the first two categories are depicted in Table 3. Exceptions to these recommendations and therapy for patients in the third category are discussed in the following paragraphs.

For infants less than 2 months of age, and for those patients more than 2 months old in whom there is reason to suspect the presence of "unusual" organisms, initial therapy must include one of the penicillins, usually ampicillin together with another drug, preferably gentamicin sulfate or kanamycin sulfate.[12, 13] (Methicillin should be substituted for ampicillin if staphylococcal disease is suspected.) After identification and specific antimicrobial susceptibility testing of an etiological organism has been accomplished, the use of two drugs should be interrupted and therapy continued with the single least toxic drug demonstrated to be effective against the organism *in vitro*. Demonstrably, bactericidal antimicrobials are to be preferred. Therapy should be continued for a minimum of 3 weeks in infants less than 2 months of age, despite earlier return of CSF to normal, because relapses requiring additional therapy are particularly frequent in this age group.

For patients older than 2 months of age in whom studies at admission fail to identify a specific etiological agent, ampicillin alone has been preferred. In a controlled study,[14] single drug ampicillin therapy was shown to be more effective, overall, than a combination of ampicillin and chloramphenicol in the three common kinds of bacterial meningitis. Indeed, analysis of the data from that same controlled study showed that, combining etiological groups, antibiotic antagonism probably existed in the treatment group who received combination therapy with chloramphenicol plus ampicillin.[15]

Recently, ampicillin-resistant *H. influenzae* organisms have been recognized in several regions of the United States and in Europe.[16, 17] The mechanism of resistance appears to be the production, by a few specific strains, of a beta-lactamase which inactivates ampicillin.[18] There is no evidence as yet of a general increase in resistance of *H. influenzae* strains to this antibiotic.[19] In regions in which ampicillin resistance has been reported or suspected, combined initial therapy utilizing both ampicillin and chloramphenicol may be preferred, particularly for rapidly progressive disease, at least until the susceptibility of isolated strains of *H. influenzae* has been determined.[20]

TABLE 3 Suggested Therapy for Meningitis in Patients Without Evident Immunological or Mechanical Defect or Underlying Disease

Age of Patient	Initial Therapy (Before Organism Identified)	Definitive Therapy (After Organism Identified)
<2 mo	Ampicillin,* 75–150 mg/kg/day IV plus gentamicin sulfate 5 mg/kg/day (or kanamycin sulfate, 15 mg/kg/day)	Dependent upon specific susceptibilities of organisms (see text)
2 mo and older	Ampicillin 150 mg/kg/day IV**	Meningococci — Penicillin G or ampicillin Pneumococci — Penicillin G or ampicillin *H. influenzae* — Ampicillin or chloramphenicol Purulent unknown — Ampicillin

*Must be given intravenously. One third of estimated daily dose by rapid IV infusion, followed by one sixth of daily dose by rapid IV infusion at 4-hour intervals. Dose is 75 mg/kg/day during the first week of life, 150 mg/kg/day thereafter.

**Combined with chloramphenicol (100 mg/kg/day to maximum of 4 gm) if *H. influenzae* that are resistant to ampicillin are suspected (see text).

For patients who have known meningococcal or pneumococcal disease, penicillin G remains the drug of choice because of relative cost and ease of administration, but ampicillin is an equivalent alternate.[21] For patients with proved susceptible *H. influenzae* meningitis, ampicillin is presently the drug of choice; chloramphenicol or tetracycline is an acceptable alternate for patients unable to tolerate penicillin, despite the hematological toxicity of chloramphenicol and the toxicities and difficulty in administration of tetracycline.[22] Inadequate response has been seen in patients with meningococcal disease who have received cephalothin therapy.

For patients in whom unusual organisms are suspected or identified, other drugs may be required. Selection of the appropriate antimicrobial agent, or agents, for initial therapy should be based upon the overall evaluation of the patient at the time of admission. Selection of final therapy should be based upon demonstrated *in vitro* efficacy and knowledge of the relative toxicities of the available agents.

Due to the prevalence in recent years of sulfonamide-resistant groups A, B, and C meningococci,[23, 24, 25] there is no reason to include sulfonamides in any antibiotic regimen used in bacterial meningitis, except for the very rare entity of central nervous system nocardiosis. There is no evidence that sulfonamides increase the efficacy of penicillin, ampicillin, chloramphenicol, or tetracycline therapy in the common kinds of meningitis, and there is ample evidence that drug fever or other manifestations of sulfonamide toxicity frequently complicate the clinical management of the disease.

Routine intrathecal or intraventricular administration of antibiotics is not necessary. In neonatal meningitis caused by gram-negative organisms, delayed response to therapy may occur. Supplemental intrathecal gentamicin or kanamycin therapy, 1 mg daily by barbotage until cultures are negative, is recommended.[13] Similarly, ventriculitis due to relatively resistant organisms may require direct instillation of gentamicin into the ventricle in doses of 0.5 to 1 mg.[26] After negative cultures have been obtained, the frequency of intrathecal or intraventricular injections may be reduced to alternate days or every third day for the remainder of the course of therapy.

Monitoring Antimicrobial Therapy

A CSF specimen should be examined 24 hours following the initiation of therapy. The gram stain of the sediment at this point usually will not contain demonstrable microorganisms, and cultures should be negative. CSF of neonates, particularly those with gram-negative organisms, may remain positive on both smear and culture. If organisms persist for 2 or 3 days, intrathecal therapy (see earlier) may be indicated. The white cell count and protein level may be increased over determinations at admission. Such increases, considered alone, are not causes for alarm. The CSF glucose concentration should be greater than that observed initially, provided therapy is effective. (It should be noted that such rapid CSF responses may not occur in young infants with meningitis due to bacteria of enteric origin. Responses are often delayed—at times for several days.)

With the exception of early infancy, when therapy must be continued for a minimum of 3 weeks, treatment is continued until the patient has been afebrile for a minimum of 5 days. At that time, another repeat CSF specimen is obtained, and, if the cell count is less than 30 cells, the glucose is normal, the protein is normal, or almost normal, and no microorganisms are seen, therapy may be discontinued. It is well to observe the patient for 2 additional days, as relapses, although very rare, do occur. If these criteria are not met, it is desirable to reevaluate the patient for signs of subdural effusion, brain abscess, sinusitis, mastoiditis, and other foci of infectiion which might be causing continued reseeding of the meninges. Occasionally, the cell count and protein level criteria are not achieved, despite 3 or 4 days of additional therapy and a search for underlying problems. If adequate clinical response has been achieved, antimicrobial therapy may be discontinued; we recommend 2 additional days of observation with careful evaluation of possible sequelae. Relapses, although rare, are seen most frequently in young infants with meningitis due to enteric bacteria; we have observed none in meningococcal disease, regardless of age.

During the present uncertainty as to the future prevalence of ampicillin-resistant *H. influenzae*, it should be noted that several case reports have discussed "failure" or "relapse" of *H. influenzae* meningitis despite ampicillin therapy.[27-31] In one patient orbital cellulitis with positive blood cultures for *H. influenzae*, type b, occurred after therapy was stopped; there was no recurrence of meningitis.[27] In another, the initial treatment was probably inadequate as a consequence of oral administration of the drug.[28] A third patient had subdural effusions.[29] The remaining two reports are quite brief, and reasons for treatment failure are not obvious.[30, 31] It is important to emphasize that such "treatment failures" occur with other drugs. *H. influenzae* may persist or recur in the CSF despite therapy with chloramphenicol or tetracycline.[15, 21, 22] During a 22-month period when we were conducting controlled trials of ampicillin versus "conventional therapy," six instances of persistence or recurrence of *H. influenzae,* type b, were observed after 24 hours of treatment among 107 patients who received chloramphenicol, or penicillin G plus chloramphenicol.[15, 21] Among 66 patients who received ampicillin only, none had persistence or recurrence of *H. influenzae,* type b, in the CSF after 24 hours.[15, 21] It is also important to emphasize that routine disc susceptibility testing of *H. influenzae,* type b, against ampicillin may yield misleading results. In our experience with

H. influenzae, type b, most strains reported as "resistant" by the disc technique have been susceptible when tested by tube dilution. Occasionally (less than 1 per cent), *H. influenzae* isolates have been found to be relatively resistant in tube dilution tests. The response to therapy has not correlated completely with *in vitro* testing, even with well standardized laboratory techniques.

PROPHYLAXIS

Secondary cases of *H. influenzae* meningitis occasionally occur in young siblings of patients, but the low incidence does not justify attempts at prophylaxis. In contrast, the frequency and severity of coprimary and secondary cases among household associates of patients with meningococcal disease[23, 24, 32] suggest that prophylaxis might be useful. The current prevalence of sulfonamide-resistant meningococci limits the usefulness of sulfonamides; these drugs have been shown to eradicate susceptible strains from the nasopharynges of carriers.[23, 24] Rifampin has shown promise in terminating the nasopharyngeal carrier state, although emergence of resistant strains may present problems in the future.

Close observation of household associates of index cases and other close contacts is indicated. Prompt clinical evaluation and systemic therapy should be provided if symptoms suggestive of clinical diseases are reported.[33] Rifampin is currently the only acceptable method of eradication of meningococci from carriers.[34, 35] Oral penicillin prophylaxis (one million units daily for 4 days) or parenteral procaine penicillin G (600,000 units daily for 4 days) may be useful to suppress the bacteremia expected during the period of greatest risk, although neither one will be effective in clearing the nasopharyngeal carrier state. Rifampin represents the only approach for contacts who are allergic to penicillin. The vestibular reactions associated with minocycline limit its use among associates of patients with meningococcal disease.[36, 37]

There is no satisfactory evidence that hospital personnel caring for patients with meningococcal disease are at increased risk, but strict medical aseptic technique is recommended.

Three meningococcal polysaccharide vaccines are available for clinical use. These include monovalent A, monovalent C, and bivalent A–C vaccine. These vaccines are derived from bacterial cell wall polysaccharide, and the antigens represent polymers with specific serogroup antigenic characteristics.[38] Although routine immunization with these vaccines is not generally recommended, they may be useful to control outbreaks of meningococcal disease caused by organisms of serogroup A or C. Also, they may be useful for travelers to countries in which there is either serogroup A or C epidemic disease, and for household or neighborhood contacts in whom cases of either group may have occurred. Although the majority of household associates will not be benefited, it is possible that neighborhood and more distant contacts might be immunized in advance of infection.[39] Unfortunately, these vaccines do not appear to be effective in children younger than 2 years of age,[38] and no group B vaccine has been developed. Vaccines prepared from *H. influenzae* type b polysaccharide have received considerable attention, but are not likely to become available in the near future. A particular problem is the failure to stimulate adequate antibody response among immunized infants, the age group at greatest risk from the infection.

SURGICAL CONSIDERATIONS

Although relatively few subdural effusions require surgical intervention, it should be noted that about 10 per cent of infants and young children with acute purulent meningitis will develop clinically significant effusions. Daily removal of subdural fluid to a maximum of 20 ml from each side is recommended. If significant quantities of fluid continue to form after 2 weeks of daily removal, despite continuation of antibiotic therapy, surgical intervention should be considered. However, surgery should be deferred until after at least 3 weeks of antimicrobial therapy with daily fluid removal. Antibiotics should be continued during surgery and for at least a week thereafter.

Brain abscesses, although virtually unknown with meningococcal disease and uncommon with *H. influenzae*, occur occasionally as concomitants of meningitis due to pneumococci or "unusual" organisms. Brain abscesses are especially common in the patient with acute or chronic mastoiditis. A brain scan or cerebral angiogram is indicated to localize the lesion. Surgical therapy is customarily delayed until convalescence, as in the case of acute mastoiditis, unless progressive localizing signs necessitate an emergency procedure.

Repeated episodes of pneumococcal meningitis suggest a skull fracture, usually communicating with the mastoid, middle ear, a frontal sinus, or the ethmoid sinus through the cribriform plate. If the dural defect tract can be located during convalescence, surgical repair is indicated.

Other surgical therapy includes skin grafts for patients with extensive loss of tissue following the development of large cutaneous infarctions of ecchymotic areas after acute meningococcal disease.

REHABILITATIVE MEASURES

Although some patients have readily demonstrable sequelae during convalescence after bacterial meningitis and other acute central nervous system infections, the necessity for proper rehabilitative measures frequently is overlooked. During convalescence, careful serial evaluations of motor, sensory, and intellectual functions should be made. These evaluations should be repeated approximately 2 months after discharge from the hospital. For infants and young children, in whom specific evaluations of central nervous system functions (particularly the sensory and intellectual) may be more difficult, the evaluations should be repeated at 3- or 4-month intervals for a year or more. It is important to note that proper recognition and attention to such defects as hearing loss, impairment of vision, and motor disability are necessary if optimal function is to be achieved, and if necessary skills are to be developed for the future.

CONCLUSIONS

The presently available, effective antimicrobial therapy has substantially decreased the frequency of disability due to meningitis and has been even more effective in reducing mortality. Optimum therapeutic results are dependent upon prompt clinical recognition of disease, the specific identification of the infectious agent, the prompt administration of bactericidal drugs by the intravenous route, and proper monitoring of the patient with acute illness. Indeed, rapid diagnosis, monitoring the patient for shock with prompt restoration of effective circulation, early detection of complications, and proper concern for rehabilitative measures are features of therapy of equal importance to the selection of a particular antimicrobial agent.

REFERENCES

1. Mace, J. W., Peters, E. R., and Mathies, A. W., Jr.: Cranial bruits in purulent meningitis in childhood. N. Engl. J. Med., 278:1429, 1968.
2. Hand, W. L., and Sanford, J. P.: Post-traumatic bacterial meningitis. Ann. Int. Med., 72:869, 1970.
3. Robinson, M. G., and Watson, R. J.: Pneumococcal meningitis in sickle cell disease. N. Engl. J. Med., 274:1006, 1966.
4. Jones, S. R., Luby, J. P., and Sanford, J. P.: Bacterial meningitis complicating cranial-spinal trauma. J. Trauma, 13:895, 1973.
5. Fox, H. A., Hagen, P. A., Turner, D. J., Glasgow, L. A., and Connor, J. D.: Immunofluorescence in the diagnosis of acute bacterial meningitis: A cooperative evaluation of the technique in a clinical laboratory setting. Pediatrics, 43:44, 1969.
6. Weil, M. H., Shubin, H., and Carlson, R.: Treatment of circulatory shock: Use of sympathomimetic and related vasoactive agents. J.A.M.A., 231:1280, 1975.
7. Goldberg, L. I.: Dopamine—clinical uses of an endogenous catecholamine. N. Engl. J. Med., 291:707, 1974.
8. Migeon, C. J., Kenny, F. M., Hung, W., and Voorhess, M. L.: Study of adrenal function in children with meningitis. Pediatrics, 40:163, 1967.

9. Abildgaard, C. F., Corrigan, J. J., Seeler, R. A., Simone, J. V., and Schulman, I.: Meningococcemia associated with intravascular coagulation. Pediatrics, *40*:78, 1967.

10. McGehee, W. G., Rapaport, S. I., and Hjort, P. F.: Intravascular coagulation in fulminant meningococcemia. Ann. Int. Med., *67*:250, 1967.

11. Hardman, J. M.: Fatal meningococcal infections: the changing pathologic picture in the '60's. Milit. Med., *133*:951, 1968.

12. Leedom, J. M., Wehrle, P. F., Mathies, A. W., Ivler, D., and Warren, W. S.: Comments about the role of gentamicin in the treatment of meningitis in neonates. Adapted from discussion presented at Gentamicin Conference, University of Illinois College of Medicine, Chicago, Illinois, October 31, 1968.

13. McCracken, G. H., Jr.: The rate of bacteriologic response to antimicrobial therapy in neonatal meningitis. Am. J. Dis. Child., *123*:547, 1972.

14. Wehrle, P. F., Mathies, A. W., Jr., Leedom, J. M., and Ivler, D.: Bacterial meningitis. Ann. N.Y. Acad. Sci., *145*:488, 1967.

15. Mathies, A. W., Jr., Leedom, J. M., Ivler, D., Wehrle, P. F., and Portnoy, B.: Antibiotic antagonism in bacterial meningitis. *In* Antimicrobial Agents and Chemotherapy—1967. Proceedings, Seventh Interscience Conference on Antimicrobial Agents and Chemotherapy, Chicago, Illinois, October, 1967. Ann Arbor, Michigan, Amer. Soc. Microbiol., 1968, pp. 218–224.

16. Tomeh, O. M., Starr, S. E., McGowan, J. E., Terry, P. M., and Nahmias, A. J.: Ampicillin-resistant *Hemophilus influenzae* type b infection. J.A.M.A., *229*:295, 1974.

17. Kahn, W., Ross, S., Rodrigues, W., Controni, C. T., and Saz, A. K.: *Hemophilus influenzae* type b resistant to ampicillin. J.A.M.A., *229*:298, 1974.

18. Farrar, E. W., and O'Dell, N. M.: Beta-lactamase activity in ampicillin-resistant *Haemophilus influenzae*. Antimicrob. Agents Chemother., *6*:625, 1974.

19. Overturf, G. D., Wilkins, J., Leedom, J. M., Ivler, D., and Mathies, A. W.: Susceptibility of *Hemophilus influenzae*, type b, to ampicillin at Los Angeles County-USC Medical Center. A reappraisal after 10 years. J. Pediatr., *87*:297, 1975.

20. Katz, S., Klein, J. O., Yow, M. D., Barret, F. F., Feldman, R. S., Fleming, P. Overturf, G., Wehrle, P. F., and Wilfert, C.: Ampicillin resistant strains of *Hemophilus influenzae* type b. Pediatrics, *55*:145, 1975.

21. Mathies, A. W., Jr., Leedom, J. M., Thrupp, L. D., Ivler, D., Portnoy, B., and Wehrle, P. F.: Experience with ampicillin in bacterial meningitis. *In* Antimicrobial Agents and Chemotherapy—1965. Proceedings, Fifth Interscience Conference on Antimicrobial Agents and Chemotherapy and Fourth International Congress of Chemotherapy, Washington, D.C., October, 1965. Ann Arbor, Michigan, Amer. Soc. Microbiol., 1966, pp. 610–617.

22. Lepper, M. H., and Spies, H. W.: Nontuberculous bacterial infections of the central nervous system. GP, *25*:83 (Feb.), 1962.

23. Leedom, J. M., Ivler, D., Mathies, A. W., Thrupp, L. D., Portnoy, B., and Wehrle, P. F.: Importance of sulfadiazine resistance in meningococcal disease in civilians. N. Engl. J. Med., *273*:1395, 1965.

24. Leedom, J. M., Ivler, D., Mathies, A. W., Jr., Thrupp, L. D., Fremont, J. C., Wehrle, P. F., and Portnoy, B.: The problem of sulfadiazine-resistant meningococci. *In* Antimicrobial Agents and Chemotherapy—1966. Proceedings, Sixth Interscience Conference on Antimicrobial Agents and Chemotherapy, Philadelphia, Pennsylvania, October, 1966. Ann Arbor, Michigan, Amer. Soc. Microbiol., 1967, pp. 281–292.

25. Jacobson, J. A., Weaver, R. E., and Thornberry, C.: Trends in meningococcal disease. J. Infect. Dis., *132*:480, 1975.

26. Moellering, R. C., Jr., and Fischer, E. G.: Relationship of intraventricular gentamicin levels to cure of meningitis; Report of a case of *Proteus meningitis* successfully treated with intraventricular gentamicin. J. Pediatr., *81*:534, 1972.

27. Young, L. M., Haddow, J. E., and Klein, J. O.: Relapse following ampicillin treatment of acute *Hemophilus influenzae* meningitis, Pediatrics, *41*:516, 1968.

28. Cherry, J. D., and Sheenan, C. P.: Bacteriologic relapse in *Hemophilus influenzae* meningitis. N. Engl. J. Med., *278*:1001, 1968.

29. Sanders, D. Y., and Garbee, H. W.: Failure of response to ampicillin in *Hemophilus influenzae* meningitis. Am. J. Dis. Child., *117*:331, 1969.

30. Greene, H. L.: Failure of ampicillin in meningitis (Letter to the Editor). Lancet, *1*:861, 1968.
31. Hall, B. D.: Failure of ampicillin in meningitis (Letter to the Editor). Lancet, *1*:1033, 1968.
32. Munford, R. S., Taunay, A. E., Morais, J. S., et al.: Spread of meningococcal infection within households. Lancet, *1*:1275, 1974.
33. Artenstein, M. S.: Prophylaxis for meningococcal disease, commentary. J.A.M.A., *231*:1035, 1975.
34. Eickhoff, T. C.: In vitro and in vivo studies of resistance to rifampin in meningococci. J. Infect. Dis., *123*:414, 1971.
35. Munford, R. S., de Vasconcelos, Z. J. S., Phillips, C. J., et al.: Eradication of carriage of *Neisseria meningitidis* in families: A study in Brazil. J. Infect. Dis., *129*:644, 1974.
36. Devine, L. F., Johnson, D. P., Hagerman, C. R., et al.: The effect of minocycline on meningococcal nasopharyngeal carrier state in naval personnel. Am. J. Epidemiol., *93*:337, 1971.
37. Vestibular reactions to minocycline: Follow-up, Center for Disease Control. Morbid. Mortal. Wkly. Rep., *24*:55, 1975.
38. Goldshneider, I., Gotschlich, E. C., and Artenstein, M. S.: Human immunity to the meningococcus. J. Exp. Med., *129*:1307, 1969.
39. Meningococcal polysaccharide vaccines. Recommendation of the Public Health Service Advisory Committee on Immunization Practices. Morbid. Mortal. Wkly. Rep., *24*:381, 1975.

Chapter Eight

THE CARE OF THE INFANT IN CARDIAC FAILURE

DAVID GOLDRING, M.D.,
ANTONIO HERNANDEZ, M.D.,
ALEXIS F. HARTMANN, JR., M.D.

Cardiac failure in the infant is a medical emergency, and the responsible physician must be able to make this diagnosis with confidence and institute immediate treatment if the patient is to be salvaged. The physician must, therefore, have an understanding of the generally accepted hypothesis of the pathogenesis and etiology of cardiac failure. He also must be able to recognize and appreciate the significance of the signs and symptoms. Finally, he must be well versed in the general and special aspects of treatment of this life-threatening cardiovascular derangement.

PATHOGENESIS OF CARDIAC FAILURE

The fundamental pathophysiological mechanism underlying heart failure has been the subject of intensive research and can be treated only briefly here. The reader who wishes to review the subject in greater depth is referred to standard texts[1, 2] and other published studies which discuss special aspects of heart failure, such as myocardial energetics and biochemical derangements[3, 4, 5] and the roles of the sympathetic nervous system[6] and peripheral circulation[7] in this condition.

From the Washington University School of Medicine: The Edward Mallinckrodt Department of Pediatrics, Division of Cardiology, and St. Louis Children's Hospital, St. Louis, Missouri. Aided in part by the Arthur Fund, St. Louis Children's Hospital Heart Mother Fund, Scott Gentsch Memorial Fund, William T. Beauchamp Memorial Fund, John Clay Seier Fund, and the John Brewer Fund.

105

Any single definition of cardiac failure may be open to criticism because of the complex nature of this disorder and the controversial aspects of the subject. However, most cardiologists would agree that heart failure may be defined simply as the inability of the heart to pump blood commensurate with the body's needs. Cardiac failure may result from a primary abnormality of the heart muscle caused, for example, by inflammatory disease (rheumatic fever), or may be secondary to structural defect, such as a stenotic valve which produces a pressure overload, or volume overload, as in a left to right shunt (ventricular septal defect). When the right ventricle fails, it cannot eject as much blood as it does under normal conditions. The output of that chamber therefore is diminished and its residual blood volume is increased. The end-diastolic pressure rises, and there is a corresponding rise in the right atrial and venous pressure. In a similar fashion, when the left ventricle fails, there is an increase in the end-diastolic pressure of that chamber as well as in the left atrium and pulmonary veins. In most instances, right-sided failure results from and is associated with left-sided failure. In an effort to preserve cardiac output and accommodate the larger volume of residual blood, cardiac dilatation occurs, in accordance with the Frank-Starling concept, which states that the contractile force of the heart muscle is a function of the length of the muscle fibers, or the more the heart is filled in diastole, the greater the force of the following contraction. This principle operates until the optimum degree of myocardial fiber length is reached. Thereafter, further dilatation stretches the fibers beyond the length for optimal function, and the force of contraction declines.

The sympathetic nervous system has been shown to play a vital role in reflexly initiating compensatory mechanisms in heart failure. The increase in venous pressure mentioned is an example of this, as is tachycardia, which helps preserve or increase cardiac output. Arteriolar vasoconstriction tends to preserve blood pressure in the face of a falling cardiac output.

In advanced heart failure the rate of blood flow to the kidneys and skin is reduced so that blood can be diverted to the heart, brain, and skeletal muscle, which have high metabolic requirements. The decrease in renal blood flow is thought to stimulate aldosterone secretion by way of the renin-angiotensin system,[8, 9] which then causes renal retention of sodium and water. This, in turn, increases the circulating blood volume and thus helps to preserve cardiac output. Therefore, the elevations of pressures, the disturbances in blood flow, and the abnormal distribution of water and electrolytes which characterize heart failure may be looked upon as homeostatic mechanisms whereby the body attempts to preserve cardiac output. The clinician who can recognize the signs and symptoms that appear in the wake of these compensatory mechanisms will be able to diagnose heart failure.

Etiology of Cardiac Failure in Infancy

The experience at most pediatric cardiology centers has shown that about 20 per cent of infants and children with organic heart disease develop cardiac failure at some time. Ninety per cent of these children develop failure during the first year of life, and the majority have congenital cardiac malformations.[10] This presentation therefore will be focused on the recognition and treatment of heart failure during the first year of life.

According to Keith,[10] the cardiac malformations most commonly complicated by heart failure are, in order of frequency, transposition of the great vessels, coarctation of the aorta, ventricular septal defect, aortic atresia, endocardial fibroelastosis, atrioventricularis communis, total anomalous pulmonary venous return, single ventricle, and patent ductus arteriosus.* These defects account for more than 80 per cent of all cases of heart failure due to cardiovascular malformations. Ostium secundum atrial septal defects and tetralogy of Fallot, though relatively common defects, seldom are complicated by congestive failure. The reason for this is not entirely understood.

Characteristically, infants with congenital defects, such as aortic atresia or hypoplasia of the left ventricle and aortic arch, usually will develop cardiac failure in the first week of life. In contrast, the infant with a large interventricular septal defect may not develop heart failure until 1 to 6 months of age. A newborn infant with aortic atresia will be in difficulty soon after birth because of the mechanical obstruction to the outflow of blood from the left ventricle and the constriction of the ductus arteriosus in the first 24 to 48 hours. An infant with a large interventricular septal defect will not develop failure for the first 4 to 6 weeks because the pulmonary vascular resistance is sufficiently high, initially, to prevent excessive blood flow from the left to the right ventricle. However, as pulmonary vascular resistance normally falls with age as a result of dilation of the pulmonary arterioles, the left to right flow progressively increases. If the capacity of the pulmonary vasculature is exceeded, as well as that of the left atrium and left ventricle, cardiac failure will result. This mechanism of left ventricular failure which is seen in relation to the postnatal decrease in pulmonary vascular resistance applies to other congenital heart defects that involve a large communication between the ventricles or great vessels, i.e., atrioventricularis communis, patent ductus, and others.

---

*Attention recently has been focused on patency of the ductus arteriosus leading to congestive heart failure, especially in prematures with respiratory distress syndrome. This condition may well rank first in the preceding list. Whether aggressive surgical ligation of the ductus or intensive medical therapy (indomethacin) is the treatment of choice is an unsettled issue at present.[11]

Signs and Symptoms[12, 13, 14]

The common signs and symptoms in the infant with congestive heart failure (combined right and left ventricular failure) are tachypnea, tachycardia, cardiomegaly, hepatomegaly, pulmonary rales and rhonchi, feeding difficulties, growth failure, and cyanosis. Less common manifestations include peripheral edema, ascites, and gallop rhythm. Large, clinically demonstrable pleural and pericardial effusions rarely have been seen in our experience.

The purpose of the following discussion on the pathogenesis of the signs and symptoms is to develop a picture of the distinct clinical syndrome which the physician can recognize as cardiac failure.

Cardiomegaly. Since 90 per cent of infants who present in heart failure will have a congenital structural defect of the heart (either on the basis of pressure or volume overload), compensatory hypertrophy of the heart is to be expected as a result of the chronic stress imposed upon the heart muscle by the altered hemodynamics. If congestive heart failure is superimposed, there will be, in addition, compensatory dilatation of the heart muscle.

There are some types of congenital heart malformations which do not present with cardiomegaly by physical examination or roentgenography, such as total anomalous venous drainage below the diaphragm, cor triatriatum, and pulmonary venous atresia. In these conditions there is pulmonary venous obstruction which results in pulmonary arterial hypertension and right ventricular pressure overload but not volume overload; the left heart may be hypoplastic. The clinical picture is that of congestive heart failure, cyanosis, marked right ventricular hypertrophy shown by electrocardiography but a normal overall heart size, and pulmonary vascular congestion detected by chest roentgenography.

Tachypnea and Dyspnea. Tachypnea during sleep, with rates that range from 50 to 100 per minute, is commonly seen in infants in failure. Dyspnea, especially while sucking the bottle, is also frequently observed.* Both tachypnea and dyspnea are primarily manifestations of left ventricular failure, and are thought to be due to pulmonary congestion and increased pulmonary capillary pressure which result in pulmonary interstitial, alveolar, and bronchiolar edema. The viscoelastic properties of the lung are altered, and this results in diminished compliance, with consequent restrained inspiration and expiration, i.e., shal-

---

*The paroxysmal dyspnea, tachypnea, and increased cyanosis ("blue spells," "syncopal episodes") occasionally seen in patients with tetralogy of Fallot usually subside spontaneously or respond to oxygen administration and morphine sulfate. These spells are not a consequence of heart failure, but are thought to result from a sudden transient increase in right to left flow or an increased demand of the tissues for oxygen, as occurs with fever, excitement, or exercise.

low breathing. An increased respiratory stimulus, most probably neurogenic (exaggerated Hering-Breuer reflex),[15] and occasionally hypoxemia increase ventilation by increasing the rate. Pulmonary rales will be heard when the failure is severe. Very often there is an associated *pulmonary infection*[16] which usually precipitates congestive heart failure. Under these circumstances, the rales may be a result of the infection or failure, or both. In the face of elevated left ventricular end-diastolic pressure, left atrial and pulmonary venous pressure, pulmonary edema may be seen,[1] and the chest will be filled with rales and rhonchi, although bloody, frothy sputum is not commonly seen.

Hepatomegaly. The elevation in the atrial, central, and peripheral venous pressure has been attributed to heightened venous tone, probably induced by reflex stimulation of the sympathetic nervous system and secretion of norepinephrine.[6, 7] In infants, the evidence of increased venous pressure is not as obvious as in adults. Distention of the external jugular vein rarely is observed in infants because of their short necks and the marked compliance or vascular distensibility of the liver. *Hepatomegaly* is, therefore, regularly seen in infants with heart failure, although liver tenderness, so frequently observed in adults and older children, is not commonly seen.

Tachycardia. This is almost always present in cardiac failure. The rate may be as high as 200 per minute. This is a major compensatory response which initially helps preserve or increase cardiac output. The pathogenesis of this response is thought to be the increased level of circulating catecholamines commonly observed in heart failure. The compensatory effect of the tachycardia is limited by the shortening of diastole and consequent reduction in coronary and ventricular filling as the rate increases.

Edema. In infants edema is not readily apparent. The first indication may be a sudden weight gain (200 to 300 gm) in 24 hours. Upon close inspection there may be puffiness on the dorsum of the hands or feet and around the eyes. The pathogenesis of peripheral edema is incompletely understood, but it is thought to result from the increased venous and, therefore, capillary hydrostatic pressure, as well as sodium-water retention. (See earlier discussion of *Pathogenesis of Cardiac Failure.*)

Feeding Difficulties. Feeding difficulties with resultant growth failure commonly are seen in infants with heart failure. The tachypnea, dyspnea, and cough, especially if there is a superimposed lower respiratory infection, will make it difficult for the infant to suck, and the calorie and fluid intake will fall below the daily requirements. Growth failure therefore will result.

Gallop Rhythm. The presence of an *accentuated* third heart sound should make one suspect heart failure in an infant. This is a protodiastolic sound which appears 0.10 second after the second sound, and it has been attributed to the sudden distention of the ventricles during the rapid filling phase of diastole. This same mechanism is believed to produce the third heart sound normally heard in most infants, though sometimes very faintly.

Cyanosis.   Varying degrees of cyanosis may be seen in infants who present in severe congestive heart failure. One or a combination of the following three mechanisms may be responsible. The first type is seen in congenital heart disease with a right to left shunt. The second type is central cyanosis, which is caused by inadequate oxygenation of the blood in the lungs on account of congestion, infection, or both. The third type is caused by an excessive extraction of oxygen from the capillary blood in the tissues. This last type is observed especially in severe congestive failure when the circulation time is prolonged beyond the normal range of 6 to 12 seconds for the infant or young child.[1]

Diseases Confused with Heart Failure

There are a number of disease states which may be confused with congestive heart failure, for example: the respiratory distress syndrome, severe acute bronchiolitis, pneumonia, tracheoesophageal fistula, diaphragmatic hernia, hypoglycemia, renal disease, sepsis, central nervous system disorders (trauma, hemorrhage, infection), neonatal polycythemia, and idiopathic persistence of the fetal circulation.[17] Indeed, in some cases it may be difficult to rule out primary cardiac disease without resorting to cardiac catheterization and angiocardiography. In most instances, however, the correct diagnosis can be made after a careful history, physical examination (presence of a murmur), demonstration of single or biventricular enlargement by the electrocardiogram, and the finding of cardiomegaly and pulmonary congestion by chest roentgenography.

TREATMENT[1, 2, 12, 13]

Cardiac failure in infants has a very serious prognosis, and the reported mortality ranges from 50 to 85 per cent, because a significant number of the deaths occur in babies born with inoperable cardiac malformations. Although the mortality is high, the spectrum of congenital cardiac malformations which are amenable to either palliative or corrective surgical therapy is ever increasing. An aggressive and enthusiastic approach to medical treatment is therefore vital if a baby is to be salvaged by surgical therapy. Since most infants in cardiac failure have congenital structural malformations of the heart, the initial medical therapy should be aimed at expeditious stabilization of the hemodynamic state so that the sick infant can be studied by cardiac catheterization and angiocardiography as soon as possible. A definitive anatomical diagnosis can thus be made, and the plan for therapy outlined, be it immediate surgical intervention or continued medical treatment. At times, cardiac catheterization and angiocardiography may have to be done on an emergency basis. For example, a baby with complete transposition of the great vessels will need, in most instances, a balloon septostomy at the time of catheterization, for sheer survival.[18]

The salvage rate of critically ill infants in cardiac failure will be improved if the diagnostic studies are done at a medical center which has the necessary equipment and trained medical personnel. If a physician's practice is some distance from a medical center, he or she can initiate treatment at the office which will improve the probability of survival of the patient. If the doctor suspects congestive heart failure, the patient should be given one half the digitalizing dose of digoxin parenterally (see following section on *Digoxin* for dosage schedule), placed in oxygen, and sent to the hospital. If the patient is restless, a dose of morphine sulfate should be given (see later discussion of *morphine sulfate* for dosage schedule), and if bacterial infection is suspected, antibiotic therapy is strongly recommended (see later discussion on *antibiotics*).

Monitoring

At the hospital, the infant should be admitted to a well-equipped and well-staffed *intensive care unit* where he or she can be monitored, i.e., *daily weights, recorded intake* and *output*. The vital signs should be monitored carefully with regard to *respiratory rate, electrocardiographic changes,* and *blood pressure.* (We have used the Doppler ultrasound method which measures the systolic and diastolic pressures. This method is uniquely suited for the infant under 6 months of age.)[19] In addition, the *blood gases* Pa_{O_2}, Pa_{CO_2}) as well as the serum pH should be followed at regular intervals, and periodic determinations of the *serum electrolytes* are vital guides to rational fluid therapy. All these data should be kept on a daily chart at the bedside.

Digoxin

Although the mechanism of action of digitalis is still imperfectly understood, there is universal agreement that it is the most valuable drug in the treatment of cardiac failure because digitalis increases the force of contraction of the failing myocardium, thereby increasing cardiac output. The most popular glycoside of digitalis for pediatric use has been digoxin. Numerous dosage regimens have been proposed, depending upon the age of the patient, and different dosage schedules have been proposed for oral and parenteral routes. There is questionable basis for both practices. Digoxin is absorbed equally well when given orally or parenterally, and there is questionable evidence that premature and newborn infants are more sensitive to the drug than older children.[20] We prefer to start with a digitalizing dosage of 0.04 mg per kg of body weight. One half the dose is given immediately, and one fourth in 6 hours and the other fourth again in 6 hours. A maintenance dose of 10 per cent of the total digitalizing dosage is then given every 12 hours. We prefer to give the drug parenterally to a critically ill infant because of the probability of vomiting. If the initial dose is found to be inadequate, the amount of glycoside may be increased to as much as 0.1 mg per kg as a total digitalizing dose. It should be emphasized that each patient has to be managed individually, and the treatment of each patient should be carried out as a biological titration. One is not as apt, therefore, to encounter digoxin intoxication with this regimen.*

Since infants rarely vomit with digoxin intoxication, one has to rely upon electrocardiographic monitoring for evidence of overdosage. This is not a sensitive method for detecting digoxin intoxication, but the appearance of a significant prolongation of the AV conduction time (0.04 second or greater) when compared with the predigitalization electrocardiogram and the appearance of premature ventricular contractions should be looked for as signs of intoxication. The recent availability of a method for the determination of serum digoxin concentration may be helpful for additional monitoring of a critically ill baby.[21]

Diuretics

Essentially all diuretic agents function by suppressing the resorption of sodium by the kidney, with subsequent decrease in the edema. The mercurial diuretic, meralluride, has largely been replaced by furosemide. The dose of furosemide is 1 mg per kg of body weight for intravenous use, and this may be repeated in 12 hours, if necessary. One may expect a response in 15 minutes to an hour. This drug also may be given orally (3 mg/kg/day). Because of the danger of urinary potassium loss and possible ototoxicity,[22] treatment with furosemide should be limited to the emergency situation, and maintenance diuretic therapy should be continued with chlorothiazide (20 to 30 mg/kg/day) and spironolactone (1 to 3 mg/kg/day).

---

*Higher doses of digoxin have been recommended,[1, 12, 13] but we feel the regimen recommended in this discussion provides the greatest factor of safety to the patient.

Atmospheric Environment and Posture

The administration of *oxygen* (oxygen concentration in incubator, 30 to 40 per cent) to the infant is of benefit, especially if there is super-imposed bacterial infection or atelectasis. In addition, the relative humidity in the incubator should be 40 to 50 per cent. The *temperature* inside the incubator should be adjusted so that the infant's rectal temperature is maintained at 37°C. A hot, humid environment should be avoided because an infant in congestive heart failure cannot initiate the compensatory mechanisms, such as an increase in cardiac output, increase in dermal blood flow, and increase in perspiration, which a normal infant calls into play for thermal regulation.[23] The *posture* of the patient should be adjusted so that his or her head and chest are on an incline of 10 to 30 degrees. In the recumbent position the shift of blood to the thorax from the lower extremities and splanchnic viscera increases the degree of pulmonary congestion which is already present as a result of congestive heart failure. This undesirable effect is lessened in the semisitting position. Also, by elevation of the head and chest the work of breathing will be reduced because the compression on the diaphragm by the abdominal viscera will be decreased.

Feeding and Metabolism

Critically ill infants should be supported by parenteral fluids. Small feedings or gavage may provoke vomiting and aspiration. A fluid containing 10 per cent glucose (on rare occasions an infant in heart failure may be hypoglycemic), with sodium, 1 to 4 mEq/kg/24 hours, and potassium, 0 to 3 mEq/kg/24 hours, depending upon the serum electrolytes, may be used. The total fluid administered in 24 hours should be 50 to 100 ml per kilogram. If the baby has rales and obvious edema, the lower figure should be used. When the baby has improved, small oral feedings may be started. A low salt formula, such as Similac PM 60/40 (Ross Laboratories), may be used for several days, but infants tolerate the conventional formulas quite well without aggravation of the edema.

Respiratory and metabolic acidosis may be seen in infants with heart failure. There are alveolar and bronchiolar transudates which compromise gas exchange at the alveolar level and are reflected in a low Pa_{O_2} and elevated Pa_{CO_2}. In extremely severe heart failure the hypoxemia encourages anaerobic metabolism, with a consequent increase in the production of lactic acid. Under these circumstances, cautious treatment with sodium bicarbonate is indicated. One may calculate, in the conventional manner, the amount of bicarbonate level (20 to 25 mEq/L) minus the patient's actual bicarbonate level × 0.6 × kg body weight is equal to mEq of bicarbonate to be given. We usually give one fourth to one half of this amount during a 6- to 8-hour period to reduce the possibility of untoward reactions such as hypernatremia, water retention, and alkalosis, because the initially high serum lactic acid content may be metabolized quickly with reduction in the metabolic acidosis if the heart function improves after digitalization. Thus the full dose of bicarbonate initially determined may not be needed.

Additional Therapeutic Measures

Morphine sulfate is a valuable drug in the treatment of heart failure, especially for the extremely restless infant, as well as the patient who presents with either impending or overt pulmonary edema. The benefit of the drug in pulmonary edema is its effect upon the peripheral circulation. The capacity of the total vascular bed is increased, thereby encouraging venous pooling and thereby decreasing venous return.[24] The recommended dose is 0.5 to 1 mg per 5 kg of body weight. This dose may be repeated in 3 to 4 hours.

Antibiotics usually are indicated in patients with acute heart failure because of the high incidence of superimposed pulmonary infection. After appropriate cultures are obtained, initial broad coverage should be instituted. For infants (birth to 3 months) ampicillin, 100 to 200 mg/kg per 24 hours, and kanamycin sulfate, 10 to 15 mg/kg per 24 hours, or gentamycin, 5 to 7.5 mg/kg per 24 hours, should be given intramuscularly. For infants (3 to 12 months), ampicillin, 100 to 200 mg/kg per 24 hours, and methicillin, 100 mg/kg per 24 hours, should be given intramuscularly or intravenously.[25] If a specific infecting organism is isolated, the appropriate antibiotic drug then can be substituted.

Anemia (Hgb <7 gm per 100 ml), if present, should be corrected so that there is an optimum hemogloblin level for oxygen transport. A packed red blood cell solution should be given cautiously and slowly (5 ml/kg) so that the hemoglobin is raised to 10 gm per 100 ml or higher. This should be administered after the baby has had the benefit of the treatment outlined previously.

Emergency measures sometimes are indicated for the infant who presents with heart failure in a moribund state. Because one can presume that the baby has severe metabolic acidosis, a rapid intravenous or, in desperate circumstances, intracardiac infusion of *sodium bicarbonate* (2 to 5 mEq/kg) may be given. An *Isuprel* drip is also indicated (0.2 μg/kg/min) and preferably should be given by an infusion pump while the heart rate and blood pressure are monitored continuously. This drug is especially useful in bradycardia and has an added advantage because of its positive inotropic effect. On occasion, a mechanical ventilator will be necessary if the patient cannot maintain adequate gas exchange, as is seen commonly in the immediate post-operative period after cardiac surgery. Since most of these infants in congestive failure are weak and have superimposed pulmonary infection with increased or changing lung compliance, a volume-limited ventilator is the instrument of choice.[26] In cases with extreme bradycardia or cardiac arrest, the physician has to resort to *external cardiac massage* and *assisted respiration* with an endotracheal tube.

SUMMARY

Heart failure may be defined simply as the inability of the heart to pump blood commensurate with the body's needs. Although it is possible for the right or left ventricle to fail separately, it is much more common for infants to present with failure of both chambers. When a ventricle fails, the end-diastolic pressure in that chamber rises and the pressure in the atrium and central and peripheral veins is increased. There is a decrease in blood flow to the kidney, and this decrease is thought to be responsible for the renal retention of sodium and water which, in turn, increases blood volume. Thus, the elevations in pressure, the disturbances in blood flow, and abnormal distribution of water and electrolytes are homeostatic mechanisms which help preserve cardiac output. Because of these compensatory mechanisms, signs and symptoms develop which the clinician recognizes as heart failure.

Infants under 1 year of age account for 90 per cent of pediatric patients who develop congestive heart failure, and the majority of these have congenital heart disease.

Although the mortality in infants with congestive heart failure is high (50 to 85 per cent), the spectrum of congenital cardiac malformations which is amenable to corrective surgery is ever increasing. The physician must, therefore, be able to make the diagnosis of heart failure with confidence and institute immediate therapy. The patient, ideally, should be transferred to a medical center and admitted to a well-equipped and well-staffed intensive care unit in which 24-hour monitoring is available and therapy can be initiated.

Since most of the infants will have congenital structural malformation of the heart as the basis for their failure, the treatment should be aimed at expeditious stabilization of the hemodynamic state so that the patient can then be evaluated by cardiac catheterization and angiocardiography as soon as possible. A definitive anatomical diagnosis thus can be made, and the plan for therapy decided, whether it be immediate surgical intervention or continued medical treatment.

The approach just outlined will continually improve the salvage rate of infants in congestive heart failure.

REFERENCES

1. Keith, J. D., Rowe, R. D., and Vlad, P.: Heart Disease in Infancy and Childhood. New York, Macmillan, 1967.
2. Friedberg, C. K.: Diseases of the Heart. 3rd ed., Philadelphia, W. B. Saunders Co., 1966.
3. Braunwald, E., Ross, J., and Sonnenblick, E. H.: Mechanism of Contraction of the Normal and Failing Heart. Boston, Little, Brown, 1967.
4. Spann, J. F., Jr., Mason, D. T., and Zelis, R. F.: Recent advances in the understanding of congestive heart failure (I). Mod. Concepts Cardiovasc. Dis., 39:73, 1970.
5. Spann, J. F., Jr., Mason, D. T., and Zelis, R. F.: Recent advances in the understanding of congestive heart failure (II). Mod. Concepts Cardiovasc. Dis., 39:79, 1970.
6. Braunwald, E.: The sympathetic nervous system in heart failure. Hosp. Prac., 31:31, 1970.
7. Mason, D. T.: Control of peripheral circulation in health and disease. Mod. Concepts Cardiovasc. Dis., 36:25, 1967.
8. Haber, E.: The renin-angiotensin system in curable hypertension. Mod. Concepts Cardiovasc. Dis., 38:7, 1969.
9. Romero, J. C., and Hoobler, S. W.: The renin-angiotensin system in clinical medicine. Am. Heart J., 80:701, 1969.
10. Keith, J. D.: Congestive heart failure. Pediatrics, 18:491, 1956.
11. Lees, M. H.: Patent ductus arteriosus in premature infants—a diagnostic and therapeutic dilemma. J. Pediatr., 86:132, 1975.
12. Lees, M. H.: Heart failure in the newborn infant. J. Pediatr., 75:139, 1969.
13. Nadas, A. S., and Hauck, A. J.: Pediatric aspects of congestive heart failure. Circulation, 21:424, 1960.
14. Braunwald, E.: Physiology of congestive heart failure. Ann. Intern. Med., 64:904, 1966.
15. Marshall, R., and Widdecombe, J. G.: The activity of the pulmonary stretch receptors during congestion of the lung. Qt. J. Exp. Physiol., 43:320, 1958.
16. Laforce, F. M., Mullane, J. F., Boehme, R. F., Kelly, W. J., and Huber, G. L.: The effect of pulmonary edema on antibacterial defenses of the lung. J. Lab. Clin. Med., 82:634, 1973.
17. Brown, R., and Pickering, D.: Persistent transitional circulation. Arch. Dis. Child., 49:883, 1974.
18. Rashkind, W. J., and Miller, W. W.: Creation of an atrial septal defect without thoracotomy. J.A.M.A., 196:991, 1966.
19. Hernandez, A., Hartmann, A. F., and Goldring, D.: Measurement of blood pressure in infants and children by the Doppler ultrasonic technique. Pediatrics, 48:788, 1971.
20. Hernandez, A., Burton, R. M., Pagtakhan, R. D., and Goldring, D.: Pharmacodynamics of ^{3}H-digoxin in infants. Pediatrics, 44:418, 1969.
21. Hayes, C. J., Butler, V. P., Gersony, W. M.: Serum digoxin studies on infants and children. Pediatrics, 52:561, 1973.
22. Cooperman, L. B., and Rubin, I. L.: Toxicity of ethacrynic acid and furosemide. Am. Heart J., 85:831, 1973.
23. Burch, G. E., and Giles, T. D.: The burden of a hot humid environment on the heart. Mod. Concepts Cardiovasc. Dis., 39:115, 1970.
24. Vasko, J. S., Henney, R. P., Oldham, H. N., Brawley, R. K., and Morrow, A. G.: Mechanism of action of morphine in the treatment of experimental pulmonary edema. Am. J. Cardiol., 18:876, 1966.
25. J. Neal Middelkamp: Personal communication.
26. Smith, R. M.: The critically ill child: Respiratory arrest and its sequelae. Pediatrics, 46:108, 1970. (See also Chapter 11, this book.)

Chapter Nine

ACUTE HEPATIC FAILURE

CHARLES TREY, M.B., CH.B., M.D.

The clinical syndrome of acute liver failure is the manifestation of severe hepatic dysfunction or massive hepatic necrosis. The child usually presents with a history suggestive of viral infection. There may have been exposure to hepatitis, blood products, or presumed hepatotoxins. Progressive jaundice is usual, except in the liver failure of Reye's syndrome; other symptoms include fetor hepaticus, decrease in liver size, and asterixis ("liver flap"). Mental confusion or coma may develop as the disease progresses. The biochemical abnormalities usually include elevated serum bilirubin and glutamic-oxaloacetic transaminase (GOT). Increased serum alpha-amino-nitrogen and blood ammonia, and a prolonged prothrombin time, unaffected by parenteral vitamin K administration, are useful indications of increasing severity of the disease. Hypoglycemia can occur in severe liver failure and is common in Reye's syndrome. Serum albumin decreases as the failure progresses. The patient's course may fluctuate, and improvement or recovery is possible at almost any stage.[1-3]

While the underlying cause may not be immediately apparent, diagnosis usually is not difficult if other varieties of coma, such as those from metabolic or intracranial causes, are excluded. In encephalopathy and fatty degeneration of the liver and viscera (Reye's syndrome), the child is not jaundiced and the diagnosis may be confused with other forms of toxic encephalitis.[4, 5] Reye's syndrome thus must be suspected in non-icteric children in coma with high levels of serum GOT and other enzymes, increased blood ammonia, and prolonged prothrombin time. These laboratory measurements should be performed at frequent intervals in the child in whom the diagnosis is suspected, as the abnor-

From New England Deaconess Hospital, New England Baptist Hospital, Children's Hospital Medical Center, and Harvard Medical School, Boston, Massachusetts.

malities may not be evident at first but can become manifest during the course of illness.

Histological examination of the liver in acute hepatic failure shows severe hepatocellular necrosis. In Reye's syndrome and in tetracycline-associated liver disease, the hepatocytes are infiltrated diffusely by small fat droplets without displacement of the nucleus, and only a few cells are necrosed. Liver biopsy, if the child's coagulation studies are normal, is useful in differentiating these two conditions and also in detecting granuloma, lymphoma, and other systemic diseases which can present with acute hepatic failure. Usually the hepatic failure is part of the systemic involvement.[6]

In children who have been presumed to have normal liver function prior to liver failure, infectious hepatitis can be suspected. The demonstration of hepatitis B surface antigen is useful in the confirmation of hepatitis B (serum) hepatitis. The presence in the patient's serum of the Dane particle can confirm the diagnosis of hepatitis B antigenemia at an earlier stage of the disease. While hepatitis A (infectious) hepatitis antibody testing is now available, tests for the determination of hepatitis A virus in excreta or blood are still being elaborated.[7] An "e" antigen, which seems not to be a viral particle, has been demonstrated in the serum of patients with chronic active or persistent hepatitis.[8] There are many patients in whose serum the antigens or antibodies of various forms of hepatitis are absent. The hepatitis of these patients may be due to infectious mononucleosis, Coxsackie virus, or viruses yet to be determined. Appropriate tests for the agents should be done.

In the patient who shows a combination of hepatitis and hemolytic anemia, or whose hepatitis runs a protracted course, Wilson's disease is an important diagnostic possibility. Its prompt detection allows early treatment with penicillamine or similar agents.

Drugs that can cause acute hepatitis need to be considered in every case, since in many instances their removal can lead to clinical improvement. Tetracycline, as a dose-related hepatotoxic agent,[9] is an example. On rare occasions salicylates can cause hepatitis, especially in children with rheumatoid arthritis, and ingestion of an overdose of acetaminophen (Paracetamol) has caused serious and at times fatal hepatitis. This has been treated successfully with intravenous cysteamine, if given within 8 to 10 hours of ingestion of acetaminophen.[10, 11]

Table 1 shows the presumed causes, and outcomes, in our experience with 24 children up to 14 years of age in the Fulminant Hepatic Failure Surveillance Study (FHFSS).[1] Patients who did not progress to severe hepatic coma (unresponsiveness, except in a reflex manner, to painful stimuli) had a much better chance of survival. Of 318 FHFSS patients of all ages in hepatic failure with hepatic coma, 42 (13 per cent) were children up to 14 years. Twenty-six of these 42 children sur-

TABLE 1   Presumed Causes and Outcome of Fulminant
Hepatic Failure in Children

	Author's Experience		Fulminant Hepatic Failure Surveillance Study	
Cause	Number of Cases	Number Surviving	Number of Cases	Number Surviving
Infectious hepatitis	12	6	26	16
Serum hepatitis	2	2	5	2
Halothane	1	1	2	2
Drugs	2	2	0	0
Reye's syndrome	6	3	7	4
Others	1	1	2	2
TOTAL	24	15	42	26

vived; 38 of the 42 were in severe hepatic coma, and 13 of these survived. Four children who had infectious hepatitis did not progress to that state; of these, three survived and one died of septicemia and subacute hepatic necrosis. The overall experience is similar to that with our own 24 patients (Table 1), 11 of whom also are included in the Surveillance Study. The others were seen either before the initiation of that study or since the third report to members of FHFSS.

PREVENTION

Prevention of acute liver failure may be possible; early recognition can improve the prognosis. Prophylaxis, by the early administration of gamma globulin to children who have been in contact with patients with infectious hepatitis, may prevent or attenuate that infection.[12] The dangers of drug abuse should be stressed, since this constitutes the second commonest cause of fulminant hepatic failure in the age group over 14. In two of our patients, prolonged intravenous administration of tetracycline may have led to fulminant hepatic failure.[13, 14] Generalized allergic reaction and hepatic disease have been reported with para-aminosalicylate.[15] In such patients the discontinuance of the medications in the early stages of reaction may prevent hepatic failure.

The clinical entity of halothane-associated hepatic disease should be considered in a child who develops unexplained fever and jaundice after repeated exposure to this anesthetic agent. These events sometimes are confused with the diagnosis of postoperative infection or cholestatic jaundice and thus can lead to further surgery. No test detects the occasional child at risk from this complication of the use of halothane. Thus, unexplained and unexpected fever following surgery should be a relative contraindication to further use of halothane, and postoperative jaundice should be an absolute contraindication.[1, 16]

On occasion, patients with chronic liver disease can present in hepatic coma. This usually is precipitated by infections, gastrointestinal bleeding, or electrolyte imbalance which might have been preventable. The child has signs of chronic liver disease, such as spider angioma, palmar erythema, or portal hypertension. As in the investigation of comatose patients with fulminant hepatic failure, other causes of coma must be excluded. The principles of therapy are similar in both groups.

TREATMENT

General Principles

The purposes of treatment are to alleviate the systemic effects of hepatic failure and to promote liver cell regeneration. Our knowledge of the latter is so limited that therapy is aimed essentially at supporting the patient in the hope that sufficient hepatic regeneration to sustain life will occur. The rationale of treatment is based on clinical observations and experimental studies. In regard to the central nervous system, the response of the child in hepatic coma will depend on the severity of the liver disease and the presence of complications. In the mild form agitation and confusion are noted, while in the severe stage the child may be unresponsive to painful stimuli and in decorticate or decerebrate posture.[17] Mental confusion and restlessness are not indications for sedation, but rather they are warnings that the patient may lapse into severe hepatic or hypoglycemic coma, which will be discussed later. Sedatives metabolized in the liver, such as morphine or paraldehyde,[18] are contraindicated. If sedation is necessary, drugs excreted in the kidneys, such as long-acting barbiturates or meperidine, should be chosen.

In patients or animals with liver disease and portal-systemic shunts, high protein diets or ammonia salts can precipitate or aggravate hepatic coma. The mechanism of these effects is not clear. The practical application of these observations to children with liver failure is that protein intake or degradation in the intestinal tract should be reduced. Protein is either eliminated entirely from the diet during the acute disease or markedly restricted; protein degradation by intestinal bacteria is decreased by altering the intestinal flora with antibiotics (such as neomycin), and its products are removed by frequent enemas. Lactulose, a disaccharide, is useful as a cathartic because the body has no enzyme to digest it. Its administration not only decreases ammonia (by reducing intracolonic pH) but also diminishes the coliform bacteria of the gut. The early detection or prevention of gastrointestinal bleeding, should it develop, is important, as the added protein in the gastrointestinal tract can aggravate the coma, while the shock from volume depletion can endanger the life of the patient.

Hypoglycemia can be a manifestation of severe liver dysfunction and frequently is seen in Reye's syndrome. Blood sugar should be estimated frequently and an adequate blood glucose concentration should be maintained. We have encountered hypoglycemia despite the administration of intravenous glucose, in cases in which the quantity administered has been inadequate.[19] Frequent bedside estimation of blood glucose by Dextrostix,* as well as laboratory determination, can aid in detecting this complication.

Ascites is seen in both acute and chronic liver disease. While peritoneal fluid should be aspirated for diagnostic tests and cultures, the only indications for removal of larger volumes are respiratory embarrassment or esophageal variceal bleeding in the presence of tense ascites. In patients with chronic liver disease, injudicious use of diuretics and inadequate replacement of lost potassium can result in severe depletion. Electrolyte imbalance, especially hypokalemia, can aggravate or precipitate hepatic coma. Supplementary potassium (as potassium chloride) may need to be given intravenously or orally.

The effects of hepatic failure on the kidney apparently are unrelated to organic lesions.[20] The characteristically low urinary sodium (e.g., 5 mEq/L) and the high urinary potassium (e.g., 35 mEq/L) do not suggest renal tubular malfunction or acute tubular failure. The 24-hour urinary potassium is useful in calculating the minimum potassium requirement. The serum creatinine level rises, and oliguria occurs in the late stages. Treatment is aimed at maintaining normal serum electrolyte concentrations, intravascular volume, and colloid osmotic pressure. The intravascular volume can be roughly estimated by the central venous pressure (CVP); if the CVP is low, colloid is given as salt-poor human albumin or plasma. The liver cannot adequately maintain the serum albumin.

The child in severe liver failure is prone to infection, the site and organism of which may be difficult to detect. The temperature may not be elevated; in severe illness it actually may be lower than normal. If intravascular coagulation (as manifested by thrombocytopenia and low fibrinogen) occurs, it usually is due to septicemia rather than liver disease *per se*. Sputum, urine, blood, and cerebrospinal fluid cultures, as well as chest roentgenograms, may be necessary to detect the site and extent of infection. If there is indication of infection, an appropriate antibiotic should be given. If the child cannot cope with his or her oral secretions or has respiratory distress, a cuffed endotracheal tube will be

---

*Ames Company, Elkhart, Indiana, 46514.

required. Loss of swallowing reflex usually precedes respiratory depression.

Steroids frequently are used in patients with acute hepatic failure, but it is difficult to judge their value.[21, 22] Contraindications to their use are infection and gastrointestinal hemorrhage, which is commonly due to superficial gastritis and usually responds to fresh blood replacement and intravenous posterior pituitary (Pituitrin), although it occasionally requires surgery.

The results of the approach described here have been good in the child with chronic liver disease and superimposed strain on the decreased liver metabolism. As these patients improve, protein slowly is reintroduced in the diet and oral antibiotics are reduced. The initial addition of protein is only 10 gm or less daily. If the child does not become very drowsy or confused, low salt milk (8 oz of whole milk contains 9.1 gm protein) is then tried as an addition and, if tolerated, that quantity of protein is included in the diet. In this way the response to increased protein intake can be assessed. The hypoalbuminemia which usually occurs during the course of acute liver failure may need to be combatted by intravenous administration of salt-poor albumin, especially if the serum albumin is under 2 gm per 100 ml. When ascites and peripheral edema cause discomfort the diuretic spironolactone (Aldactone) should be tried, but many patients usually require the concomitant use of benzothiadiazides such as chlorothiazide. If these are used, they should be supplemented with potassium chloride.

Specific Procedures

Fulminant hepatic failure has a high mortality.[1] Procedures such as hemodialysis, peritoneal dialysis, and blood and plasma exchange transfusions therefore have been advocated to eliminate or dilute the unknown metabolites and thus reduce the degree of encephalopathy and other systemic effects of severe disease.[23-29]

Exchange transfusion with whole blood and plasmapheresis, and return of packed cells and platelets with fresh plasma, have been the most common procedures used. These can be performed in most medical centers. The indications are severe hepatic coma without response to treatment after about 24 hours, or rapid deterioration with respiratory distress. Because the child is usually in a high cardiac output state and sensitive to volume depletion, the blood pressure, CVP, and blood volume should be stable before the procedure is begun. About 150 per cent of the calculated blood volume is exchanged by administration and withdrawal of blood simultaneously into and from two vessels, with the patient's vital signs monitored. The procedure is repeated about every

24 hours if the patient does not improve. Fresh blood must be used in order to replace platelets. If heparinized blood is used, clotting time is estimated following the replacement and protamine sulfate is administered to maintain a normal clotting time.

Although such transfusions often are used, their therapeutic value is difficult to gauge. In our experience over 60 per cent of children so transfused awoke sufficiently to talk, but many of these children subsequently died of complications or relapsed into coma. The survival of about 40 per cent may be related to the ability of the liver to regenerate. We have demonstrated improvement in cardiac output and prothrombin time after exchange transfusion. In the third report of the Fulminant Hepatic Failure Surveillance Study,[1] 33 of 38 children with deep hepatic coma had exchange transfusion and of these 33, 30 died; the five children who were not so treated all died. We have seen one patient with Reye's syndrome who was in coma for 1 day survive without replacement, and there are other reports of such patients. In experiments on rhesus monkeys, repeated exchange transfusions have been shown to reverse hepatic coma and significantly prolong life.[29] While exchange transfusions are recommended for liver failure in humans, more experience is necessary to define their value.

In one randomly allocated and controlled trial, conducted with few adult patients, greater mortality occurred in the treated group.[27] On the other hand, most centers report transient improvement in the level of consciousness with treatment, although patients tend to relapse into coma.[28] Increase of survival time has been observed in animals treated by exchange transfusion, but its role has not yet been defined in facilitating regeneration of the liver. Age is a significant factor in the prognosis of fulminant hepatic failure, for patients under 15 years old have a 30 per cent survival rate,[29] although this may be explained in part by differences of etiology associated with different ages. A supposed "hepatotrophic" effect of insulin and glucagon has been noted, but any therapeutic application to patients in hepatic failure still needs investigation.[30, 31]

Once facilities and blood are available for transfusions, it is difficult to discontinue such supportive therapy in the child who does not respond. Continual improvement in prothrombin time and appearance of alpha fetal globulin are useful signs, whereas the lowering of serum GOT, or of other enzymes, and of blood ammonia does not necessarily indicate good prognosis. The electroencephalogram is useful mainly in terminal events, in which flat voltage may be a sign of permanent brain damage. Complications such as renal failure, respiratory failure, and sepsis (which can occur at any stage) need not be indications for stopping such a program of therapy. There have been reports of survival despite all these complications.[30, 31] On the other hand, hepatic coma is only one manifestation of liver failure, and patients who have recovered from coma can succumb to any of the other complications mentioned.

Treatment by human cross circulation has been used in adult patients, but ethical considerations and the risk of transmitting the disease to the normal volunteer add special difficulties. Cross circulation with a baboon has been reported,[32] but is still in experimental stages. It may be noted that repeated cross circulation between two normal baboons usually results in severe reactions.[33] Pig or bovine livers have been used in extracorporeal perfusions in the treatment of hepatic failure. There are reports of improvement in consciousness while the patient is connected to the human donor or animal liver, but long-term cures are few. Artificial liver support systems are being investigated. Hemodialysis through columns with resin coated with albumin or activated charcoal is now in use. The former is efficient in clearing bilirubin and has been used in patients who suffer from the Crigler-Najjar syndrome. The latter is effective in absorbing acetaminophen (Paracetamol).[28] In patients who have not responded to usual conservative treatment and in whom liver failure is fulminant, such procedures may be indicated, though they must be performed in specially equipped centers. Especially for pediatric patients, the overall results are difficult to assess, as are those of any of these procedures performed on adult patients

TABLE 2   Regimen for Treatment of Hepatic Failure

Acute Phase
 Diet
  Stop protein.
  Add glucose and carbohydrate.
  Administer parenterally vitamins K, B complex, folic acid, and ascorbic acid.
 Antibiotics
  Oral, and poorly absorbed (e.g., neomycin, 1 to 4 gm daily).
  Combat infection if present.
 Purgation and Enema
  Use if indicated.
To Prevent Precipitating or Aggravating Factors
  1. Protein restriction.
  2. Treat gastrointestinal bleeding.
  3. Fluid and electrolyte correction.
  4. Avoid diuretics—except spironolactone.
  5. Avoid paracentesis.
  6. Maintain adequate blood glucose.
  7. Sedation, if necessary, by drugs excreted by the kidney.
Ascites

  Diagnostic tap
  Spironolactone (Aldactone 25 mg, tid)
  Salt-poor albumin
Further Procedures (possibly indicated in rapid deterioration or severe hepatic coma not responding to other treatment)
  1. Exchange blood or plasma transfusion (one and one-half to two times blood volume).
  2. Cross circulation with human or primate donors.
  3. Perfusion with *ex vivo* liver.
  4. Liver transplantation.

---

whose chronic liver disease tends to have a highly variable course, partly because of its many causes.

SUMMARY

The aim of treatment in liver failure in children is to maintain the child until the liver function is improved. (See accompanying chart for outline of suggested regimen.) Possible causes of coma other than liver failure must be investigated; hypoglycemia, infection, electrolyte imbalance, or gastrointestinal hemorrhage must be prevented if possible or promptly recognized and treated if they occur. Dietary protein is restricted and alimentary protein breakdown by bacteria is decreased by oral antibiotics and purgatives. Glucocorticosteroids may be administered. If the deeply comatose child does not improve or deteriorates rapidly, procedures such as exchange blood transfusions should be used. All aspects of therapy may be required in the child recovering from the acute phase or in the child with chronic liver failure. The mortality is high, and prevention or early detection of this syndrome is important.

REFERENCES

1. Trey, C., Lipworth, L., Chalmers, T. C., Davidson, C. S., Gottlieb, L. S., Popper, H., and Saunders, S. J.: Fulminant hepatic failure. Presumable contribution of halothane. N. Engl. J. Med., 279:789, 1968.
2. Trey, C., Burns, D. G., and Saunders, S. J.: Treatment of hepatic coma by exchange blood transfusion. N. Engl. J. Med., 274:473, 1966.
3. Ritt, D. J., Whelan, G., Werner, D. J., Eiglerbrodt, E. H., Schenker, S., and Combes, B.: Acute hepatic necrosis with stupor or coma: An analysis of thirty-one patients. Medicine, 48:151, 1969.
4. Reye, R. D. K., Morgan, G., and Baral, J.: Encephalopathy and fatty degeneration of the viscera. A disease entity in childhood. Lancet, 2:749, 1963.
5. Smith, A. L.: Ammonia disposal in Reye's syndrome. N. Engl. J. Med., 294:897, 1976.
6. Sherlock, S.: Diseases of the Liver and Biliary System. 5th ed., Philadelphia, F. A. Davis Co., 1975, p. 490.
7. Symposia on viral hepatitis. Am. J. Med. Sci., 270:1, 1975.
8. Eletheriou, N., Heathcote, G., Thomas, H. C., and Sherlock, S.: Incidence and clinical significance of α antigen and antibody in acute and chronic liver disease. Lancet, 2:1171, 1975.
9. Klatskin, G.: Toxic and drug induced hepatitis. In Schiff, L., ed.: Diseases of the Liver. 4th ed., Philadelphia, J. B. Lippincott Co., 1975, p. 604.
10. Editorial, Paracetamol hepatotoxicity. Lancet, 2:1189, 1975.
11. Rumack, B. H., and Matthew, H.: Acetaminophen poisoning and toxicity. Pediatrics, 55:871, 1975.
12. Pollock, T. M., and Reid, D.: Assessment of British gamma globulin in preventing infectious hepatitis. A report to the Director of the Public Health Laboratory Service. Br. Med. J., 2:451, 1968.
13. Lepper, M. H., Wolfe, C. K., Zimmerman, H. G., Caldwell, E. R., Spies, W. H., and

Dowling, H. F.: Effects of large doses of aureomycin on human liver. Arch. Int. Med., *88*:271, 1951.

14. Schultz, J. C., Adamson, J. S., Workman, W. W., and Horman, T. D.: Fatal liver disease after intravenous administration of tetracycline in high dosage. N. Engl. J. Med., *269*:999, 1963.

15. Lederman, R. J., Davis, F. B., and Davis, P. J.: Exchange transfusion as treatment of acute hepatic failure due to anti-tuberculous drugs. Ann. Int. Med., *68*:830, 1968.

16. Gottleib, L. S., and Trey, C.: The effects of fluorinated anesthetics on the liver and kidneys. Ann. Rev. Med., *25*:411, 1974.

17. Plum, F., and Posner, J. B.: The Diagnosis of Stupor and Coma. Philadelphia, F. A. Davis Co., 1966, p. 138.

18. Hayward, J. N., and Boshell, B. R.: Paraldehyde intoxication with metabolic acidosis. Report of 2 cases, experimental data and critical review of the literature. Am. J. Med., *26*:965, 1967.

19. Sampson, R. I., Trey, C., Timme, A. H., and Saunders, S. J.: Fulminant hepatitis with recurrent hypoglycemia and hemorrhage. Gastroenterology, *53*:291, 1967.

20. Baldus, W. P., and Summerskill, W. H.: Liver-kidney interrelationships. *In* Schiff, L., ed.: Diseases of the Liver. 4th ed., Philadelphia, J. B. Lippincott Co., 1975, p. 445.

21. Katz, R., Velasco, M., Klinger, J., and Alessandri, H.: Corticosteroids in treatment of acute hepatic coma. Gastroenterology, *42*:258, 1962.

22. Gregory, P. B., Knaller, C. M., Kempson, R. L., and Miller, R.: Steroid therapy in severe viral hepatitis: A randomized trial. N. Engl. J. Med., *294*:681, 1976.

23. Neinhuis, L. I., Mulmed., E. T., and Kelley, J.: Hepatic coma, treatment emphasizing merit of peritoneal dialysis. Am. J. Surg., *106*:980, 1963.

24. Krebs, R., and Flynn, M.: Treatment of hepatic coma with exchange transfusion and peritoneal dialysis. J.A.M.A., *199*:430, 1967.

25. Lee, C., and Tink, A.: Exchange transfusion in hepatic coma; report of a case. Med. J. Aust., *1*:40, 1958.

26. Burnell, J. M., Thomas, E. D., Ansell, J. S., Cross, H. E., Dillard, D. H., Epstein, R. B., Eschbach, J. W., Jr., Hogan, R., Hutchings, R. H., Motulsky, A., Ormsby, J. W., Poffenbarger, P., Scribner, B. H., and Volwiler, W.: Observations on cross circulation in man. Am. J. Med., *38*:832, 1965.

27. Redeker, A. G., and Tamahiro, H. S.: Controlled trial of exchange transfusion in fulminant viral hepatitis. Lancet, *1*:3, 1973.

28. Williams, R.: Fulminant viral hepatitis. Clin. Gastroenterol., *3*:419, 1974.

29. Trey, C.: The fulminant hepatic failure surveillance study. Brief review of effects of presumed etiology and age on survival. Can. Med. Assoc. J., *106*:525, 1972.

30. Starzl, T. F., Lee, I. Y., Porter, K. A., and Putman, L. G.: The influence of portal blood upon lipid metabolism in normal and diabetic dogs and baboons. Surg. Gynecol. Obstet., *140*:381, 1975.

31. Trey, C., Garcia, F. G., King, N. W., Lowenstein, L. M., and Davidson, C. S.: Massive liver necrosis in the monkey. The effects of exchange blood transfusion on fulminant liver failure. J. Lab. Clin. Med., *73*:784, 1969.

32. Trey, C., and Davidson, C. S.: The management of fulminant hepatic failure. *In* Popper, H., and Schaffner, F., eds.: Progress in Liver Diseases. Vol. III, New York, Grune & Stratton, 1970, pp. 282–298.

33. Bosman, S. C. W., Lerblanche, J., Saunders, S. J., and Harrison, G. G.: Cross circulation between man and baboon. Lancet, *2*:583, 1968.

34. Starb, R., Buckner, C. D., Epstein, R. B., Graham, T., and Thomas, E. D.: Clinical and hematologic effects of cross circulation in baboons. Transfusion, *9*:23, 1969.

Chapter Ten

ACUTE RENAL FAILURE

SHELDON ORLOFF, M.D.,
DONALD E. POTTER, M.D.,
MALCOLM A. HOLLIDAY, M.D.

Acute renal failure has many causes (Table 1). The prognosis of any episode is dependent on the cause, the associated findings, and the reversibility of the damage. Major advances in the treatment of critically ill children have led to an increase in the incidence of acute renal failure, but the survival rate from both acute and prolonged renal failure appears to have improved.[1, 2] Three developments may account for this improvement. Physicians are more alert to the causes, early signs, and the proper treatment of acute renal failure; experienced teams of nephrologists, nurses, and technicians now provide expert care; and treatment of chronic renal failure by dialysis and transplantation is more widely accessible. Pediatric nephrology has emerged as a working subspecialty of pediatrics. This paper describes the causes, prevention, and treatment of acute renal failure in children, as studied at the University of California over the last ten years.

DEFINITION AND DIAGNOSIS

Acute renal failure is defined by oliguria, i.e., urine output less than 300 ml/m²/day (< 20 ml/100 kcal/day—see page 138), or by laboratory findings of azotemia, i.e., blood urea nitrogen (BUN) greater than 80 mg/100 ml and creatinine greater than 1.5 mg/dl developing in a child who previously had satisfactory kidney function. Its potential for development should be recognized when there is a predisposing condition, e.g., hypotension, myoglobinuria, hemoglobinuria, or use of a nephrotoxic drug.

From the Department of Pediatrics, University of California, San Francisco, and San Francisco General Hospital, San Francisco, California. Supported by Training Grant HD 00182 from the National Institute of Child Health and Human Development.

The authors are indebted to Dr. Carolyn Piel, house staff, fellows, and nurses on the renal service at the University of California, San Francisco, and San Francisco General Hospital. We gratefully acknowledge their assistance in the medical management of these patients.

TABLE 1   Causes of Acute Renal Failure in Infants and Children*

Prerenal (decreased perfusion)
  Hypovolemia:
    Hemorrhage (internal or external)
    Gastrointestinal losses (vomiting and/or diarrhea, nasogastric tubes)
    Sequestration (local injury, trauma or disease; burns; postsurgery)
    Malnutrition
    Anemia
  Decreased cardiac function (congestive heart failure):
    Pericardial tamponade
    Myocardiopathy
    Congenital abnormality
    Arrhythmia
    Acute anemia (hemolytic crises, sickle crises)
  Peripheral vasodilatation:
    Sepsis
    Drug-induced (antihypertensives, anesthetics)
  Increased vascular resistance:
    Anesthesia
    Surgery
    Hepatorenal syndrome
  Renal vascular obstruction:
    Embolus or thrombus (renal vein thrombosis)
    Narrowing of renal artery(ies) (congenital stricture, fibromuscular hyperplasia)
    External compression (tumor)

Renal
  Glomerular:
    Acute glomerulonephritis (poststreptococcal, rapidly progressive, etc.)
    Chronic glomerulonephritis (familial, hereditary)
    Structural abnormalities (cysts, dysplasia)
    Intravascular coagulation (sepsis, hemolytic-uremic syndrome)
  Glomerular or Tubular:
    Nephrotoxins (drugs, chemicals, radiographic dyes?)
    Necrosis (cortical, tubular medullary, i.e., extended prerenal)
    Tumors (compression, invasion, radiation)
  Tubular:
    Intravascular hemolysis (hemoglobinuria)
    Injury (myoglobinuria)
  Vascular:
    Systemic vasculitis (lupus, other collagen-vascular diseases)
    Compression (stricture, tumor)
    Acute and/or chronic rejection
  Other:
    Obstructive, i.e., extended postrenal

Postrenal
  Urethral (foreign body, meatal stenosis)
  Bladder neck:
    Functional (neurogenic, ganglionic blocking drugs, antihistamines)
    Tumor
    Infection
    Foreign body
    Pregnancy

---

*Modified from Schrier, R. W.: Acute renal failure. Diagnosis, Management and Pathogenesis. Calif. Med., *115*:28, 1971.

**TABLE 1   Causes of Acute Renal Failure in Infants
and Children** — (*Continued*)

Ureteral:
  Internal
    Sulfa or uric acid crystals (especially post–antineoplastic drug therapy)
    Blood clots (sickle cell, hemorrhagic cystitis)
    Infection (stricture and/or debris and/or edema)
    Calculi (oxalosis, cystinuria)
    Edema (surgery, infection)
  External
    Surgical (adhesions, edema, ligation)
    Tumor

The causes of acute renal failure are listed in Table 1. Many of these entities can be diagnosed from the history and physical examination. They are reviewed in detail elsewhere and are not considered individually here.[3] They are grouped into three major categories — prerenal, renal, and postrenal — because therapy is different for each group. Early detection and prompt treatment of prerenal and postrenal causes of acute renal failure may limit or prevent damage and the need for extended treatment.[4, 5] Renal causes, however, usually either are irreversible or require prolonged therapy, since direct renal damage has occured. The classification above, although helpful in treatment and prognosis, is somewhat arbitrary since both pre- and postrenal causes of acute renal failure can also lead to either reversible or irreversible renal parenchymal damage.

Prerenal

Prerenal causes of acute renal failure are the most common in children. The physiological mechanism is decreased renal perfusion secondary to absolute or relative hypovolemia. Diarrheal dehydration is the most common cause in children. Surgical shock and trauma are also common causes. Hypovolemia and decreased renal perfusion result in decreased glomerular filtration rate and stimulate secretion of renin, aldosterone, and antidiuretic hormone, which further decrease urine flow. Extended hypoperfusion of the kidney results in renal damage — tubular or cortical necrosis — so that there may be progression from prerenal to renal failure. Irreversible damage seldom occurs in children with diarrheal dehydration but is not uncommon in newborn infants who have shock associated with hypoxia, infection, or major surgery.

Prerenal acute renal failure usually is apparent from clinical signs of extracellular fluid volume (ECFV) depletion. It is quickly responsive to volume restoration. However, significant renal damage can occur when signs of extracellular fluid volume depletion are not obvious, particularly in a child sequestering extracellular fluid volume in an injured site, e.g., after extensive surgery or trauma, or with gastrointestinal obstruction or peritonitis.[6]

The distinction between prerenal failure and acute tubular necrosis (ATN) or cortical necrosis (ACN) may be difficult to make. Prerenal failure is the presumptive diagnosis when clinical signs of dehydration or shock are present. An adequate diuretic response to rehydration confirms this impression. However, in situations in which signs are equivocal or fluid volume apparently has been restored but oliguria persists, certain laboratory indicators are helpful in distinguishing prerenal failure from acute tubular necrosis. The response to decreased perfusion includes a urinary sodium concentration less than 15 mEq/L; urinary potassium concentration greater than 40 mEq/L; and a ratio of urine: plasma urea greater than 10:1.[7]

Further aids helpful in differentiating prerenal azotemia from acute tubular necrosis are direct measurement of plasma volume, measurement of central venous pressure, and a trial of fluid or diuretic therapy, or both (see section on Hypoperfusion).

Postrenal

The mechanism in postrenal acute renal failure is obstruction of both ureters, bladder or urethra. Such obstructions are uncommon in children except in the first year of life, but because their relief may restore urine flow and good function, they should be considered when the diagnosis is not readily apparent.

There is usually little history to suggest obstruction except in newborns. Its presence may be suspected from physical examination. Failure of newborns to urinate within 48 hours after birth or the presence of oligohydramnios may be signs of obstruction. The most common situation in older children is the partial obstruction that may be associated with poor growth and enuresis. An intercurrent urinary tract infection may then cause acute renal failure in these children. Multiple congenital anomalies commonly are associated with renal anomalies and obstruction. Rectal and abdominal or pelvic masses due to hydroureter, hydronephrosis, enlarged bladder, tumor, and dysplastic or cystic kidney also are common.

An intravenous pyelogram or renal scan may be useful in determining whether obstruction exists.[8] Renal biopsy, retrograde pyelography, or cystoscopy are only occasionally necessary.

Treatment for postrenal acute renal failure is relief of obstruction. Frequently this is followed by a diuresis of water or salt and water which can persist for 2 to 14 days. Maintaining good extracellular fluid volume and renal perfusion during this period often results in surprising restoration of function.

Renal

Renal causes of acute renal failure comprise the largest number of cases that require extended management. This group includes diseases and toxic agents that directly damage glomeruli, tubules, and renal vasculature. Glomerular damage is most commonly due to one of the glomerulonephropathies, while tubular damage is more commonly a result of ischemia or nephrotoxins. Vascular damage is an uncommon cause of acute renal failure in children. The degree and type of damage determine the degree and duration of renal insufficiency.

In cases of renal injury, treatment of the underlying cause is often unsatisfactory. Exceptions include steroid or immunosuppressive therapy, or both, for collagen-vascular diseases and certain glomerulonephropathies. The primary goal of therapy is supportive care for the patient with renal failure until renal function returns or the damage is deemed irreversible. In the event of the latter, the advisability of treatment for chronic end-stage renal failure—dialysis and transplantation—must be considered.[9-11]

DETECTION AND TREATMENT OF MANIFESTATIONS OF RENAL FAILURE

The treatment of acute renal failure includes the treatment of the underlying cause(s), the management of the complications of renal failure, and the provision of appropriate supportive therapy—fluid and nutritional—within the constraints imposed by the renal failure.

Hypoperfusion and Restoration of Extracellular Fluid Volume (ECFV)

The most urgent task in acute renal failure is the recognition of any deficit in "effective" extracellular fluid volume and rapid restoration of this deficit if detected. Poor perfusion may be caused by decreased vascular tone, loss of blood volume, loss of extracellular fluid volume, or sequestration of extracellular fluid volume (third space loss) into an injured area. In all cases effective plasma volume (PV) is reduced. History and physical examination with reference to weight changes, urinary patterns, skin turgor, dryness of mucous membranes, vital signs (especially increased pulse and decreased blood pressure), and evaluation of respiratory and cardiovascular function usually are adequate for judging whether extracellular fluid volume, plasma volume, and renal perfusion are adequate.

TABLE 2   Extracellular Fluid-Expanding Solutions

Solution	Na	Cl	HCO₃	K
			mEq/L	
0.9% saline (isotonic)	154	154	0	0
Ringer's lactate	130	110	28 (as lactate)	4
0.5 liter 0.45% saline + 40 ml 10% NaHCO₃*	144	70	74	0

*This solution used only in acidotic patients.

If a volume deficit is suspected, 20 ml/kg of an isotonic solution suitable for expanding extracellular fluid volume (Table 2)[12] is infused every 20 to 60 minutes until circulation and skin turgor are restored as judged from examination. Sixty to 120 ml/kg total fluid usually are required. In trauma or burns, the required fluid may be as high as 200 ml/kg.[13] Bladder catheterization may be necessary in order to monitor urinary response. A venous catheter should be inserted to the level of the right atrium to monitor central venous pressure (CVP) in patients in whom it is difficult to assess cardiovascular status. In this situation, fluid is given to maintain central venous pressure at 10 to 15 cm H₂O.[14, 15]

Colloid solutions seldom are necessary unless there has been a loss of plasma protein or unless malnutrition exists. Colloid solutions may be used in treating patients with hypoproteinemia due to nephrosis, enteritis, or malnutrition. When colloid is given because of an acute loss of plasma into an area of injury or burn, intravascular volume may become overexpanded as healing occurs and the proteins are recovered into the vascular space. Pulmonary edema, heart failure, or hypertension may result.

Oliguria and Use of Mannitol and Diuretics

When renal perfusion has been impaired and circulation has been restored, oliguria may persist. At this point the distinction between "poor perfusion" oliguria and acute tubular necrosis is obscure. In some cases of extreme oliguria or anuria in which perfusion seems adequate, it is useful to establish whether there is significant glomerular filtration. Intravenous mannitol alone or with diuretics has been recommended in these circumstances.[16-18] Once filtered, mannitol is not reabsorbed. When perfusion and filtration have improved but urine flow has not, giving mannitol will result in an increase in urine flow. The osmotic effects of mannitol also may affect glomerular filtration rate. "Loop-type" diuretics, such as furosemide and ethacrynic acid also may initiate a diuresis in renal failure. Used improperly, mannitol may cause disturbances in volume distribution, or osmolality of body fluids. Used in excess, diuretics may cause specific toxicities.

If urine formation is poor after extracellular fluid volume restoration, or if hemo- or myoglobinuria is present and there is no obstruction, 0.5 to 1 gm/kg mannitol (2.5 ml/kg of a 20 per cent solution) may be given intravenously over 20 to 30 minutes. This can be followed by furosemide or ethacrynic acid, 1 mg/kg, intravenously every 2 to 4 hours. This should generate 6 to 10 ml/kg urine in 1 to 3 hours. If renal response is adequate, 4 per cent mannitol in 0.2 per cent saline may be given to match urine output each 4 to 8 hours for 24 to 36 hours. This solution is approximately equal to the composition of urine in mannitol diuresis; therefore significant electrolyte imbalances are unlikely. However, it is important to monitor serum sodium, weight, intake, output and, if appropriate, central venous pressure.

Hyperkalemia

Hyperkalemia should be suspected in any patient in whom the diagnosis of acute renal failure has been made. Serum potassium (K_s) should be measured and an electrocardiogram obtained. Hyperkalemia occurs primarily as a result of decreased excretion but is accentuated by metabolic acidosis, hemolysis, infection, increased tissue catabolism, gastrointestinal bleeding, and trauma. When K_s is greater than or equal to 7 mEq/L or when there are electrocardiographic abnormalities such as prolonged QRS, depressed ST, high T waves, bradycardia or heart block, a medical emergency exists.

The priorities for acute treatment of hyperkalemia are:

1. Intravenous injection of 2.5 mEq/kg $NaHCO_3$ to increase the pH of serum and rapidly and temporarily lower K_s. Hypocalcemia, tetany, and extracellular fluid volume overload may result. Repeat doses are not recommended.

2. Intravenous injection of 0.5 ml/kg 10 per cent calcium gluconate over 2 to 4 minutes. Infusion of calcium does not decrease serum potassium but counteracts the effects of hyperkalemia on the heart. Infusion should be monitored by electrocardiogram and slowed or discontinued if severe bradycardia develops. The effect of calcium is likewise rapid and transient, and it should be followed by other measures that have more prolonged action.

3. Injection over 30 to 60 minutes of 1 ml/kg 50 per cent glucose (0.5 gm/kg). When glycogen has been depleted, glucose and potassium move into cells. Subsequent infusion of hypertonic glucose at 1.5 gm/kg and 1 unit insulin/3 gm glucose at a rate equal to calculated fluid needs can then be started until dialysis is begun. The effect can be noted in 1 to 2 hours.

4. An exchange resin may be used in conjunction with any of the preceding measures or alone if K_s is between 5.5 and 7 mEq/L. Sodium polystyrene sulfonate (Kayexelate, a sodium-potassium exchange resin), 1 gm per kg orally or rectally (1 gm dissolved in 2 to 4 cc water, 10 per cent dextrose or sorbitol) has been effective (sorbitol is less well retained rectally). Retention for 30 to 60 minutes is necessary to decrease K_s by 1 mEq/L within 2 to 4 hours. The dose may be repeated as often as necessary; however, frequent use may result in rectal irritation or gastrointestinal bleeding. Since Kayexalate exchanges sodium for potassium, its use entails a gain in body sodium.

5. Adequate nutrition will help to control K_s by reducing catabolism and increasing uptake with new cell growth (see section on Nutrition).

If these measures fail to keep K_s below 6.5 mEq/L, dialysis should be initiated.

Seizures

Seizures, which occur rather commonly when renal failure has progressed to uremia, may, however, be the first sign of such failure. One or more factors may be responsible: (1) underlying disease causing seizures, e.g., hemolytic-uremic syndrome, lupus erythematosus; (2) azotemia and the nonspecific central nervous system alterations associated with it; (3) hypocalcemia; (4) hyponatremia; and (5) hypertension.

Treatment is directed to the specific cause when known (see appropriate section for recommendations). When the cause is obscure or specific treatment has been ineffective, anticonvulsant drugs, diazepam (0.25 to 0.33 mg/kg intravenously), or barbiturates (5 to 8 mg/kg every 6 to 8 hours intramuscularly or orally) are given. If seizures are poorly controlled with these measures, appropriate treatment is then dialysis.

Underlying Disease. Treatment of seizures associated with the hemolytic-uremic syndrome, lupus erythematosus, or other systemic diseases requires nonspecific control of seizures and specific therapy to control the disease when possible.

Hypocalcemia. Hypocalcemia associated with seizures is treated with 10 per cent calcium gluconate, 0.5 ml/kg given intravenously over 2 to 5 minutes. Hypocalcemia is usually a consequence of hyperphosphatemia and the latter is treated with phosphate-binding antacids, 5 to 60 ml four times a day. Unless required for the treatment of seizures, calcium should not be given intravenously if the serum phosphorus level exceeds 7 mg/dl.

Azotemia. When azotemia is believed to be a factor in causing seizures, dialysis is indicated. When BUN exceeds 100 mg/dl, as is common in acute renal failure, care must be taken in lowering the BUN so that the rate of reduction does not exceed 15 mg/dl/hr (see p. 139). Reduction of BUN too rapidly may be a factor in causing seizures.

Hyponatremia.   When Na_s is less than 130 mEq/L without hyperglycemia, there is a relative retention of water. Treatment by restricting water allows Na_s to increase, since insensible losses from the body are not replaced. In patients with seizures, or with Na_s less than 120 mEq/L, hypertonic salt solutions may be used. Three per cent saline at a dose of 12 ml/kg, given over 1 hour, will increase Na_s approximately 10 mEq/L. This usually will control seizures caused by hyponatremia. The use of hypertonic solutions incurs the risk of extracellular fluid volume overload, heart failure or hypertension, or all three. Dialysis may therefore be necessary as a follow-up when hypertonic solutions are administered.

Hypertension.   Hypertension is a common cause of seizures in acute renal failure. The most common cause of hypertension is hypervolemia or overexpansion of extracellular fluid and plasma volume. This occurs when salt intake exceeds excretory capacity. Renal vascular pathology which results in cortical ischemia and hypersecretion of renin, may also cause hypertension.

Treatment of volume overload consists of sodium and water restriction, the use of diuretics and other hypertensive drugs, and if these measures are ineffective, dialysis. Fluid intake should be limited to calculated insensible water loss (20 to 30 ml/100 kcal/day) plus replacement of urine output measured every 4 to 24 hours, depending on the rate of flow. Sodium intake should be limited to measured urine losses. In the child with severe oliguria, no sodium should be given. Furosemide 1 to 2 mg/kg may be given intravenously and repeated every 6 hours if effective. If as much as 2 mg/kg is ineffective, it should not be repeated.

For the treatment of moderately severe hypertension (diastolic pressure 90 to 120 mm), the most useful drug is hydralazine, 0.25 to 0.5 mg/kg up to 20 mg per dose intravenously or intramuscularly. When given intravenously, its antihypertensive effect begins in 5 minutes, reaches a peak at 20 to 40 minutes, and lasts for 2 hours. The dose may be repeated every 2 hours if necessary. Complications are reflex tachycardia, the development of tachyphylaxis, and rarely, atrial flutter. Alpha methyldopa, in a dose of 6 to 20 mg/kg given intravenously every 4 to 6 hours is less effective than hydralazine, but can be a useful substitute.

For severe hypertension, diastolic pressure greater than 120 mm, or for the treatment of hypertensive encephalopathy, either intravenous hydralazine or the more potent vasodilator, diazoxide, should be given. If hydralazine is ineffective, it should be followed by diazoxide, which rarely fails to lower blood pressure. Diazoxide can cause reflex tachycardia and, occasionally, severe hyperglycemia. In our hands it has proved to be a safe and effective agent at a dose of 5 to 7 mg/kg given rapidly over 15 to 30 seconds. Its effect begins within 5 to 10 minutes, and lasts from 4 to 36 hours.[20]

After hypertension has been controlled with parenteral medication, treatment with alpha methyldopa (5 to 25 mg/kg given orally every 6 hours) should be instituted. Hydralazine, 0.2 to 2 mg/kg given orally every 6 hours may be required in addition, and if hypertension is accompanied by high plasma renin levels, propranolol may be a useful drug.[21] The effective dose of propranolol in children has varied from 1 to 24 mg/kg/day; it usually is given in four divided doses.[22, 23]

Cardiac Failure and Pulmonary Edema

Pulmonary edema and other signs of congestive heart failure are almost always the result of hypervolemia and not of a failing myocardium. In addition, hypertension, uremia, and electrolyte abnormalities may secondarily affect myocardial contractility. Treatment again consists of sodium and water restriction and administration of diuretics, as outlined in the previous section. Since digitalis is usually ineffective and can be hazardous in patients with electrolyte abnormalities, its use is seldom indicated. If pulmonary edema is severe and these above measures are ineffective, morphine 0.1 mg/kg should be given and peritoneal dialysis instituted. While this is being set up, a phlebotomy of approximately 10 per cent of the child's blood volume may be lifesaving. Treatment of severe pulmonary edema should be monitored by measurements of central venous pressure.

Acidosis

Acidosis develops because of renal impairment in acidification, i.e., decreased excretion of hydrogen ion, decreased reabsorption of bicarbonate, and the increased acid production of various catabolic states associated with acute renal failure.

Acute symptomatic acidosis (pH less than 7) should be treated with 2 to 3 mEq/kg sodium bicarbonate given intravenously over 5 to 10 minutes. Rapid correction of acidosis decreases serum ionized calcium and can result in tetany. Also, the amount of sodium infused may aggravate preexisting hypervolemia, or hypertension, or both. In such situations the persistence of severe acidosis is an indication for dialysis.

When acute renal failure is associated with significant urine formation, "high output failure," and there is a significant excretion of bicarbonate, i.e., bicarbonate wasting, bicarbonate therapy may be indicated. Bicarbonate wasting is suggested by the presence of hypochloremia. Usually in acute renal failure small doses of bicarbonate suffice—2 to 4 mEq/kg/day.

Therapy also may be directed to decreasing formation of organic acid by treatment of the catabolic states associated with uremia, e.g., fever, infection, and malnutrition. When dialysis and nutritional support are adequate, pH normally will be greater than or equal to 7.2 (see section on Nutrition).

Anemia

Anemia is frequently associated with acute renal failure. Transfusions usually are given only in response to symptoms or in situations in which hemoglobin is dropping rapidly. Blood should be fresh, to limit the hazard of hyperkalemia, and packed cells should be used in most situations. Because there is an incidence of hypertension and seizures with transfusions in oliguric children, exchange rather than direct transfusion is recommended.

Infection

Patients with acute renal failure are particularly susceptible to infection.[24] Careful observation for early signs of infection is important. Antibiotics should be reserved for treatment of either specifically identified or life-threatening infections only, and then given in modified doses because of the limited excretory capacity in uremia. The use of drugs in uremia is reviewed in a recent monograph.[25]

Azotemia

Azotemia is the accumulation of nonprotein nitrogenous (NPN) substances in the blood. The substances most commonly measured are urea nitrogen (BUN), creatinine, and uric acid. Other substances such as guanines and indican, and some amines or amino acids also accumulate and may be important. Nonprotein nitrogenous retention of substances other than urea is thought to be a factor in causing pericarditis, peripheral neuropathy, and clotting disorders. Although there is little evidence that urea nitrogen is the primary toxin, BUN levels correlate with the signs and symptoms of uremic toxicity and serve as a guide to the severity of the clinical situation. In acute renal failure, elevated BUN is a consequence not only of decreased renal function but also of increased catabolism of body protein. This results from poor dietary intake and may be accentuated by infection, trauma, gastrointestinal bleeding, acidosis, and hemolysis.

Body protein catabolism may be modified with parenteral nutrition by giving carbohydrate and amino acids.

Water and Electrolytes

The child with minimal or no excretory function requires a special control of intake. Minimum needs must be met, needs for excretion of excess. While this directly relates to water and electrolytes, calories become almost as important. Intake should maintain zero water balance, with water of intake + that of oxidation + that of endogenous breakdown equal to urine (if any) + insensible loss. With urine output negligible, zero balance will require water intake of 30 ml/kcal (or 400 ml/m²)/day.* If weight is maintained, fat and muscle will decrease: to keep body water proportionate to solids will then require only 20 to 25 ml intake/100 kcal, as weight drops 1 to 2 per cent per day.[6] Water should be given as a 10 to 15 per cent dextrose solution intravenously or orally as high caloric fluids to try and minimize fat and muscle breakdown (ketosis and negative nitrogen balance) (see section on Nutrition). Insensible losses of electrolytes are negligible and need not be replaced. If urine volume is small, its replacement becomes optional.

On the other hand, in renal failure with polyuria or extensive extrarenal losses, water and electrolytes should be monitored directly and replaced in equal amounts provided that hypervolemia and electrolyte abnormalities are not present.

Nutrition

Children with acute renal failure rarely have their nutritional needs met. Acute illness, by itself, leads to both a decreased intake of and increased need for calories and protein nitrogen. The occurrence of a negative balance of each in acute disease has been well established.[26, 27]

In a mildly stressed individual, providing approximately 20 per cent of estimated needs will minimize muscle and fat breakdown (used for energy and essential nitrogen). In acute disease these basic needs are increased. Acute renal failure poses problems in meeting these needs. Decreased excretion limits the amount of water, electrolytes, and protein that can be tolerated. The frequent association of a variety of complicating clinical conditions leads to a "hypercatabolic" state. This progressive cycle of azotemia and catabolism aggravates the "uremic" state. Recent evidence has shown that early and aggressive attention to nutritional management can moderate this cycle.[28, 29]

The aim of nutritional therapy is, therefore, provision of optimal calories and protein nitrogen in order to: (1) decrease catabolism of

---

*Calculation of calorie expenditure is as follows: 1 to 10 kg:100 kcal/kg/day; 11 to 20 kg:1000 kcal + 50 kcal/kg/day; > 20 kg:1500 kcal + 20 kcal/kg/day (e.g., 30 kg = 1700 kcal/day); 30 kg or 1700 kcal = 1 sq m.

body protein and improve nutritional state; (2) lower BUN and the degree of uremia; (3) prevent development of acidosis, hyperphosphatemia, hypocalcemia, and hyperkalemia; (4) decrease the need for dialysis; (5) improve the immune response and healing; and (6) decrease morbidity and mortality.

In acute renal failure specific nutritional requirements are poorly defined. It has been shown that uremic patients can utilize endogenous urea nitrogen for protein synthesis.[30] Efficient nitrogen utilization is dependent both on energy intake and the biological value of the protein provided.[31, 32]

Since 1963, various authors have shown that orally administered essential amino acids, either alone or as a supplement to normal diets, and with adequate calorie intake, can suppress urea formation and improve nutritional status,[26, 29, 33, 34] i.e., body protein nitrogen balance. This positive balance not only decreases urea production but also increases uptake of potassium and phosphate into new cells and decreases acid release.

Improved nutrition also has been associated with increased ability to control infection and improve tissue repair, and with decreased morbidity and mortality.[35, 38]

Usually the patient presenting with acute renal failure has been fed a high calorie-carbohydrate mixture or given 10 to 15 per cent dextrose by vein in an attempt to meet basic needs and minimize body protein and fat breakdown with its resultant BUN and ketone formation. With the restricted intakes dictated by renal failure, only 15 to 25 per cent of needed calories and little nitrogen can be given. Glucose polymers, e.g., Polycose,* provide 2 kcal/ml in a solution having an osmolality of 600 mOsm/L. Combined with cream and amino acid solutions, e.g., Aminade,† these have been used with limited success in acute disease. The nausea, vomiting, and gastroenteritis associated with uremia or the underlying illness usually leads to either physical inability or psychological unwillingness to take oral feedings.

For these reasons, parenteral nutrition via central catheter may be the preferred method for providing adequate nutrition. Techniques for this procedure, and its limits when used in acute renal failure, are described elsewhere.[36] (Parenteral nutrition has also proved useful in acute renal failure in the newborn.[37]) The disadvantages of total parenteral nutrition include: the incidence of infection from the catheter (less than 10 per cent when cared for appropriately),[38] and the risk of hyperglycemia, fluid, and/or electrolyte imbalance. Providing adequate calories and protein to achieve zero or positive nitrogen balance may require giving excess fluid, which in turn necessitates dialysis to correct volume expansion.

---

*Polycose, made by Ross Laboratories, Columbus, Ohio 43216.
†Aminade, made by McGraw Laboratories, Glendale, Calif. 91201.

Dialysis

The use of dialysis has been the major reason for the increased survival rate in acute renal failure.[39, 40] Peritoneal dialysis, which can be instituted quickly in a child requires a minimum of equipment and is relatively simple and safe to perform, has been the preferred treatment in most institutions.[41] Although hemodialysis is more efficient and therefore preferable in severely catabolic patients, its use requires access to the circulation, which is time-consuming and may be difficult in small children, and it is technically more demanding than peritoneal dialysis. Whichever form of treatment is used, a team experienced in pediatric dialysis will ensure the best results and the fewest complications.

Until recently, indications for dialysis were central nervous system symptoms (lethargy, coma, irritability, seizures); congestive heart failure; severe hypertension; gastrointestinal or skin bleeding; uncontrollable hyperkalemia, hyponatremia, or acidosis; or, in the absence of symptoms, a BUN higher than 80 to 100 mg/dl. Any one or a combination of symptoms can be observed and treated in a single patient.

Recently, "prophylactic dialysis" (instituted after 24 to 48 hours of severe oliguria regardless of symptoms or BUN level) has been associated with decreased morbidity and mortality in a variety of settings.[42, 43] Early and frequent dialysis also has the added advantage of permitting improved nutrition with relaxed fluid, salt, and protein restrictions. The combination of frequent dialyses and improved nutrition work together to reduce the complications of acute renal failure.[44]

REFERENCES

1. Stott, R. B., Cameron, J. S., Ogg, C. S., and Bewick, M.: Why the persistingly high mortality in acute renal failure? Lancet, 2:75, 1972.
2. Meadow, S. R., Cameron, J. S., Ogg, C. S., and Saxton, H. M.: Children referred for acute dialysis. Arch. Dis. Child., 46:221, 1971.
3. Schrier, R. W.: Acute renal failure—diagnosis, management and pathogenesis. Calif. Med., 115:28, 1971.
4. Hall, J. W., Johnson, W. J., Maher, F. F., and Hunt, J. C.: Immediate and long-term prognosis in acute renal failure. Ann. Int. Med., 73:515, 1970.
5. Merrill, J. P.: Acute renal failure. J.A.M.A., 211:289, 1970.
6. Williams, G. S., Klenk, E. L., and Winters, R. W.: Acute renal failure in pediatrics. In Winters, R. W., ed.: The Body Fluids in Pediatrics. Boston, Little Brown, 1973.
7. Handa, S. P., and Morrin, P. A. F.: Diagnostic indices in acute renal failure. Can. Med. Assoc. J., 96:78, 1967.
8. Fry, I. K., and Cattell, W. R.: The I. V. P. in renal failure. Br. J. Hosp. Med., 3:67, 1970.
9. Wilson, C. J., Potter, D. E., and Holliday, M. A.: Treatment of the uremic child. In Winters, R. W., ed.: The Body Fluids in Pediatrics. Boston, Little Brown, 1973.

10. Potter, D., Belzer, F. O., Ranes, L., Holliday, M. A., Kountz, S. L., and Najarian, J. S.: Treatment of chronic uremia in childhood: I. Transplantation. Pediatrics, *45*:432, 1970.
11. Potter, D., Larsen, D., Leumann, E., Perin, D., Simmons, J., Piel, C. F., and Holliday, M. A.: Treatment of chronic uremia in childhood: II. Hemodialysis. Pediatrics, *46*:178, 1970.
12. Dobrin, R. S., Larsen, C. D., and Holliday, M. A.: The critically ill child: Acute renal failure. Pediatrics, *48*:286, 1971.
13. Moyer, C. A., Margraf, H. W., and Oonafo, W. W.: Burn shock and extravascular sodium deficiency—treatment with Ringer's solution with lactate. Arch. Surg., *90*:799, 1965.
14. Cohn, J. N.: Central venous pressure as a guide to volume expansion. Ann. Int. Med., *66*:1283, 1967.
15. Weil, M. H., Shubin, H., and Rosoff, L.: Fluid repletion in circulatory shock: Central venous pressure and other practical guides. J.A.M.A., *192*:668, 1965.
16. Luke, R. G., Briggs, J. D., Allison, M. E., and Kennedy, A. C.: Factors determining the response to mannitol in acute renal failure. Am. J. Med. Sci., *259*:168, 1971.
17. Repetto, H. A., Lewy, J. E., Braudo, J. L., and Metcoff, J.: The renal functional response to furosemide in children with acute glomerulonephritis. J. Pediatr., *80*:660, 1972.
18. Auger, R. G., Dayton, D. A., Harrison, C. E., Jr., Zucker, F. M., and Anderson, C. F.: Use of ethacrynic acid in mannitol-resistant oliguric renal failure. J.A.M.A., *206*:891, 1968.
19. Lieberman, E. L.: Management of acute renal failure in infants and children. Nephron, *11*:193, 1973.
20. McLaine, P. N., and Drummond, K. N.: Intravenous diazoxide for severe hypertension in childhood. J. Pediatr., *79*:829, 1971.
21. Zacest, R., Gilmore, E., and Koch-Weser, J.: Treatment of essential hypertension with combined vasodilation and β-adrenergic blockade. N. Engl. J. Med., *286*:617, 1972.
22. Potter, D. E., Schambelin, M., Salvatierra, O., Jr., Orloff, S., and Holliday, M. A.: Treatment of high-renin hypertension with propranolol in children after renal transplantation. (Accepted for publication, J. Pediatr.)
23. Buerth, R. C.: Effect of propranolol in the treatment of hypertension in children (Abst.). Pediatr. Res., *10*:328, 1976.
24. Montomerie, J. Z., Kalmanson, G. M., and Guze, L. B.: Renal failure and infection. Medicine, *47*:1, 1968.
25. Anderson, R. J., Gambertoglio, J. G., and Schrier, R. W.: Clinical Use of Drugs in Renal Failure. Springfield, Ill., Charles C Thomas, 1976.
26. Moore, F. D.: Metabolic Care of the Surgical Patient. Philadelphia, W. B. Saunders Co., 1959.
27. Richards, P.: Protein metabolism in uremia. Nephron, *14*:134, 1975.
28. Holliday, M. A.: Management of the child with renal insufficiency. *In* Liberman, E. L., ed.: Clinical Pediatric Nephrology. Philadelphia, J. B. Lippincott Co., 1976.
29. Abitbol, C. L., and Holliday, M. A.: Total parenteral nutrition in anuric children. Clin. Nephrol., *5*:153, 1976.
30. Giordano, C.: Use of exogenous and endogenous urea for protein synthesis in normal and uremic subjects. J. Lab. Clin. Med., *62*:231, 1963.
31. Abitbol, C. L., and Holliday, M. A.: Calorie and amino acid supplementation in uremic children. (Submitted for publication.)
32. Miller, C. S., and Payne, A.: Theory of protein metabolism. J. Theor. Biol., *5*:398, 1963.
33. Bergström, J., Fürst, P., and Norée, L. O.: Treatment of chronic uremic patients with protein-poor diet and oral supply of essential amino acids. I. Nitrogen balance studies. Clin. Nephrol., *3*:187, 1975.
34. Dudrick, J. J., Steiger, E., and Long, J. M.: Renal failure in surgical patients. Treatment with intravenous essential amino acids and hypertonic glucose. Surgery, *68*:180, 1970.
35. Abel, R. M., Beck, C. H., Abbott, W. M., Ryan, J. A., Burnett, G., and Fisher, J. E.: Improved survival from acute renal failure after treatment with intravenous essential L-amino acids and glucose. Results of a prospective, double blind study. N. Engl. J. Med., *288*:696, 1973.

36A. Winters, R. W., and Hasselmeyer, E. G.: Intravenous Nutrition in the High Risk Infant. New York, John Wiley, 1975.

36B. Filler, R. M., Das, J. B., and Coran, A. G.: Intravenous Alimentation, Chapter 21 in this book.

37. Arnold, W., Pokroy, M., and Holliday, M. A.: Acute renal failure in the newborn. (Submitted for publication.)

38. Copeland, E. M., MacFadyen, B. V., Jr., and Dudrick, S. J.: Prevention of microbial catheter contamination in patients receiving parenteral nutrition. South. Med. J., 67(3):303, 1974.

39. Kleinknecht, D., Jungers, P., Chanard, J., Barbanel, C., Ganeval, D., and Rondon-Nucete, M.: Factors influencing immediate prognosis in acute renal failure with special reference to prophylactic hemodialysis. Adv. Nephrol., 1:207, 1971.

40. Parsons, F. M., Hobson, S. M., Blagg, C. R., and McCracken, B. H.: Optimum time for dialysis in acute reversible renal failure. Lancet, 2:129, 1961.

41. Cameron, J. S.: Peritoneal dialysis in hypercatabolic acute renal failure. Lancet, 2:1188, 1967.

42. Teschan, P. E., Baxter, C. R., O'Brien, T. F., Freyhof, J. N., and Hall, W. M.: Prophylactic hemodialysis in the treatment of acute renal failure. Ann. Int. Med., 53:922, 1960.

43. Fischer, R. F., Griffin, W. O., Reiser, M., and Clark, D. S.: Early dialysis in the treatment of acute renal failure. Surg. Gynecol. Obstet., 123:1019, 1966.

44. Asbach, H. W., Stoeckel, H., Schüler, H. W., Conradi, R., Wiedermann, K., Möhring, K., and Röhl, L.: The treatment of hypercatabolic acute renal failure by adequate nutrition and haemodialysis. Acta Anaesthesiol. Scand., 18:255, 1974.

Chapter Eleven

RESPIRATORY ARREST AND ITS SEQUELAE

ROBERT M. SMITH, M.D.

The term respiratory arrest is at once an admission of inaccuracy and confusion, since it can only stand for the chaos of a bad accident, or worse, the unhappy occasion when a patient has been allowed to slip through the measurable stages of respiratory failure because of neglect, poor judgment, or inadequate therapy.

Unfortunately, we do find ourselves confronted by children in respiratory arrest all too frequently. Regardless of the cause, saving many of them depends not only upon management of the emergency itself, about which there has been considerable discussion, but also upon management of the sequelae, an area that deserves more attention. Actually, the two phases are markedly different: the emergency period demands instant action, rapid thinking, and efficient organization, while the recovery period requires more sophisticated evaluation and grueling observation, and sometimes ends in painful decision.

MANAGEMENT OF EMERGENCY PHASE

The two principal factors in emergency care of children in respiratory arrest are: (1) the preparation for such incidents, and (2) an organized response to emergency when it occurs.

From the Department of Anesthesia, Children's Hospital Medical Center, Boston, Massachusetts.

Preparation

Suitable Treatment Areas. In modern hospitals emergency care plays a role of increasing importance. To meet the varied demands for treatment of acute illness and severe trauma there should be suitably equipped medical and surgical emergency areas for outpatient and accident care, and intensive therapy for critically ill hospitalized patients.[1] Furthermore, every ward or nursing division should be equipped to handle immediate resuscitative and other emergency measures.[2]

Equipment. In each of the aforementioned areas suction apparatus, oxygen, airways, laryngoscopes, endotracheal tubes, self-inflating breathing bags, masks, syringes, needles, and suitable drugs should be stocked, easily available, and ready for use (Table 1). Mechanical ventilators seldom are necessary for emergency use, but they should be available in intensive care units along with more extensive monitoring and diagnostic equipment. Since tracheostomy rarely is performed as a primary measure, this equipment may be stored in operating theaters.

Personnel. Most important and most difficult to establish is an around-the-clock coverage by suitably trained personnel. A properly prepared individual should have the diagnostic competence of a pediatrician and an internist, the technical skills of an anesthesiologist and a surgeon, and the organizational ability of a gang boss. Because of the

TABLE 1   Basic Resuscitation Equipment

Suction apparatus: Immediately available. Sterile plastic catheters, sizes 6, 8, 10, 12 French. Wooden tongue blades

Oropharyngeal airways: Sizes 0, 1, 2, 3

Self-inflating (Ambu type) bags: Child and adult sizes

Masks: Newborn, infant, child, small adult sizes

Anesthesia non-rebreathing T-systems with 1.5- and 2.0-liter bags

Laryngoscope: Standard handle. Blades: Miller no. 1, Flagg no. 2, Miller no. 2, and Macintosh no. 3

Endotracheal tubes: Plastic Magill sizes 2.5 through 5.0 uncuffed, sizes 5.5 through 8.0 cuffed (all with straight connectors)

Magill endotracheal forceps: Small and adult sizes

Drugs: Epinephrine (1:1000), calcium chloride (10%), dextrose (50%), isoproterenol, dopamine, diazepam, digitoxin, heparin, and saline

Defibrillator with 5-cm and 10-cm diameter paddles

Intravenous apparatus and *surgical equipment* available

---

rarity of such a combination in any one person, it is customary to rely upon teams and hope that the cumulative talents of the team will be sufficient to meet the situation.

Of the preceding requirements, diagnostic acuity usually is the most important. Though treatment must be immediate, each step should be determined by previous accurate diagnosis. That which is life-saving in one situation (strong positive pressure respiration in respiratory distress syndrome)[3] may be fatal in another outwardly similar situation (diaphragmatic hernia).[4]

The importance of early diagnosis in these emergencies cannot be overemphasized. Although the possible causes of respiratory arrest are innumerable, there are several basically different clinical situations. The differential diagnosis can be narrowed considerably, depending upon whether the stricken child is encountered in (1) the delivery room or newborn nursery, (2) the outpatient emergency room, (3) the postoperative room or surgical ward, or (4) the medical ward. In the operating room respiration is usually under the control of the anesthesiologist and respiratory arrest seldom constitutes an emergency. Table 2 suggests a few of the more common causes of respiratory arrest in each of the situations mentioned. The physicians involved should keep these in mind and should have a practical knowledge of their diagnosis and early treatment. While sorting out the proper diagnosis and organizing emergency care, one must bear in mind three important precepts: (1) Don't harm the patient by using wrong methods. (2) Don't waste time with useless diagnostic or therapeutic procedures. (3) Don't initiate a costly effort to prolong dying when the situation is irreversible.

Therapeutic Action Pattern in Response to Respiratory Arrest

The physician's response to respiratory arrest is multiphasic and includes simultaneously scanning the scene, calling for assistance and information, and starting therapy. As previously stated, there is no standard routine to be followed.

Assuming that an infant unexpectedly has become apneic and pulseless, one must attempt to restore ventilation and circulation, but with definite precautions.

An anoxic patient's last act often is that of regurgitation. Immediate attempts at mouth-to-mouth resuscitation can fill his or her trachea with vomitus and end all hope of survival.

The first step in resuscitation should be to *clear the airway*. This can be done most effectively with a laryngoscope and a suction catheter, which would be at hand only in specially equipped areas. By turning the infant's head to one side, however, and sweeping out his or her mouth

**TABLE 2   Hospital Locations of Common Causes of
Respiratory Distress**

Delivery Room and Newborn Nursery

Prematurity[5]
Hyperbilirubinemia
Sepsis
Central nervous system lesions[6]
   developmental pathology
   birth injuries
   drug overdosage[7]
Respiratory lesions[9]
   airway obstruction
   respiratory distress syndrome[10]
   diaphragmatic hernia[11,12]
   spontaneous pneumothorax[13]
Cardiovascular lesions[14,15]
   hypoplastic left heart
   aortic stenosis

Emergency Room

Trauma
   head, chest, or abdominal injury[16,17]
   drowning,[18] burns[19]
   foreign body in airway[20]
Respiratory infection
   epiglottitis[21,22]
   tracheobronchitis[23]
   pneumonia
   status asthmaticus[24]
Central nervous system disease
   encephalitis[25]
   epilepsy[26]
   Reye's syndrome[8]
   tumor
Cardiovascular disease
   hemorrhagic shock
   acute cardiac failure[27]
   arrhythmias

---

with one's finger, a passage usually can be made. Keeping the child's head turned to the side to prevent accumulation of material in the hypopharynx, one should then carry out a brisk *5-second cardiac massage.*[38]

At such times closed or external cardiac massage is often most effective when both hands are used, thumbs at mid-sternum, squeezing forcibly enough to halve the anterior-posterior diameter of the infant's chest at each compression (Figs. 1 and 2). To avoid rupture of the stomach, it is best to stand above the infant's head, as shown in Figure 2, so that the hands do not encompass the abdomen. A series of

TABLE 2   Hospital Locations of Common Causes of Respiratory Distress (*Continued*)

Surgical Ward and Recovery Room

General surgery
    shock, hypovolemia, hypothermia[17]
    aspiration of blood and vomitus[28]
    pneumothorax
    atelectasis, pneumonia
Cardiac surgery[29]
    hemothorax
    pulmonary hypertension[30]
    cardiac failure
    arrhythmia
Neurosurgery
    increased intracranial pressure[6]
    coma[25]
Ear, nose, and throat surgery
    postoperative hemorrhage[28]
    tracheostomy obstruction or displacement[31]

Medical Ward

Respiratory
    pneumonia
    cystic fibrosis[32]
    status asthmaticus
Central nervous system
    encephalitis
    Guillain-Barré disease[33]
    epilepsy
    tetanus[34]
Cardiac
    cardiac failure, arrhythmias
    digitalis poisoning
Acute hepatic failure[35]
Acute renal failure[36]
Metabolic
    hypoglycemia[37]
    endocrine disorders

15 compressions in 5 seconds matches the 180 per minute rate of an active infant heart and initiates both ventilation and circulation.

Having thus used the first 10 seconds, one next ventilates the child gently with mouth-to-mouth or bag-and-mask method. Neonates require only small 20-ml respiratory "puffs," and forceful ventilation easily causes pneumothorax. One should watch or auscultate the chest for adequate expansion on both sides, and also rule out the presence of diaphragmatic hernia before increasing ventilatory pressure in distressed neonates.

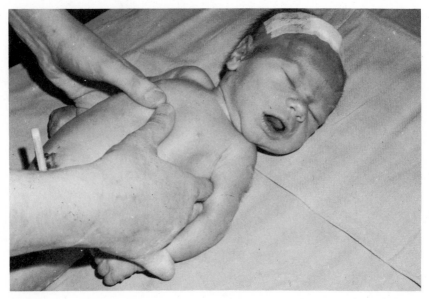

Figure 1. Closed cardiac massage. Thumbs press at mid-sternum, but hands may compress stomach or liver.

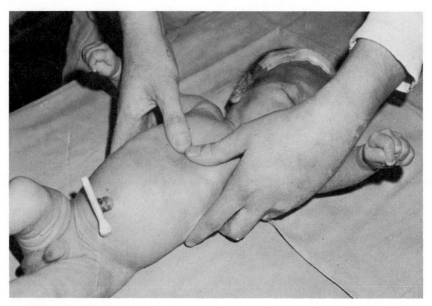

Figure 2. Closed cardiac massage applied from above child's head to avoid compression of abdomen.

For continued resuscitation, one worker should perform the cardiac massage and another attend to ventilation.

If mouth-to-mouth and mask methods fail to establish satisfactory exchange, endotracheal intubation should be carried out at once. If it is obvious that recovery will require an extended period of time, it is preferable to administer 100 per cent oxygen for 3 or 4 minutes before proceeding with the intubation.

Tracheostomy is indicated as an emergency procedure only in rare instances of total occlusion of the trachea. As an alternative to tracheostomy a large bore (12- to 16-gauge) needle may be inserted through the cricothyroid ligament and oxygen then forced through the needle under pressure. It must be emphasized, however, that a child cannot be expected to suck air through such a needle unassisted. This erroneous assumption has been known to have resulted in death.

When ventilating by mask, the Ambu and other self-inflating bags are of value chiefly for their ability to function without the support of oxygen tank or pipeline. Ventilation with room air thus administered may be adequate, but additional oxygen often is necessary. Attaching an oxygen line to an Ambu-type system increases the potential oxygen concentration, but for maximal levels one should use an anesthesia circle or non-rebreathing system by which 100 per cent oxygen is assured.

One is never certain of a clear airway during the use of mask ventilation, and there is an ever-present danger of gastric distention which increases in proportion to the severity of the child's condition. It may be necessary to relieve the distention by manual pressure on the stomach or by passage of a nasogastric tube.

The essential maneuvers of endotracheal intubation should be mastered by any physician before he or she assumes the responsibility for care of small patients. Fortunately intubation of the trachea is least difficult when a child is weak and flaccid. Positioning the child is of primary importance. The head should be slightly elevated and the nose tilted upward so that the head is in a "sniffing" position (Fig. 3). The once popular method of hyperextending the child's head over the edge of the bed justifiably has been abandoned.

Detailed descriptions of intubation techniques are available in basic texts,[2, 39] but actual experience is mandatory. Suffice it to say here that the most common errors in emergency endotracheal intubation are passing the tube beyond the carina into the right main bronchus, and into the esophagus. The latter mistake is easily made and may be very difficult to recognize. The position of the tube should be checked by stethoscope immediately and promptly confirmed by x-ray if intubation is to be prolonged.

To promote return of spontaneous respiration the use of stimulating drugs has never been considered effective, but narcotic antagonists

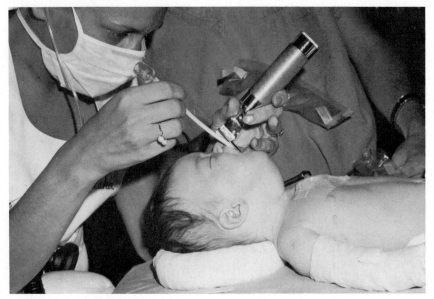

Figure 3. Endotracheal intubation; head is raised in "sniffing" position to provide best exposure of glottis.

should be used if narcotic overdosage seems probable. In this role naloxone (Narcan) is believed most advantageous at present, the dose being 0.01 mg per kilogram of body weight by intravenous or intramuscular route.

While the essential measures of cardiorespiratory support are being started, numerous details of diagnosis and supportive therapy must be considered. Cardiac massage is continued until spontaneous cardiac beat is evident and output is adequate to maintain oxygen delivery to the tissues. Until that time cardiac massage must be carried on with sufficient force to produce palpable pulsation of femoral arteries. The pupils should return to normal size but may remain dilated following a prolonged period of anoxia, or following use of epinephrine.

Cardiac stimulants (epinephrine and calcium chloride by direct intracardiac injection) are indicated if heart action is not restored promptly; hypertonic glucose, isoproterenol, dopamine, and buffering agents can be added by intravenous route (Table 3).[1]

Within the first 10 minutes after the onset of a major catastrophe, assistants should be directed to aid cardiac massage, start infusions, check breath sounds, attach an electrocardiograph, and check initial diagnosis, early and recent history, operative and postoperative course, last oral intake, medication, sensitivity, hyperactivity, seizure, respiratory problems, fever, weakness, and other relevant data. Chest x-ray is taken, and blood is drawn for cross-matching, culture, cell counts,

TABLE 3   Drugs for Cardiorespiratory Emergencies

		Dosage			
Drug	Concentration	Under 5 Kg	5 Kg and Over	May be Repeated	Interval
Epinephrine	1:1000 (0.1%)	0.2 ml	0.25 ml/10 kg	2–3 ×	5–10 min
Calcium					
gluconate	100 mg/ml (10%)	1 ml	1.0 ml/10 kg	2–3 ×	5–10 min
chloride	100 mg/ml (10%)	0.5 ml	0.5 ml/10 kg	2–3 ×	5–10 min
Sodium bicarbonate	44 mEq/50ml (1 mEq/ml)	3–4 ml	2 mEq/kg slowly	Twice at 5-min intervals, then as indicated by pH and Pa_{CO_2}	
THAM	200 mg/ml (1.5 M)	3–4 ml	1 ml/kg	As above	
Isoproterenol (Isuprel)	As infusion with precision (Harvard) pump; 0.5 mg (2.5 ml 1/5000) in 100 ml saline, avoid small vessels, regulate as needed.				
Dopamine	As infusion with precision (Harvard) pump; dilute to give 5–10 μg/kg/min, and regulate as needed.				
Glucose	500 mg/50 ml (50%)	1 ml	1 ml/5 kg	Not repeated	

hematocrit, glucose level, electrolytes, Pa_{O_2}, Pa_{CO_2}, and pH. The umbilical artery is cannulated in neonates, while the radial artery may be cannulated in older children. A thermistor is attached for continuous temperature recording, and a warming lamp and blankets are used to preserve body temperature in infants.[40] Lumbar puncture, pupillary and fundus examination, and other neurological procedures are in order for diagnosis of nervous system lesions. The bladder is catheterized for urinary specimens and subsequent monitoring of renal function.

To reduce the dangers caused by confusion and overenthusiastic helpers, it is highly advisable to post one intelligent observer at an early stage as coordinator and recorder, to list each drug and procedure, and to assist in overall organization. Otherwise the chaos that results after 30 minutes of resuscitative efforts makes further therapy grossly inaccurate.

MANAGEMENT OF SEQUELAE

Although treatment of later stages of respiratory arrest is less frantic and allows time to sort out and evaluate some of the problems, many of the answers are extremely elusive.

Management of these children varies considerably, depending upon whether they are among those who recover promptly, those in whom recovery is delayed, or those in whom recovery does not occur.

Group 1: Prompt Recovery Following Respiratory Arrest

A child who chokes on a peach stone or who is submerged underwater for 1 or 2 minutes may develop respiratory arrest and then, after a few minutes of effective treatment, start to breathe spontaneously, move, gag, cough, open his or her eyes, awaken, and regain full mental and physical control.

Recovery is actually 100 per cent in many of these children, and no subsequent therapy is indicated; however, some precautions are always advisable, and serious errors may occur. As soon as a patient begins to breathe spontaneously after a period of apnea, there is a tendency to withdraw assistance and let him do it all by himself. This is a grave error, for there is usually an appreciable period when spontaneous respiration is present but inadequate, and marked hypoxic damage and respiratory acidosis may result. Respiration must be assisted until the patient's respiratory exchange is active and adequate.

If the child has had endotracheal intubation, extubation should be preceded by careful clearing of the pharynx, mouth, and nose of any foreign material that could be aspirated.

Following any use of positive pressure ventilation and cardiac massage, it is advisable to rule out by chest x-ray pneumothorax or rib cage fracture. Even when children appear to recover promptly, it should be noted that any period of hypoxia may be followed by hyperexcitability, fever, visual disturbance, memory loss, incoordination, seizures, renal shutdown, and other complications. Immediately following any hypoxic episode, a child should be kept under continuous observation for 3 or 4 hours and released only when the parents have been adequately alerted. The child should return for reexamination within 2 weeks.

Group 2: Delayed Recovery Following Respiratory Arrest

Days or weeks of supportive therapy may be required during recovery from severe hypoxic damage caused by the respiratory arrest, or from a prolonged underlying process such as Guillain-Barré disease or encephalitis.

When acute hypoxia has caused tissue damage, all efforts are centered upon supportive care and reduction of oxygen requirements by control of muscular activity and body temperatures. If there is a specific disease process in addition, definitive antibiotics, medication, and other measures are added.

The problems of prolonged support are related chiefly to ventilation. Although this aspect has been discussed widely, several points are controversial and remain unsettled. On two points there is general agreement. The first is the importance of moving all patients who require prolonged respiratory care to an area especially designed and equipped for this purpose.[41] Equipment includes resuscitation apparatus, ventilators, and monitoring devices, plus laboratory facilities for 24-hour blood gas analysis. The second feature is the necessity of staffing this area, or unit, with physicians, nurses, and technicians who will render top-level care on a continuous basis.

Indication for Mechanical Ventilation. The decision of when to turn to mechanical ventilation is often a difficult one to make. If the child remains apneic after the arrest, the answer is obvious. When respiration fails gradually, or returns only partially after arrest, the decision may be guided by clinical and laboratory standards such as those shown in Table 4 as adapted from Wood and Downes.[24]

Choice of Ventilatory Support. In establishing mechanical ventilatory support there is an ever-widening variety of devices and techniques from which to choose. Attempts to ventilate children by "negative pressure" ventilators without endotracheal intubation or tracheostomy have been made by Chernick,[42] Cox,[43] and others, but airway obstruction and gastric distention have been difficult to avoid. Establishment of a reliable airway is essential, and for this the endotracheal tube currently is preferred by many workers because of greater ease of placement and fewer complications, especially in infants.

An endotracheal tube passed through the nose is secured more easily, and its presence is less disturbing than one passed through the mouth. It may, however, be necessary to use the easier oral route when intubating a critically hypoxic child, changing to a nasal tube after the child's condition has become stabilized.

Endotracheal tubes may cause tissue irritation unless manufactured according to strict standards.[44] Only those should be used that bear the mark IT or Z79, signifying that they have been tested by tissue implantation. Plastic, uniform-bore Magill endotracheal tubes are preferable to the tapered Cole tubes, which put added pressure on the vocal cords. Earlier belief that tracheostomy should be performed after 3 days of intubation generally has given way to the acceptance of prolonged intubation.[45]

TABLE 4 Indications for the Use of Mechanical Ventilation

Clinical Signs	Arterial Blood Gases
Prolonged apneic spells	Pa_{O_2} less than 50 mm Hg in 100 per cent oxygen
Retraction with rising heart rate	Pa_{CO_2} more than 75 mm Hg, pH less than 7.15
Fatigue or hyperexcitability	
Cyanosis in 40 per cent oxygen	
Coma	

Several ventilators now are available for use with infants and children.[1, 43] As shown in Table 5, these are differentiated chiefly on the basis of being controlled by the volume delivered (volume limited) or by the amount of pressure developed (pressure limited). The type chosen for individual patients varies with the size of the child, the pathological physiology involved, and the particular experience of the responsible personnel.

For children with normal lungs either type may be used successfully. When pulmonary disease causes reduction or variability in lung compliance, however, the volume-limited ventilators are more dependable than the pressure-limited ones.[46]

Important modifications in delivery of mechanical ventilation have been introduced, including intermittent positive pressure breathing (IPPB),[47] positive end-expiratory pressure (PEEP),[48] continuous positive airway pressure (CPAP),[49] and intermittent mandatory ventilation (IMV).[50] These have greatly increased the potentiality of ventilatory assistance, and one should be aware of the advantages and limitations of each. In spite of these advances it has been constantly evident that success in mechanical ventilation rests far less upon the machine than upon those directing the care of the child.

Starting Patient on Ventilator. Use of a mechanical ventilator should not be initiated when the patient's condition is obviously irreversible (seldom an easy decision), since once committed, it is much more difficult to discontinue this form of treatment. When ventilatory care clearly is indicated, the ventilator must be adjusted to provide proper respiratory rate, tidal volume, pressure, inspiratory-expiratory ratio, oxygen concentration, and humidification, and the choice must be made between assisting or controlling ventilation. Initial settings are calculated from physiological data such as the Radford nomogram[51] with practical modification,[52, 53] and subsequently altered as indicated by clinical signs and blood gas determinations.

If patients are hyperactive, or fail to breathe with the ventilator,

---

TABLE 5   Mechanical Ventilators Used for Pediatric Patients*

Volume Limited	Pressure Limited
Bennett MA-1	Baby Bird
Bourns	Bennett PR-2
Draeger Spiromat	
Engstrom	
Emerson	
Servo 900†	

*Adapted from Downes, J. J., Fulgencio, T., and Raphaely, R. C.: Recent clinical advances. Pediatr. Clin. North Am., *19*:423, 1972, with permission of the authors and the publishers.

†Servo 900 (Schönander) can be regulated by minute volume or pressure settings.

their activity may be controlled by morphine or *d*-tubocurarine in small repeated intravenous or intramuscular doses (0.1 mg/kg and 0.3 mg/kg, respectively).

Strict sterile precautions must be employed when suction is used with endotracheal or tracheostomy tubes, since infection is commonplace and dangerous. Good humidification is an essential factor in ventilating devices, not only for physiological and anti-inflammatory effects but also because it prevents secretions from drying and occluding endotracheal tubes. With adequate humidification, endotracheal tubes may be left in place indefinitely without fear of such occlusion. Antibiotics should be used if sufficient indications are present.

Careful attention must be given to fluid therapy and the maintenance of nutrition. Fluid therapy is rendered considerably more complex during ventilator therapy. Marked increase in body fluid has been related to use of humidified oxygen and to increase of antidiuretic hormone due to pressure-related responses in the right atrium. On the other hand, in those patients in whom increased expiratory resistance is used to promote oxygenation, it may be necessary to induce hypervolemia temporarily in order to prevent hypotension.[54]

To regulate fluid and electrolyte balance, urinary catheterization usually is advisable, along with careful daily weighing of the patient.

For nutrition, a nasogastric tube may suffice for short periods, or a feeding gastrostomy for longer treatment. Total parenteral alimentation, as developed by Filler and others,[55] can save many children who could not otherwise survive. (See also Chapter 21 in this book.)

Problems of Continuing Ventilator Care. Once ventilatory support has been initiated, many clinical signs are lost, and numerous parameters must be followed to maintain a correct physiological course. It is extremely helpful to start a large time-flow chart that can be posted on the wall with interim recordings of important vital functions, including temperature, pulse rate, blood pressure, respiratory rate, minute volume, maximum inspiratory pressure, dead space/tidal volume ratio, inspired oxygen concentration, oxygen flow in liters, arterial pH, Po_2, Pco_2, electrolytes, hematocrit, white blood count, urinary specific gravity, volume, osmolality, fluid in and out volumes, and medications. Demonstrations of these values will give all personnel an easy and rapid summary of the patient's progress and greatly facilitate management.

Space in this chapter allows for only a minimum of suggestions on ventilatory management. Of special importance are avoidance of (1) rapid change in acid-base balance, and (2) the belief that respiratory alkalosis is a safer state than respiratory acidosis. Actually, it is preferable to hold the patient in a slight respiratory acidosis with arterial pH near 7.25 and Pco_2 40 to 45 mm Hg.

Acute respiratory failure (ARF) requiring ventilatory assistance usually is associated with severe metabolic and respiratory acidosis. Emphasis has been placed upon the danger of rapid correction of acidosis by use of sodium bicarbonate, or tris(hydroxymethyl)aminomethane (THAM), or both. Finberg,[56] Simmons,[57A] and others[57B] have stated repeatedly that the resultant hyperosmolality caused by these buffering agents introduces increased incidence of intracranial hemorrhage in neonates as well as renal pathology and excessive pH changes in older children. Finberg suggests that sodium bicarbonate be administered either in isotonic solution or by hypertonic bolus, and if by the latter means that the limit be 6 mEq per kg per 12 hours.[56] It is also essential when either buffer is used that ventilation be augmented, since sodium bicarbonate releases additional carbon dioxide while THAM acts as a respiratory depressant.

Another consideration has been brought forward by Garella and co-workers[58] who have found that when patients are severely acidotic there is significant expansion of the extracellular fluid space, and that more buffering agent is required than standard formulae suggest. The reasonable answer is to use isotonic fluid, go slowly, and rely on direct measurement of serum pH and clinical signs rather than formulae or preconceived rules.

An error frequently made is to allow the hemoglobin to fall to levels that reduce the oxygen-carrying power of the blood. In critical conditions a transfusion will make it possible to avoid the use of dangerously high oxygen concentrations.

Vigorous supportive care should include moving and turning the child, intermittent positive pressure respiration, suctioning of the airway with the aid of irrigating saline as indicated, and addition of aerosols for bronchodilation. Manual compression and thumping of the rib cage also are helpful. X-rays are taken at frequent intervals.

Monitoring of critically ill infants and children demands skill and judgment. Enough information should be obtained to ensure optimal care of the child, but invasive techniques should be held to a minimum. Monitoring by stethoscope, electrocardiogram, and apnea and pulse alarms is free of hazard, as is blood pressure determination by cuff and sonic sensor. Thermometer and temperature control and intra-arterial instrumentation may lead to a variety of hazards.[40, 59] Their use should be indicated clearly, and requires meticulous attention. Central venous pressure lines, while seldom dangerous, are difficult to maintain in small children and the information is apt to be unreliable.

Termination of Ventilator Care.   Problems related to termination of ventilator support and removal of endotracheal tubes have been reduced considerably but not entirely eliminated. Earliest possible discontinuation is desirable in view of potential hazards.

Complicated methods of weaning formerly included on-and-off trials, and shifting from controlled to assisted ventilation. With the introduction of intermittent mandatory ventilation such intermediary techniques may be eliminated. Prerequisites for withdrawal of ventilatory support still include mental clarity, adequate nutritional status, acceptable chest x-ray, neuromuscular adequacy, and normal results of electrolyte, hematological, and blood gas determinations (Cox,[60] Vidyasagar and Wai[61]).

As described by Downes and Raphaely,[1] weaning or discontinuation of mechanical ventilation can be started when the Pa_{CO_2} remains less than 50 mm Hg and the Pa_{O_2} more than 100 mm Hg at 50 per cent inspired oxygen concentration with peak inflating pressures less than 25 cm H_2O.

The process of weaning must be controlled scrupulously, and attended by specially trained personnel. For this reason it is seldom advisable to attempt this phase of care after 3 P.M. or on weekends, when less supervision is usually available.

After discontinuation of ventilatory support the endotracheal tube should be left in place for several hours, during which time mild expiratory resistance is provided by continuous positive airway pressure (CPAP), to prevent atelectasis. Extubation is performed only by those skilled in airway management, with provision for immediate reintubation at hand should the need arise.

Complications of Long-Term Ventilator Care. Many of the problems associated with the first use of mechanical ventilators have been solved only to be replaced by new ones. As noted by Stern,[62] it may be difficult to decide whether some complications are caused by the ventilating device or are a result of the primary disease. Better construction of ventilators finally has made it possible to adapt the machine to the child rather than the original approach of attempting to fit the child to the machine. Now an infant of any size can be sustained for prolonged periods with little expectation of injury. Some important features here are better understanding or use of endotracheal tubes, their fixation without movement, and especially the use of tubes that avoid pressure, a slight leak around the tube now being considered the greatest insurance against injury.

Fortunately, many complications caused by the use of cuffed endotracheal and tracheostomy tubes are eliminated since cuffs rarely are employed in tubes for infants and small children.

The regularity with which severe tracheal ulceration has been found at autopsy of patients who have been intubated even for brief periods and the rarity with which such lesions have been found in patients following recovery after relatively prolonged ventilation strongly suggest that inadequate circulation of tissues under moderate pressure is of most critical importance.

Earlier concern over granulomata following intubation has waned because of their rarity and easy removal, but the occasional tracheal stricture remains a real threat and may cause respiratory obstruction.

Pathological lesions of brain and lung ascribed to ventilatory therapy have been examined carefully. The marked softening of brain tissue found at postmortem examination after prolonged ventilatory support has been pointed to as one of the evils of mechanical respirators. It now seems probable that factors underlying the so-called "ventilator brain" have been due to prolonged hyperventilation coupled with the fact that many patients have been supported so long after clinical death that the brain has undergone early decomposition.[63]

Additional causes of concern have been uncovered, including the possible washout of surfactant by continuous positive pressure, interference with protein-binding of bilirubin with resultant hyperbilirubinemia, and alteration of water metabolism through antidiuretic hormone response to pressure changes in atrial receptors.

The danger of retrolental fibroplasia (RLF) continues to worry all who treat premature infants, and becomes more of a problem as survival of these infants increases.[64A] The level of safe oxygen concentration has not yet been established, and one is left in fear of avoiding RLF at the cost of anoxia, or avoiding anoxia at the risk of blindness.

Pulmonary lesions associated with oxygen and ventilatory therapy remain a major problem; they are varied in nature and involve considerable morbidity and mortality. The mechanism of their production is not clear and prevention has been unsuccessful. High concentration of oxygen by itself is undoubtedly one factor,[64] and increased ventilatory pressure probably has additional damaging effects; both act in proportion to the degree and duration of their use.[65] The response of the lungs includes hyperemia, atelectasis, and consolidation of the pulmonary tissue; the initial defect probably is damage and swelling of the endothelial lining of pulmonary capillaries.[66] A vicious cycle is thus begun, in which the reduced oxygen uptake makes continued oxygen administration necessary. The process leads to complete consolidation of the lungs and an anoxic death.[67]

Because of the dangers involved, the general beliefs are that when possible, inspiratory pressure should be less than 40 mm Hg, Po_2 less than 125 mm Hg, and inspired oxygen concentration less than 40 per cent.

Group 3: The Child Who Cannot Recover

This group offers the unhappy problem of the decision to terminate support. In the emergency phase, in case of obvious brain trauma, rigor mortis, agonal stages of irreversible disease, or with the patient who has had repeated cardiac arrests without hope of recovery, the decision may be easy. Ventilatory support should not be initiated in these patients. Those whose outcome was uncertain at first and who fail to recover have been the source of much professional and ethical concern. Diagnosis of irreversible brain damage is still difficult, and, if made, must be followed by the more harrowing decision of what to do next. Recently it was stated that a patient whose depressed responses were not under the effect of temperature change or drugs, whose pupils remained fully dilated and unreacting, and who remained unresponsive to all stimuli and repeatedly showed a flat electroencephalogram might be considered to have irreversible brain damage.[68] Establishment of such criteria appeared to open the way for rational action to terminate hopeless therapy. Subsequently, however, widely contested cases have brought the issue into such sharp focus that one must scrutinize all legal restrictions with extreme care before taking any such action.[69, 70]

REFERENCES

1. Downes, J. J., and Raphaely, R. C.: Pediatric intensive care. Anesthesiology, *43*:238, 1975.
2. Smith, R. M.: Anesthesia for Infants and Children. 3rd ed., St. Louis, C. V. Mosby Co., 1968.
3. Reid, D. H. S., and Tunstall, M. D.: Treatment of respiratory distress syndrome of newborn with nasotracheal intubation and intermittent positive pressure respiration. Lancet, *1*:1196, 1965.
4. McNamara, J. J., Eraklis, A. J., and Gross, R. E.: Congenital posterolateral diaphragmatic hernia in the newborn. J. Thorac. Cardiovasc. Surg., *55*:55, 1968.
5. Gregory, G. A.: Resuscitation of the newborn. Anesthesiology, *43*:225, 1975.
6. Matson, D. D.: Neurosurgery of Infancy and Childhood. 2nd ed., Springfield, Ill., Charles C Thomas Co., 1969.
7. Zelson, C.: Infant of the addicted mother. N. Engl. J. Med., *288*:1293, 1973.
8. Reye, R. D., Sydney, M. D., Morgan, G., et al.: Encephalopathy and fatty degeneration of the viscera: A disease entity in childhood. Lancet, *2*:749, 1963.
9. Avery, M. E., and Fletcher, B. D.: The Lung and its Disorders in the Newborn Infant. 3rd ed., Philadelphia, W. B. Saunders Co., 1974.
10. Farrell, P. M., and Avery, M. E.: State of the art: Hyaline membrane disease. Am. Rev. Resp. Dis., *111*:657, 1975.
11. Rowe, M. I., and Uribe, F. L.: Diaphragmatic hernia in the newborn infant. Blood gas and pH considerations, Surgery, *70*:758, 1971.
12. Raphaely, R. C., and Downes, J. J.: Congenital diaphragmatic hernia: Prediction of survival. J. Pediatr. Surg., *8*:815, 1973.
13. James, O. C., and Marx, G. F.: Spontaneous bilateral pneumothorax in a newborn infant. Anesthesiology, *28*:629, 1967.
14. Nadas, A. S., and Fyler, D. C.: Pediatric Cardiology. 3rd ed., Philadelphia, W. B. Saunders Co., 1972.
15. Rudolph, A. M.: Congenital Diseases of the Heart. Chicago, Year Book Medical Publishers, Inc., 1975.
16. DeVivo, D. C., and Dodge, P. R.: Diagnosis and management of head injury. Chapter 5 in this book.
17. Replogle, R. L., and Reyes, H. M.: Management of trauma and shock in the pediatric patient. Chapter 1 in this book.
18. Modell, J. H., Davis, J. H., Giammona, S. T., Moya, F., and Mann, J. F.: Blood gas and electrolyte changes in human near-drowning victims. J.A.M.A., *203*:337, 1968.
19. Herrin, J. T., and Crawford, J. D.: The seriously burned child. Chapter 4 in this book.
20. Robinson, C. L., and Mushin, W. W.: Inhaled foreign bodies. Br. Med. J., *2*:324, 1956.

21. Milko, D. A.: Nasotracheal intubation in the treatment of acute epiglottitis. Pediatrics, *53*:674, 1974.
22. Rapkin, R. H.: Nasotracheal intubation in epiglottitis. Pediatrics, *56*:110, 1975.
23. Adair, J. C., Ring, W. H., Jordan, W. S., et al.: Ten-year experience with IPPB in the treatment of acute laryngotracheobronchitis. Anesth. Analg., *50*:649, 1971.
24. Wood, D. W., Downes, J. J., and Lecks, H. I.: A clinical scoring system for the diagnosis of respiratory failure in childhood status asthmaticus. Am. J. Dis. Child., *123*:227, 1972. (See also Chapter 13 in this book.)
25. Plum, F., and Posner, J. F.: Diagnosis of Stupor and Coma. Philadelphia, F. A. Davis Co., 1966.
26. Hunter, R. A.: Status epilepticus: History, incidence, and problems. Epilepsia, *1*:162, 1959.
27. Goldring, D., Hernandez, A., and Hartmann, A. F., Jr.: The care of the infant in cardiac failure. Chapter 8 in this book.
28. Davies, D. D.: Reanesthetizing cases of tonsillectomy and adenoidectomy because of persistent postoperative hemorrhage. Br. J. Anaesth., *36*:244, 1964.
29. Dammann, J. F., Jr., Thung, N., Christlieb, I. J., Littlefield, J. B., and Muller, W. H., Jr.: The management of the severely ill patient after open heart surgery. J. Thorac. Cardiovasc. Surg., *45*:80, 1963.
30. Battersby, E. F., and Glover, W. T.: Management of respiratory insufficiency in infants with congenital heart disease. Anesth. Clin., *12*:141, 1974.
31. Crocker, D.: Management of tracheostomy. Chapter 12 in this book.
32. Bates, D. V., Macklem, P. T., and Christie, R. V.: Respiratory Function in Disease. Philadelphia, W. B. Saunders Co., 1971.
33. D'Souza, B. J., and McKhann, G. M.: Guillain-Barré syndrome. *In* Gellis, S. S., and Kagan, B. M., eds.: Current Pediatric Therapy. 7th ed., Philadelphia, W. B. Saunders Co., 1976.
34. Wolfsdorf, J.: The acute care of respiratory problems in the neonate, infant, and child. *In* Furman, E., ed., The Anesthesiologist's Role in Pediatric Acute Care. Int. Anesthesiol. Clin., *13*:75, 1975.
35. Trey, C.: Acute hepatic failure. Chapter 9 in this book.
36. Holliday, M. A., Potter, D. E., and Dobrin, R. S.: Treatment of renal failure in children. Pediatr. Clin. North Am., *18*:613, 1971.
37. Greenberg, R. E., and Christiansen, R. O.: Hypoglycemia. Chapter 17 in this book.
38. Kouwenhoven, W. B., Jude, J. R., and Knickerbocker, G. G.: Closed-chest cardiac massage. J.A.M.A., *173*:1064, 1960.
39. Stephen, C. R., Ahlgren, E. W., and Bennett, E. J.: Elements of Pediatric Anesthesia. Springfield, Ill., Charles C Thomas Co., 1970.
40. Smith, R. M.: Temperature monitoring and regulation. Pediatr. Clin. North Am., *16*:643, 1969.
41. Guidelines for Organization of Critical Care Units, Report of Committee, in Guidelines, J. J. Downes, Chairman. J.A.M.A., *222*:1532, 1972.
42. Chernick, V., and Vidyasagar, D.: Continuous negative chest wall pressure for HMD. Pediatrics, *49*:753, 1972.
43. Cox, J. M. R.: Review article: Prolonged pediatric ventilatory assistance and related problems. Crit. Care Med., *1*:158, 1973.
44. Stetson, J. B.: Apparatus for anesthetics for children. Endotracheal tube irritation. Paper, Fourth World Congress of Anesthesiologists, London, September 9-13, 1968.
45. Allen, T. H., and Steven, I. M.: Prolonged nasotracheal intubation in children. Br. J. Anaesth., *44*:835, 1972.
46. Fairley, H. B., and Hunter, D. D.: The performance of respirators in the treatment of respiratory insufficiency. Can. Med. Assoc. J., *90*:1397, 1964.
47. Young, J. A., and Crocker, D.: Principles and Practice of Respiratory Therapy. 2nd ed., Chicago, Year Book Medical Publishers, 1976.
48. Petty, T. L.: PEEP (positive end expiratory pressure). Chest, *61*:309, 1972.
49. Gregory, G. A., Kitterman, J. A., Phibbs, R. H., Tooley, W. H., and Hamilton, W. K.: Treatment of idiopathic respiratory distress syndrome with continuous positive airway pressure. N. Engl. J. Med., *284*:1333, 1971.
50. Downs, J. B., Klein, E. F., Desautels, D., et al.: Intermittent mandatory ventilation. Chest, *64*:331, 1973.

51. Radford, E. D., Jr.: Ventilation standards for use in artificial respiration. J. Appl. Physiol., 7:451, 1957.
52. Robbins, L., Crocker, D., and Smith, R. M.: Tidal volume losses of volume-limited ventilators. Anesth. Analg., 46:428, 1967.
53. Epstein, R. A., and Hyman, A. I.: Ventilation requirements of newborn infants in ventilatory failure. Crit. Care Med., 3:37, 1975.
54. Wilson, R. S., and Pontoppidan, H.: Acute respiratory failure; Diagnostic and therapeutic criteria. Crit. Care Med., 2:293, 1974.
55. Filler, R. M., Eraklis, A. J., Rubin, V. G., and Das, J. B.: Long-term total parenteral nutrition in infants. N. Engl. J. Med., 281:589, 1969. (See also Chapter 21 in this book.)
56. Finberg, L.: Dangers to infants caused by changes in osmolar concentrations. Pediatrics, 40:1031, 1967. (See also Chapter 20 in this book.)
57A. Simmons, M. A., Adcock, E. W., Bard, H., et al.: Hypernatremia and intracranial hemorrhage in neonates. N. Engl. J. Med., 291:6, 1974.
57B. Wigglesworth, J. S.: Relation of intraventricular hemorrhage to hyaline membrane disease. Pediatr. Res., 9:864, 1975.
58. Garella, S., Dana, C. L., and Chazan, J. A.: Severity of metabolic acidosis as a determinant of bicarbonate requirements. N. Engl. J. Med., 289:121, 1973.
59. Mortens, J. D.: Clinical sequelae from arterial needle puncture. Circulation, 35:1118, 1967.
60. Cox, J. M.: Techniques in neonatal ventilation. Int. Anesthesiol. Clin., 12:111, 1974.
61. Vidyasagar, D., and Wai, W.: Respiratory weaning of the newborn: Some practical considerations. Crit. Care Med., 3:16, 1975.
62. Stern, L.: Metabolic problems during mechanical ventilation of newborn infants. In Kreuskamp, D. H. G., ed.: Neonatal and Pediatric Ventilation. Int. Anesthesiol. Clin., 12:13, 1974.
63. Nash, G., Bowen, J. A., and Langlinais, P. C.: Respirator lung: A misnomer. Arch. Pathol., 91:234, 1971.
64. Tilney, N. L., and Hester, W. J.: Physiologic and histologic changes in the lungs of patients dying after prolonged cardiopulmonary bypass: An inquiry into the nature of post-perfusion lung. Ann. Surg., 166:759, 1967.
64A. James, L. S., and Lanman, J. T., eds.: History of oxygen therapy and retrolental fibroplasia. Supplement. Pediatrics, 57:591, 1976.
65. Welch, B. E., Morgan, T. E., Jr., and Clamann, H. G.: Time-concentration effects in relation to oxygen toxicity in man. Fed. Proc., 22:1053, 1963.
66. Kistler, G. S., Caldwell, P. R. B., and Weibel, E. R.: Development of fine structural damage to alveolar and capillary lining cells in oxygen-poisoned rat lungs. J. Cell. Biol., 32:605, 1967.
67. Veith, F. J., Hagstrom, J. W. C., Parossian, A., Nehlsen, S. L., and Wilson, J. W.: Pulmonary microcirculatory response to shock, transfusion, and pump-oxygenator procedures: A unified mechanism underlying pulmonary damage. Surgery, 64:95, 1968.
68. A definition of irreversible coma: Report of the ad hoc committee of the Harvard Medical School to examine the definition of brain death. J.A.M.A., 205:337, 1968.
69. Harp, J. R.: Criteria for the determination of death. Anesthesiology, 40:391, 1974.
70. Engel, H. L., Jacoby, J., Modell, J. H., et al.: Pull the plug? Should mechanical respiratory support be withdrawn from patients with presumed neurologic deficits? Anesthesiol. Rev., 3:25, 1976.

Chapter Twelve

MANAGEMENT OF
TRACHEOSTOMY

DEAN CROCKER, M.D.

The indications for and methods of performing a tracheostomy in children are many and varied. There is still controversy as to the size, types, and placement of the tube; the type of incision; the relative indications for tracheostomy in infants and older children; the use of prolonged endotracheal intubation in preference to tracheostomy; and even the type of instruments used to perform the tracheostomy. However, problems discussed here are mainly the proper care of the child with a tracheostomy tube, including those associated with its removal.

Whatever the disease state from which the child suffers, certain basic principles must be kept in mind during all tracheostomy care. These relate to: (1) composition of the tracheal tube, (2) inspired gas mixtures, (3) humidification in inspired gas, (4) suctioning of secretions, (5) positive pressure breathing, (6) chest physiotherapy, (7) weaning of a patient from tracheostomy, (8) home care of tracheostomy by parent, (9) prolonged endotracheal intubation as opposed to tracheostomy, and (10) complications of tracheostomy. Let us now examine these factors in detail.

Over the last 5 years many authors have mentioned rigid, metallic, or hard rubber tubes as sources of tracheal problems. Hard rubber tubes can exert enough pressure on the posterior tracheal wall to produce tracheoesophageal fistula. Secretions may be retained because of the consistency of the rubber. Metal tubes, on the other hand, aside from the possibility of occluding a main bronchus, may impinge on the anterior tracheal wall with local irritation and the possibility of partial airway obstruction at that site. Plum and Dunning have reported local

From the Departments of Anesthesia and Respiratory Therapy, Children's Hospital Medical Center, Boston, Massachusetts.

irritation by metal tubes, and a heavy collection of mucus, which was reduced by their removal.[1] Tubes of both types share the disadvantages of local discomfort.

Such drawbacks have led to research with a variety of other substances, such as soft rubber, silicone rubber, and a number of plastic materials. Polymeric compounds designed to eliminate the aforementioned problems have had a wide range of chemical, mechanical, and physical properties, from flexible to hard, from hydrophobic to hydrophilic, and from inert to highly toxic. The polymers have the advantages of a more ideal weight than metal tubes and a non-wetting surface that is resistant to incrustation and clotting. Since they are not true chemical compounds polymers may contain impurities, varying from time to time even in products from the same company.

One most commonly used polymer is polyvinyl chloride (PVC), which has a polyethylene backbone. It is a hard, amorphous, colorless thermoplastic solid, obtained when vinyl chloride is dissolved in benzoyl peroxide under heat. The resulting polymerization precipitates the PVC resin, separable from the reactants in a variety of ways. A tubing with suitable physical properties is achieved by the addition of plasticizers and stabilizers (usually epoxydized soya oil) in various concentrations to produce varied degrees of flexibility and smoothness.

Contaminants and partially polymerized material trapped in the polymer particles may possibly induce necrosis in muscle, and different manufactures may differ in composition and thus in toxic effects on living tissue. On the other hand, it may be that as additives leach out nontoxic tubing it becomes toxic in use.

In general, PVC tubes that are prepared and evaluated properly should produce no tissue reaction from chemical irritation, while the material should have most of the characteristics of an ideal airway tube. It is, however, thermolabile, so that PVC tubes deform at high temperatures and therefore cannot be resterilized with heat. Ethylene oxide sterilization poses serious toxic potentials, both in residual ethylene oxide and as other oxide reaction products. Of these, the 2-chlorethanol from interaction of chloride ion with ethylene oxide is the most seriously toxic. Qualities that may elicit tissue reactions have not yet been determined, although Oppenheimer et al. have shown that PVC may be carcinogenic, even when free of plasticizers and stabilizers.[2]

Silicon, which constitutes about three quarters of the substance of the earth around us and is thus in plentiful supply, is prepared commercially by electrothermal reduction of silica. Silicone rubber is prepared from an elastomeric gum, milled with inorganic fillers, just as in the preparation of synthetic rubber. A curing catalyst added during mixing allows the elastic mass, molded to desired shape, to be cured to an insoluble, infusible, elastic material.

Dow Corning Corporation has developed a medical-guide *silicone rubber*, a polymer of dimethyl siloxane, commonly known as "Silastic." It makes a flexible, strong tube, which is thin-walled, chemically inert, non-melting when heated in air at 300° F, and with both elasticity and softness that persist as low as −55° F without addition of any plasticizers. Compression when the neck is bent does not constrict or compress the tube; indeed, it is practically impossible to obstruct it by kinking. The tube has a single lumen and does not require an inner tube; its curve conforms to the length and shape of the child's trachea; and its lower end is cut at an angle, facilitating insertion and avoiding the need for an obturator. No cuff is necessary. The soft, pliable material eliminates the danger of perforating the tracheal wall and has a slippery surface which greatly decreases mucous plugging and facilitates suctioning. Finally, its radiopacity makes it easy to locate by x-ray.

No evidence of toxicity or irritative reaction has been observed.

INSPIRED GAS MIXTURES

Gas mixtures most commonly administered via tracheostomy are of oxygen and air, in a percentage that will maintain arterial oxygen tension (Pa_{O_2}) at near normal. Sometimes this will require 100 per cent oxygen or sometimes 100 per cent air, which is, of course, 20 per cent oxygen. Whatever the mixture, the Pa_{O_2} should never exceed 250 mm Hg; ideally, it should never approach this figure.

Immediately following tracheostomy, arterial blood gases should be measured with the patient breathing room air, provided that his or her clinical condition will tolerate this minimal oxygen percentage. If by clinical judgment additional oxygen is required, the inspired percentage should be measured carefully at the time blood is drawn for gas determination. The most common means of administering gas to a tracheostomy is via a "Briggs" adaptor, which is a "T"-shaped connector (Fig. 1). Measuring the exact oxygen percentage delivered through such a tube is difficult because this varies with the child's respiration, and each measurement requires repeated sampling of gas. It is better to calculate the percentage of oxygen by comparing liter flow from the

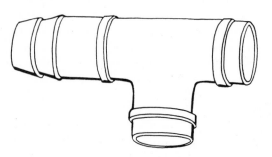

Figure 1. Briggs adaptor, for gas administration to tracheostomy.

oxygen source with minute volume of respiration, in hospitals in which this can be measured.

HUMIDIFICATION OF THE INSPIRED GAS MIXTURES

Dry gas of any composition should never be administered to a tracheostomized patient. When a tracheostomy is performed and the upper airway system (particularly the nose) is thus bypassed, the body's normal means of warming, filtering, and humidifying the inspired air is lost. The filtration effect of the extensive and moist nasal surfaces, upon which particles can settle out, can hardly be replaced artificially. Warming and humidification may be imitated, but their interrelation complicates the process.[3, 4] Nevertheless, the trachea and lungs must be supplied, if possible, with warm air of proper relative humidity.

Some definitions are necessary here since, unfortunately, many physicians fail to distinguish relative from absolute humidity, the water vapor content of air, in grams per cubic centimeter. Relative humidity expresses the ratio of the actual pressure of the water vapor in the air at a given temperature to the maximum or saturated vapor pressure possible at that temperature. Absolute humidity may remain constant, while relative humidity changes as air is warmed or cooled. Dew point is the temperature to which a gas must be cooled for moisture to condense or precipitate.

In the nose and nasopharynx, air is simultaneously warmed and moistened to a physiological relative humidity. Bypass of these areas by tracheostomy not only reduces the warmth and moisture but also removes their control, with resultant irritation of the mucous membranes of the tracheobronchial tree and predisposition to infection.[5]

Ideally, inspired gas should be warmed to near body temperature and saturated with water vapor. This can be accomplished by heating water to a vapor above body temperature at a fixed distance back on the inspiratory gas tubing. The cooling effect of the air surrounding the tubing causes a fall in temperature of the vapor to body temperature at the tracheostomy, where the temperature nevertheless must be measured in order to prevent too high an inspired gas temperature. Although water will condense in the inspiratory gas tubing as the gas stream is cooled and the vapor reaches the dew point, it is, fortunately, impossible by the administration of gas saturated to the body temperature dew point to administer too much water (i.e., too high a relative humidity) to a patient. Such a saturation should always be maintained.

However, a very different situation exists when particulate water suspended in the gas stream is administered via a tracheostomy tube. The apparatus generating liquid particles in a gas stream usually employs agitation of the liquid by a Venturi device or a spinning disc. More recently, by use of ultrahigh frequency sound, a water content supplying as much as 6 ml per minute has been nebulized into inspiratory gas mixtures; water intoxication rapidly occurred, particularly in intubated infants. Continuous ultrasonic nebulization should never be used in infants, nor, probably, in older children. It is possible to supply the entire daily water requirements of an infant or child from one of these units, but it has been found that, in children with tracheostomies and with thick or purulent bronchorrhea, the intermittent use of particulate water to provide a lavage of the tracheostomy tube is useful. The toxic properties of dry gases, particularly oxygen, have been demonstrated both experimentally and clinically.[6]

SUCTIONING OF SECRETIONS

For a procedure seemingly so easy and effortless, an infinite variety of problems occur during and after suctioning. An obvious one is the danger of infection, for it has been shown conclusively that suctioning of the airway has the immediate potential of carrying bacteria into the trachea and bronchi. Sterile technique has become of paramount importance.[7]

The use of a catheter of proper diameter relative to the lumen of the tracheostomy tube, always necessary to prevent the rapid aspiration of oxygen from the airway system with subsequent hypoxia, is especially important in infants and children. The ratio of catheter size to tube lumen is 1:3, but, as a further precaution, particularly in children with lowered Po_2, it is recommended that assisted ventilation be performed with a suitable bag and adaptor for 3 to 5 minutes prior to the suctioning episodes.

In patients with complicating hypoxia, such as those suffering from primary cardiac disease, vagal stimulation may occur with severe slowing or arrest of the heart.[8] Vagal effects are particularly active in children and, whenever problems are anticipated, suctioning should be carried out by the physician. Preoxygenation and the use of the appropriate dosage of atropine may obviate these vagal effects.

Catheters should have a "T" or side-arm opening to ambient air, and the suction should not be applied until the catheter, properly inserted into the tracheostomy tube, is being withdrawn. If the catheter does not have a side-arm opening and is closed off by kinking as it is passed down the tracheostomy, vacuum will continue to rise to maximum proximal to the catheter. When the suction then is initiated, a very high vacuum pressure will draw mucosa in at the catheter tip, performing an unintentional biopsy. Problems with bleeding and infection result. The side-arm hole should be of adequate size to allow complete air flow, thus creating no negative pressure during the time the catheter is inserted.

There is a further hazard in patients who have tracheostomy tubes with inflated cuffs. Secretions accumulate above the cuff of the tube and, upon deflation, immediately descend into the lungs, with attendant risks of atelectasis and pneumonia. To prevent this problem, the cuff of the tube should be deflated and positive pressure should be applied to the airway via the tracheostomy tube. This causes the secretions to be ejected over the vocal cords, where they may be swallowed or suctioned from the oropharynx.

The standard procedures and routines listed below and on pp. 175 and 176 should be available and familiar to anyone entrusted with suctioning and care of tracheostomy tubes.

Procedure for Tracheostomy Tube Care

Care should be taken in nursing involving a patient with a tracheostomy tube in place. Tubes are easily dislodged, leaving the patient without an airway. All nursing procedures (bath, skin care, positioning, and so forth) should be done with attention to the prevention of airway obstruction from aspiration of fluid, powder, tissue paper, and so forth, or by positioning, bed linen, patient's hands, and toys. Frequent and repeated explanations to the patient about the tube, its purpose, and the procedures being done are essential. The fact that most patients with tubes in place are inarticulate necessitates all the more reassurance and, if age and condition permit, an alternate means of communication.

The nurse should be aware of the size and type of tube the patient is using. The cuff, if in use, should be released as ordered by the physician. An extra, sterile tube of the same size and type as the one in place should be available. Extra parts and the obturator of the tracheostomy tube should be wrapped, labeled, and kept near the patient. A sterile, wrapped, and labeled Kelly clamp also should be available for emergency maintenance of the tracheostomy stoma in case of tube displacement.

It is important to remember that tracheostomy suctioning is a sterile procedure; therefore, a sterile catheter and gloves are imperative. However, during the course of the procedure, it is necessary to contaminate one hand. Indications for and frequency of suctioning are specified in the Doctors' Order Book. Prolonged suctioning, suctioning with too large a catheter, or failure to allow the patient time to ventilate between suction attempts can lead to hypoxia, predisposing the patient to cardiac arrest. The heart rate should be monitored during the suctioning procedure.

At the first sign of any respiratory distress, interrupt suctioning and provide humidified oxygen. The left main stem bronchus may be entered by positioning the head to the right, and vice versa. When the patient also requires oral or nasopharyngeal suctioning, separate, clean equipment should be used.

POSITIVE PRESSURE BREATHING

Although a number of available texts deal with this facet,[9, 10] a few basic comments relative to the use of intermittent positive pressure breathing (IPPB) devices with tracheostomy are presented here. Interconnections of standard size, usually with 15-mm tapered male and female connectors, should be employed to allow adaptation of IPPB machines, ventilators, anesthesia equipment, and resuscitative, self-inflating bags to the tracheostomy. There must be no traction or pressure from the positive pressure breathing device which might cause deviation or pressure on the tracheostomy tube. A number of swivel-type devices are available for tube and machine connection, but all of them introduce some "mechanical dead space," which may add greatly to the carbon dioxide retention of small patients.

In children, inflatable cuffs should be avoided when possible. It is better to rely upon the multiplicity of sizes of tracheostomy tubes and fit the proper size to the trachea. Nevertheless, a cuff may be required in conjunction with a positive pressure device in which the peak inspiratory pressure is high and a leak develops around the tube. A cuff also may be required to prevent aspiration of foreign material down the trachea in diseases in which the swallowing mechanism is lost.

Patients who have tracheostomies attached to positive pressure breathing devices should have frequent x-ray examinations of the chest to ensure proper location of the tip of the tube. Repeated connection and disconnection from the ventilator for suctioning, instillation, or weaning may push the tracheostomy tube in until it enters either the left or right main stem bronchus. Because of the large shunt developed in the nonventilated lung, blood gases usually will reflect this accident, as will lack of breath sounds over this area and progressive atelectasis. The peak inspiratory pressure of the ventilator will show a sudden rise, for example, from 20 cm of water to 30 cm. If this happens, the tube should be pulled back slightly after deflation of the cuff (if present), and the patient should be given periodic deep breaths and suctioned.

Steps in Procedure

1. Check suction unit and humidified oxygen for working order.
2. Be sure all necessary equipment is close at hand during the procedure.

3. Explain the procedure to the patient if his or her age and condition allow.

4. Wash hands.

5. Open gloves, catheter, and bottle of normal saline, making sure all are sterile.

6. Don gloves and remove catheter from wrapper, protecting tip while enfolding catheter in palm of sterile-gloved hand.

7. Attach suction unit tubing to the end of the catheter with gloved hand to be contaminated.

8. Moisten catheter with sterile, normal saline.

9. Turn patient's head to one side, using contaminated hand (Fig. 2).

10. With suction off, introduce catheter into tracheostomy tube until patient coughs.

11. On inspiration following cough, advance catheter to main stem bronchus and apply suction.

12. With a continuous twisting motion, remove catheter from tube while applying intermittent suction.

13. Rinse catheter with sterile, normal saline.

14. Allow patient several breaths of humidified oxygen to aid ventilation and to rest him or her between suction attempts.

15. Repeat only as necessary to clear airway.

16. Turn the patient's head to the opposite side and repeat the procedure.

17. Remove gloves and detach catheter, discarding both.

18. Check if twill or adhesive tape is too loose or tight.

19. Check tissue area around the tube for cleanliness, irritation, and broken skin. (a) Clean area carefully when necessary with a cotton applicator moistened with warm tap water. (b) Dry area carefully with a dry sponge.

20. Change tracheostomy sponge when necessary.

21. Assess patient for comfort and report any respiratory distress.

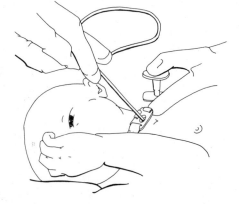

Figure 2. Suction of baby with tracheostomy. Patient's head is turned to the right for insertion of the catheter into left main bronchus. Suction is being performed while the catheter is removed. (From Young, J., and Crocker, D.: Principles and Practice of Inhalation Therapy, 1970, p. 137. Reprinted by permission of Year Book Medical Publishers, Inc.).

As has already been discussed, humidification of the ventilatory systems should be as close to 100 per cent relative humidity as possible. If the ventilator system is of the mechanical-electrical type, all connections should be via grounded plugs, and circuits should be checked periodically for integrity of grounding. With a break in the grounding system, it is possible to build up an electrical charge on the patient through the wet tubing and the tracheostomy tube; such a charge becomes particularly dangerous when associated with electrical devices (e.g., cardiac or respiratory monitors or pacemakers) because electrocution can occur.

Another problem associated with ventilatory devices centers around the water that collects in the tubing. There must be some form of trap to hold this water, and it should be drained frequently. Tubes with water in them should never be raised above the tracheostomy, as even a relatively small collection of water may drown the patient.

The respirator may be a potent source of infection and should be sterile when the patient is placed on this machine. Despite all attempts to prevent it, any ventilator will become contaminated within a period of time. Work carried out by Kundsin and Walter[11] shows that the ventilator will be infected within 24 to 48 hours, and it should be changed at or before this time. An attempt should be made to keep the water within the humidifier sterile by using acetic acid or silver nitrate solutions.[12]

CHEST PHYSIOTHERAPY

A regular regimen of assisted coughing and postural drainage should be instituted for any child with a tracheostomy. An effective cough is the most important protection against respiratory complications; without it, sputum retention may lead to atelectasis, infection, and respiratory failure. The patient may drown in his or her secretions. Even the most critically ill patient should have the benefit of positional changes from side to back to side; and, for those who will tolerate it, both head-up and head-down positions should be used as well. A pillow placed in either flank will aid in the head-down position. Clapping and cupping by an experienced therapist while these positional changes are instituted aids in raising secretions. Infants and small children often may be positioned on the therapist's knees, and chest physiotherapy thus may be carried out (Fig. 3). A combination of chest physiotherapy, suctioning, and intermittent hyperinflation produces best results. Gentle hyperinflation following removal of secretions will often reinflate areas of atelectasis, particularly in the newborn infant.

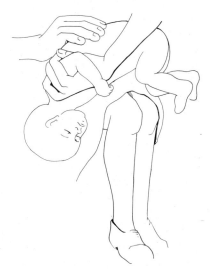

Figure 3. Clapping percussion with infant positioned across therapist's knees. This requires care but can be performed in tracheostomized child.

WEANING PATIENTS FROM TRACHEOSTOMIES

Plans to remove a tracheostomy require that the patient's disease be well under control, with no acute pulmonary infection present. Coughing mechanisms must be intact and the patency of the upper airway ensured.

Infants tracheostomized for a prolonged period of time may present the special difficulty of insufficient air flow through the upper airway, perhaps, as suggested by Gross, because lack of air movement through the larynx results in retardation of local development.[13] But patency of the airway at or below the tracheostomy site is more difficult to ensure. Obstruction by either tracheomalacia or fibrotic stenosis, well described by Cooper and Grillo,[14] occurs when a cuffed tracheostomy tube has been used. Geffin and Pontoppidan have suggested the use of prestretched inflatable cuffs to reduce this type of tracheal damage.[15] Murphy and co-workers have described stenosis following the use of an H-type incision for the tracheostomy insertion.[16] If ball-valving of the tracheostomy cartilage occurs (by in-drawing of the flap of a U-type incision, Fig. 4), the accident usually follows immediately after removal of the tracheostomy. Therefore, one should be prepared to replace the tube rapidly.

Despite the lack of clear and published proof of effectiveness, many physicians use steroids in the hope of reducing edema surrounding the tracheal lumen. Large doses of dexamethasone (Decadron) often are prescribed for 24 hours following removal of the tube.

Among the numerous types of tracheostomy tubes commercially

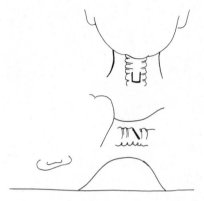

Figure 4. U-shaped incision, with ball-valving following tube removal. In some instances the incision may be an inverted U, with similar risk.

available (Fig. 5), some physicians recommend the use of progressively smaller sizes of unfenestrated tubes on successive days until the tube is removed. They point to the possible complications of ingrown tracheal mucosa into the fenestrated portion of the tube. If a fenestrated tube is used, tracheal plugs of increasing size may be inserted into the tube with the inner cannula removed (Fig. 6), and a progres-

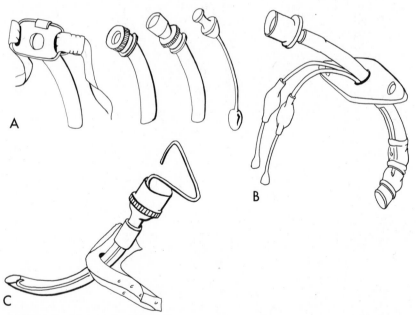

Figure 5. Types of tracheostomy tubes in common use. *A*, Metal four-part special tracheostomy tube consisting of (*left to right*) fenestrated outer cannula, regular inner cannula, special 15-mm adaptor inner cannula, and obturator. *B*, Double-cuffed tracheostomy tube of red rubber for alternation of cuffs. *C*, Lightweight, clear, inert Silon tracheostomy tube.

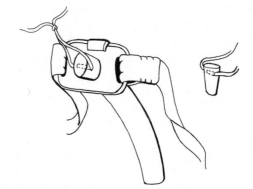

Figure 6. Fenestrated tracheostomy tube, showing plug. The type illustrated here is a complete plug.

sively greater percentage of the tidal volume thus may be diverted through the fenestration and less through the lumen of the tube. When the patient will tolerate complete plugging of the tube for 24 hours, it is removed.

Home Care of the Tracheostomized Child

Sending a child home with a tracheostomy is a most dangerous procedure. We have seen many deaths occur from acute plugging, inadvertent removal of the tube, or blockage of the lumen from external influences. Therefore, the decision to discharge such a patient must be made only after the physician is sure the circumstances warrant it. Before the child is sent home, he or she should be well adapted to the tube, and the parents should be instructed meticulously by the nursing staff in its care. Practicing of suctioning techniques, cleaning, and, ideally, replacement of the tube should be performed in the controlled situation of the hospital.

Written instructions to the parents to take home with the child should be explained carefully and studied. An example of these instructions is outlined on pages 175 and 176.

PROLONGED ENDOTRACHEAL INTUBATION AS OPPOSED TO TRACHEOSTOMY

Prolonged endotracheal intubation, defined by Davenport as the retention of the artificial airway beyond 12 hours,[17] now is recognized as a safe technique in the management of acute respiratory disorders, especially in infants.

The advantages of such intubation over tracheostomy include: (1) avoidance of an operation, (2) rapid availability in emergency situations, (3) lack of complications related to an operation such as pneumothorax, mediastinal or interstitial emphysema, and hemorrhage, (4) greater accessibility of tube in small infants with large heads and small necks, and (5) avoidance of problems of decannulation. If prolonged endotracheal intubation is to be used, handling of the larynx and the tube at initial placement should be kept to a minimum, and use of muscle relaxants in the presence of upper airway obstruction should be avoided. Tubes should be the smallest possible enabling unobstructive spontaneous respiration, absence of continuous pressure on the larynx should be assured, and good nursing and effective physiotherapy, essentials for satisfactory outcome, should be available.

Neither tracheostomy nor endotracheal intubation are without hazards in infants with acute airway obstruction and respiratory insufficiency, but Abbott[18] reports some cases in which the use of prolonged endotracheal intubation in place of tracheostomy reduced the expected complication rate. While some scarring of the trachea was described, no cases of tracheal stenosis were reported.

If larynx or trachea are already abnormal at the time of intubation, complications are more likely to occur.

Immediate complications of either intubation or extubation are: (1) death from acute obstruction of tube, (2) accidental displacement of tube, (3) partial blocking of tube by secretions, and (4) postextubation stridor.

Late complications were found in three patients in a study of 100 cases by Allen and Steven.[19] One developed subglottic stenosis, and two others had mild stenosis that responded to intermittent dilatation of the stenotic ring. However, subglottic stenosis, obstruction of the tube, and other larynx damage have been known to occur following either tracheostomy or prolonged endotracheal intubation.

COMPLICATIONS OF TRACHEOSTOMY

Many of the specified complications of tracheostomies already have been discussed in previous sections. The two complications which cause the most difficulties during the first 2 weeks following tracheostomy are mechanical problems and infections.

Mechanical problems, probably the most common cause of acute airway obstruction in tracheostomized children, should be prevented by strict attention to their common causes. The child must be positioned well at all times; he or she should never be allowed to sleep in the prone position, and his or her coverings must be placed carefully. In infants, it is wise to provide a restraint to prevent pulling at the tracheostomy. A respirator should never be connected to a tracheostomy tube unless a nurse is in constant attendance.

Probably all tracheostomies develop infection at some time. The most pressing resultant problem is to prevent pulmonary involvement, especially if there are areas of atelectasis within the lung. Routine cultures and studies of drug sensitivities are advisable during the period immediately following tracheostomy. If cultures are positive, treatment with the appropriate antibiotic should be begun. The patient eventually will develop an immunity to and symbiotic relationship with common bacteria. It is important that every attempt be made to avoid introducing any pathogens to the tracheostomy.

HOME CARE PROGRAM FOR SUCTIONING AND CARE OF TRACHEOSTOMY TUBES

Equipment

1. Suction pump
2. Y piece
3. Catheters (French rubber)
4. 3 × 3 Telfa pad
5. Four 2 × 4 Pyrex dishes with covers
6. 3 × 3 unsterile plain gauze sponges without cotton filling
7. Hydrogen peroxide, 3 per cent solution
8. Zephiran Chloride, 1:750 solution
9. Bacitracin ointment
10. Paper bag
11. Pipe cleaners
12. 2-quart covered glass jar or bottle containing boiled water
13. Metal tongs soaking in alcohol

Preparation

1. Place four boiled Pyrex dishes with covers on small tray.
2. Label each dish: (a) hydrogen peroxide, (b) water—inner tube, (c) water—flusing catheter, (d) Zephiran Chloride for soaking catheter between uses.
3. Have pipe cleaners, jar of boiled water, Telfa pads, paper bag, suction pump, and Y piece by tray.
4. Boil equipment once a day: (a) boil dishes and 2-quart bottle for 10 minutes; (b) remove containers with metal tongs; (c) fill respective containers with boiled water.
5. Change peroxide and boiled water before each use.

Procedure for Suctioning

1. Check suction pump for working condition.
2. Wash hands thoroughly.

3. Remove inner tube and place in hydrogen peroxide.
4. Remove catheter from dish labeled Zephiran Chloride—catheter marked 3 inches from tip.
5. Attach catheter to Y piece.
6. Insert catheter to marked area.
7. Apply suction and remove with a rotating motion.
8. Rinse catheter with boiled water.
9. If necessary, repeat suctioning after child has rested a minute.

Cleaning Inner Tube

1. Clean inner tube in hydrogen peroxide with pipe cleaners.
2. Rinse inner tube in container of boiled water labeled: water—inner tube.
3. Replace inner tube and lock in place.
4. Inner tube should be cleaned at least every 4 hours during the day and suctioned as necessary between cleanings.

Care of Skin Around Tracheostomy Tube

1. Cleanse area around tracheostomy tube with 3 × 3 gauze sponge moistened with Zephiran Chloride.
2. Apply small amount of Bacitracin ointment to area.
3. Apply cut Telfa pad under outer tube.

REFERENCES

1. Plum, F., and Dunning, M.: Technics for minimizing trauma to the tracheobronchial tree after tracheostomy. N. Engl. J. Med., *254*:293, 1956.
2. Oppenheimer, B. S., Oppenheimer, E. T., Danishevsky, I., Stout, A. P., and Erich, F. R.: Further studies of polymers as carcinogenic agents in animals. Can. Res., *15*:333, 1955.
3. Bang, B. G., and Bang, F. B.: Effect of water deprivation on mucous flow. Proc. Soc. Exp. Biol. Med., *106*:46, 1961.
4. Hilding, A. C.: Four physiological defenses of the upper part of the respiratory tract: Ciliary action, exchange mucin, regeneration and adaptability. Ann. Intern. Med., *6*:227, 1932.
5. Roche, H.: Air conditioning in relation to public health and to diseases of the respiratory tract. J. R. Inst. Public Health, *1*:473, 1938.
6. Lambertsen, C. J., Kough, R. H., Cooper, D. Y., Emmel, G. L., Loeschcke, H. H., and Schmidt, C. F.: Oxygen toxicity. Effects in man of oxygen inhalation at 1 and 3.5 atmospheres upon blood gas transport, cerebral circulation, and cerebral metabolism. J. Appl. Physiol., *5*:471, 1953.
7. Smith, H.: The virulence enhancing action of mucins: A survey of human mucins and mucosal extracts for virulence enhancing activity. J. Infect. Dis., *88*:207, 1951.
8. Fineberg, C., Cohn, H. E., and Gibbon, J. H.: Cardiac arrest during nasotracheal aspiration. J.A.M.A., *174*:410, 1960.
9. Mushin, W. W., Rendell-Baker, L., Thompson, P. W., and Mapleson, W. W.: Automatic Ventilation of the Lungs. 2nd ed., Philadelphia, F. A. Davis Co., 1969.
10. Young, J. A., and Crocker, D.: Principles and Practice of Inhalation Therapy. Chicago, Year Book Medical Publishers, Inc., 1970.

11. Kundsin, R. A., and Walter, C. W.: Asepsis for inhalation therapy. Anesthesiology, *23*:507, 1962.
12. Reinarz, J. A., Pierce, A. K., Mays, B. B., and Sanford, J. P.: Potential role of inhalation therapy equipment in nosocomial pulmonary infection. J. Clin. Invest., *44*:381, 1965.
13. Gross, R. E.: Personal communication, 1971.
14. Cooper, J. D., and Grillo, H. G.: The evolution of tracheal injury due to ventilatory assistance through cuffed tubes. A pathological study. Ann. Surg., *169*:334, 1969.
15. Geffin, B., and Pontoppidan, H.: Reduction of tracheal damage by the prestretching of inflatable cuffs. Anesthesiology, *31*:462, 1969.
16. Murphy, D. A., MacLean, L. D., and Dobell, A. R. C.: Tracheal stenosis as a complication of tracheostomy. Ann. Thor. Surg., *2*:44, 1966.
17. Davenport, H. T.: Prolonged endotracheal intubation in children—a perspective. Int. Anesthesiol. Clin., *8*:909, 1970.
18. Abbott, T. R.: Complications of prolonged nasotracheal intubation in infants and children. Br. J. Anaesth., *40*:347, 1968.
19. Allen, T. H., and Steven, I. M.: Prolonged nasotracheal intubation in infants and children. Br. J. Anaesth., *44*:835, 1972.
20. Wittard, B. R., and Thomas, K. E.: A new polyvinyl chloride cuffed tracheostomy tube. Lancet, *1*:79, 1964.
21. Boyd, I. A., and Pathak, C. L.: The comparative toxicity of silicone rubber and plastic tubing. Scott. Med. J., *9*:345, 1964.
22. Smith, R. M.: Diagnosis and treatment: Nasotracheal intubation as a substitute for tracheostomy. Pediatrics, *38*:652, 1966.
23. McGovern, F. H., Fitz-Hugh, G. H., and Edgemon, L. G.: The hazards of endotracheal intubation. Ann. Otol., *80*:556, 1971.
24. Harrison, G. A., and Tonkin, J. P.: Prolonged endotracheal intubation. Br. J. Anaesth., *40*:241, 1968.
25. Hatch, D. J.: Prolonged nasotracheal intubation in infants and children. Lancet, *1*:1272, 1968.
26. Dimanti, S.: Silicone rubber in surgery. Lancet, *2*:727, 1955.

Chapter Thirteen

THE MANAGEMENT OF STATUS ASTHMATICUS IN CHILDREN

GAIL G. SHAPIRO, M.D.,*
F. ESTELLE SIMONS, M.D.,†
WILLIAM E. PIERSON, M.D.,*
C. WARREN BIERMAN, M.D.†

Status asthmaticus is acute asthma that is refractory to administration of beta-adrenergic agents such as epinephrine and isoproterenol in appropriate dosages.[1,2] It is characterized by bronchial smooth muscle spasm, edematous mucosa, and tenacious secretions that obstruct air flow through bronchi and bronchioles,[3] and result in increased work and decreased efficiency of breathing. If complications ensue, such as atelectasis, pneumomediastinum, or physical fatigue, the patient may develop alveolar hypoventilation and respiratory failure. Status asthmaticus is a medical emergency. Appropriate intensive management minimizes mortality and complications and substantially reduces the length of hospitalization.

The protocol presented here evolved as a means of insuring appropriate care of children admitted to a children's hospital with status asthmaticus, and of teaching medical students and pediatric residents a therapeutic approach to this disorder. It has been employed for evaluation of various drugs, including aminophylline,[4] adrenocorticosteroids,[5] antibiotics,[6] and nebulized beta-adrenergic agents in status asthmaticus.[7] Since its initiation in 1967, no hospitalized child in this program has died of asthma and the average hospital stay for status asthmaticus has been reduced from 5.5 to 2.6 days.

From the Department of Pediatrics,* University of Washington School of Medicine and Division of Allergy, Children's Orthopedic Hospital and Medical Center, Seattle, Washington, and the Department of Pediatrics,† University of Manitoba, Winnipeg.

ADMISSION PROCEDURE

The patient should be admitted to the intensive care unit or other suitable hospital unit in which he or she can be observed closely. It is important to know certain specific historical data about the patient admitted for status asthmaticus. The history should specify the duration of the asthma and of this particular attack. Information should be obtained on names, dosages, and exact times of administration of all medications taken within the past 24 hours, such as theophylline and adrenergic agents, and of corticosteroids administered within the past 12 months, since this may modify the initial hospital drug therapy. Information concerning fluid intake, vomiting, and fever prior to admission may modify initial intravenous fluid orders.

On physical examination, special note should be taken of the patient's general appearance and level of activity, which may reflect his or her state of hypoxemia,[8] the degree of respiratory effort, duration of the expiratory phase, and presence or absence of wheezing (absence of wheezing may indicate very poor air exchange), tachycardia, and tachypnea. Presence or absence of precardiac dullness also should be noted. If present, its sudden disappearance may signify the development of a pneumomediastinum. One should look for pulsus paradoxus—a sign of impending respiratory failure[9]—and papilledema, which, if present, is associated with the presence of Pa_{CO_2} greater than 75 mm Hg.[10] Fever, otitis media, pharyngitis, or signs of pneumonia may indicate a need for bacterial or viral cultures, or both, and possible antibiotic therapy.

The pulmonary index,[8] a scoring system for quantifying physical signs of the course of status asthmaticus, has been helpful in following patients' progress (Fig. 1). Paramedical personnel (e.g., respiratory therapists) can aid the physician by quantitating clinical parameters at specific time intervals. A sudden increase in score indicates a worsening of asthma and may signal the development of a potentially serious complication that requires immediate reevaluation of the patient.

A chest x-ray is indicated in every child admitted with status asthmaticus, to rule out the possibility of pneumonia, atelectasis, pneumomediastinum, and pneumothorax. Twenty-five per cent of pediatric patients with status asthmaticus had one of these complications when admitted to the hospital.[11] Failure to obtain a baseline chest film clouds any assessment of radiological changes occurring later in the course of therapy.

Initial laboratory studies should include arterial[12] or arterialized capillary[13] blood gases, complete blood count, electrolytes, and urinalysis to provide information about the patient's physiological and metabolic derangements on admission.

Pulmonary function studies consisting of forced vital capacity (FVC), forced expiratory volume at 1 second (FEV_1), and forced ex-

PULMONARY INDEX:*

Score	Resp. Rate	Wheezing Score **	Inspir. Expir. Ratio	Accessory Resp. Musc. Utilization
0	<30	None	5/2	0
1	31-45	Terminal Expir. or c̄ Steth. only	5/3-5/4	+ −
2	46-60	Entire Expir. or c̄ Steth.	1/1	++
3	>60	Inspir. & Expir. s̄ Steth.	<1/1	++++

⇓ ⇓ ⇓ ⇓

Time	Resp. Rate	Wheezing Score	Inspir. Expir. Ratio	Accessory Resp. Musc. Use	Total
Admission					
1/2 hour					
1 hour					
3 hours					
12 hours					
24 hours					

* Pediatrics 37: 477, 1966.
** If no wheezing is audible due to minimal air exchange, score 3.

Figure 1. The pulmonary index grades physical signs in an objective manner so that the patient's progress can be followed.[8] (From Dabbons, S. A., Tkachyk, J. S., and Stamm, S. J.: Double-blind study of the effects of corticosteroids in the treatment of bronchiolitis. Pediatrics, 37:477, 1966.)

piratory flow at 25 to 75 per cent of vital capacity ($FEF_{25-75\%}$) can be obtained in children as young as 5 years of age. In those under 5 years, it is often possible to obtain peak expiratory flow rate (PEFR) on a pediatric Wright Peak Flow Meter. This aids in establishing objective measurements of pulmonary function with which serial measurements may be compared during the course of therapy.

INITIAL THERAPY

Intravenous fluids should be administered to every patient with status asthmaticus. Dehydration is almost uniformly present since many patients have been vomiting, and all have greater insensible fluid loss because of increased work of breathing. For intravascular volume repletion, the initial hydrating dose of fluids should contain isotonic sodium chloride because of the inappropriate antidiuretic hormone response demonstrated in status asthmaticus, followed by adequate fluid for maintenance and depletion repair with the addition of appropriate electrolytes. If the patient has metabolic acidosis with a pH less than 7.3 and a base deficit of more than 5 mEq/L, sodium bicarbonate should be administered for correction. A respiratory acidosis is corrected only by improving alveolar ventilation, and buffers are of little or no help in its modification.

Table 1 lists suggested dosages for fluids, which should be modified for the individual patient.

MEDICATIONS

Initial intravenous medications consist of aminophylline and adrenocorticosteroids, with antibiotics only if indicated for *bacterial* infection.

Aminophylline is an effective bronchodilator when present in serum at theophylline concentrations of 10 to 20 mcg/ml.[15] To achieve and maintain this level, a rapid infusion (15 minutes) followed by a constant infusion seems most effective (Fig. 2). The recommended doses are derived from our own trials and those of other investigators. Because our previously recommended schedule for aminophylline of 7 mg/kg loading dose followed by 15 mg/kg/24 hr[2] failed to maintain therapeutic blood levels in many children, we have increased our recommendations for the constant infusion, approximating those of Mitenko and Ogilvie.[16] Only monitoring of serum theophylline can precisely define

TABLE 1   Fluids Given in Status Asthmaticus

Intravenous Fluids (guidelines only)
1. Hydrating: initial—12 ml/kg or 360 ml/sq m for first hour[14] (normal saline).
2. Maintenance: 50 to 60 ml/kg/24 hr or 1500 ml/sq m/24 hours (5% glucose in water).
3. Depletion repair:
   Normal saline 10 to 15 ml/kg/24 hr or 300 to 500 ml/sq m.
   Water (5% glucose/water) 10 to 15 ml/kg/24 hr or 300 to 500 ml/sq m/24 hr.

Electrolytes
1. Potassium (2 mEq/100 ml of maintenance intravenous fluids).
2. Sodium (3 mEq/100 ml of maintenance intravenous fluids).

Buffers
   If pH is below 7.30 and base deficit greater than 5 mEq/L, correct to normal range with IV sodium bicarbonate as clinically indicated, administering half the calculated dosage initially and the other half after repeating blood gas determinations.

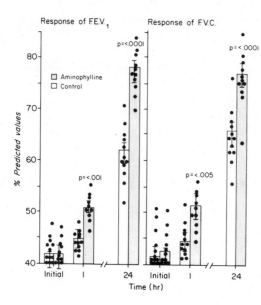

Figure 2. The effectiveness of aminophylline in status asthmaticus has been verified in a double-blind trial. Pulmonary function improved significantly faster in patients treated with aminophylline than in those treated with placebo.[4]

whether a patient is receiving optimal amounts of the medication. If signs of theophylline toxicity occur, such as CNS irritability, headache, nausea, vomiting, or abdominal cramps, the aminophylline infusion should be slowed until an emergency theophylline level can be obtained.

Aminophylline

Seven mg/kg diluted by 3 volumes of saline and given in 15 minutes as a loading dose, followed by 15 mg/kg/24 hr by continuous drip in children under 10 kg and 21 mg/kg/24 hr by continuous drip for older children. Serum theophylline levels should be monitored during therapy. Patients who have received more theophylline than 20 mg/kg in the 12 hours prior to admission should receive only one-half the loading dose of aminophylline.

Corticosteroids restore responsiveness to catecholamines *in vitro*[17] and *in vivo*.[18] Clinical trials in children with status asthmaticus show a more rapid restoration of normal O_2 tension in those who are treated with corticosteroids than in those who do not receive them (Fig. 3).[5] The advantages of corticosteroids administered early in adequate doses far outweigh any drawbacks[3] if the course does not exceed 10 days.

Dexamethasone and betamethasone appear to have advantages over hydrocortisone in status asthmaticus, since they reverse hypoxemia more rapidly. This may be due to the higher ratio of free to bound plasma steroid of patients receiving the two former preparations.

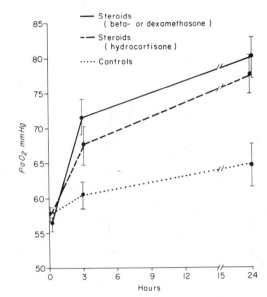

ARTERIAL OXYGEN LEVELS (mmHg)

Figure 3. Arterial oxygen levels of patients in status asthmaticus improve at a faster rate in patients treated with steroids. Betamethasone or dexamethasone seems to be more effective than equivalent doses of hydrocortisone.[5]

Adrenocorticosteroids
Dexamethasone, or betamethasone, 0.3 mg/kg stat followed by 0.3 mg/kg/24 hr by continuous intravenous infusion.

Rarely has bacterial infection been associated with status asthmaticus.[7] Antibiotics should be prescribed only in children in whom bacterial disease is strongly suggested by such clinical findings as acute otitis media, purulent pharyngitis, or pneumonia with lobular distribution of infiltrates. Because antibiotics generally are not given, careful observation and cultures are imperative so that changes suggesting bacterial infection will be noted promptly and adequate therapy begun.

Antibiotics
Only if indicated by clinical or x-ray evidence of bacterial infection. Drug and dosage should depend on the presumptive microorganism and should be adjusted on identification of the bacterial pathogen.

RESPIRATORY THERAPY

Effective respiratory therapy is extremely important in the management of status asthmaticus. The respiratory therapist who is experienced with children is a very important member of the therapeutic team in managing oxygen and aerosolized bronchodilator therapy, in the performance of postural drainage when the patient has excessive secretions, and in monitoring the clinical course.

Oxygen
Initial therapy with humidified oxygen delivered by Venturi mask is desirable until arterial blood gases have been determined. This therapy can be discontinued when the patient's oxygenation is adequate by blood gas determinations.

Sympathomimetic Agents
Isoproterenol .05 per cent[19] or metaproterenol 0.5 per cent[7] solution should be administered with O_2 for 5 to 10 minutes every half-hour for the first 2 hours of therapy by means of a low-pressure ultrasonic or Puritan wall nebulizer and repeated less frequently as the patient improves. The child's pulse rate should be monitored, and the nebulizer therapy stopped temporarily if the pulse reaches 200 beats per minute. Positive pressure ventilators (IPPB) should be avoided because of the danger of inducing further bronchoconstriction, pneumomediastinum, or pneumothorax.[20]

FURTHER THERAPY

Only by considering the information from pulmonary index scores, pulmonary function tests, and repeated blood gases can an accurate assessment of the patient's course be made. One should not be discouraged by the lag between clinical improvement and resolution of wheezing and the return of pulmonary function tests to normal. Because small airway changes may take a week or more to reverse, therapy must be adequate during and after the "critically ill" period.[21]

Clinical Evaluation

PULMONARY INDEX.   Repeat at one-half, 1, 3, 6, 12, and 24 hours after admission.

PULMONARY FUNCTION.   Repeat FVC, FEV_1, $FEF_{25-75\%}$ at 1, 3, 6, 12, and 24 hours, then every 12 hours for remainder of hospitalization.

ARTERIAL BLOOD GASES. Repeat at 1 and 3 hours, or more frequently as indicated by course.

CHEST X-RAY. Repeat chest x-ray for worsening clinical state; a sudden increase in respiratory rate or fall in blood pressure may indicate pneumomediastinum or pneumothorax.

Therapy

IN HOSPITAL. After 24 hours theophylline, corticosteroids, and antibiotics may be administered orally if the patient is improving. An overlap period of 6 to 8 hours during which the IV runs at a slow rate while oral therapy is instituted is a good way to make the transition smoothly.

Nebulized sympathomimetic agents should be used intermittently as needed. A serum theophylline level should be monitored 24 hours after switching to oral theophylline. Serum samples obtained prior to and 1.5 hours after theophylline doses are helpful and should indicate the patient's lowest and peak serum level and aid in determining more precise theophylline therapy.

ORAL THERAPY. Theophylline 5 mg/kg every 6 hours, and adjust as necessary for a serum level of 10 to 20 mcg/ml. Prednisone or methylprednisolone: 30 to 40 mg/day for 2 days, then decrease 4 to 5 mg per day until patient is off steroids.

OUTPATIENT TREATMENT. Status asthmaticus in children usually can be controlled in 24 to 48 hours, and the average hospital stay is 2.6 ± .6 days.[7] Though symptoms may be improved and wheezing absent at this time, there is a delay in return of pulmonary function to normal.[21] This makes it essential that patients be discharged on continuing therapy with theophylline, administered every 6 hours around the clock. A tapering course of A.M. prednisone should be continued for from 7 to 10 days. Prednisone or methylprednisolone should be used, since a short-acting steroid, administered in a single A.M. dose, will minimize the likelihood of iatrogenic pituitary adrenal suppression. An antibiotic course begun in the hospital should be completed.

PITFALLS IN CARE

Some common sources of complications in management that one must be careful to avoid are listed here.

1. Attempting to treat the patient with intravenous fluids and aminophylline in the emergency room. A pediatric patient sick enough to require these measures is unlikely to recover sufficiently in a few hours to be sent home safely.

2. Administering aminophylline in suppository form. Suppositories are absorbed erratically and do not provide dependable serum levels.

3. Delaying administration of therapeutic doses of adrenocorticosteroids on admission may prolong hypoxemia and unresponsiveness to beta-adrenergic agents. There are no advantages to this course.

4. Writing orders illegibly: for example, the nurse may confuse aminophylline (15 mg/kg/24 hr) with ampicillin (100 mg/kg/24 hr), with serious consequences.

5. Sedating the hypoxemic patient. The likelihood of respiratory failure increases proportionately with such medication.

6. Admitting the patient to a regular hospital ward rather than the intensive care unit. The early recognition of serious complications may be critically delayed.

7. Using antihistamines or cromolyn sodium in status asthmaticus. Neither agent has bronchodilator properties and both may affect therapy adversely.

8. Not monitoring serum theophylline levels.

9. Omitting early arterial blood gas determinations.

RESPIRATORY FAILURE

Respiratory failure occurs in a small but significant number of children admitted to the hospital with status asthmaticus. Rarely, a child experiencing an episode of severe asthma is in respiratory failure or in a state of impending respiratory arrest when first seen by a physician. More commonly, respiratory failure develops insidiously in the hospitalized asthmatic child, sometimes despite prompt optimal medical management and sometimes because failure to recognize the severity of the asthma delays appropriate therapy.

Diagnosis

Clinical criteria for diagnosis of respiratory failure in children with asthma include decreased or absent pulmonary breath sounds, severe retractions and use of accessory muscles, cyanosis in 40 per cent oxygen, depressed level of consciousness and response to pain, and poor skeletal muscle tone. The importance of frequent monitoring of arterial blood gas tensions and pH cannot be overstressed, because it is difficult to diagnose impending respiratory failure from clinical signs alone.[22]

The presence of a Pa_{CO_2} of more than 65 mm Hg confirms the diagnosis of respiratory failure, but in practice a rapid rise in Pa_{CO_2} (for example, from 40 mm Hg to 50 mm in 1 hour) in an exhausted child who is receiving optimal intravenous bronchodilator therapy is sufficient evidence for the diagnosis of respiratory failure. Carbon dioxide retention, indicating alveolar hypoventilation, occurs when airway obstruction is severe. Hypoxemia is frequently present in asymptomatic asthmatic patients, and is almost universal in acute bronchospasm. Therefore, although a Pa_{O_2} of less than 70 mm Hg in 40 per cent oxygen or greater is also said to support the diagnosis of respiratory failure, a rise in Pa_{CO_2} is the chief criterion of respiratory failure upon which the clinician depends.

Management

The treatment of respiratory failure in children with asthma is endotracheal intubation, mechanical ventilation, and continuation of bronchodilators as described in Appendix I. (See also Chapter 11, pp. 151–158.)

Intubation. Ideally, a pediatric anesthesiologist should perform intubation using a polyvinyl chloride tube of appropriate size.[23] To prevent aspiration of gastric contents, the stomach must be emptied by wide-bore tube before intubation. Orotracheal intubation generally is performed initially, but nasotracheal intubation should replace this if mechanical ventilation is required for more than 12 hours, since it causes less copious secretions and is less frequently associated with accidental extubation. A cuffed tube is not necessary in children weighing less than 20 kg despite high intra-airway pressure, and a tube with a low-pressure cuff should be used only in larger children. Tracheostomy should not be necessary, since the duration of intubation is usually less than 72 hours.

Neuromuscular Blocking Agents. Neuromuscular blocking agents such as d-tubocurarine[24] and pancuronium bromide[25] may decrease the work of breathing, prevent coughing against the ventilator, and facilitate coordination of the patient with the ventilator. These are contraindicated, however, unless the physician is trained in their use. If neuromuscular blockade is employed, a sedative must also be given, the paralyzed patient must never be left unattended, and there must be a low pressure-sensitive alarm in the inspiratory line of the ventilator.

Monitoring. Careful monitoring of the patient's clinical signs and blood gases must be continued during mechanical ventilation (see Appendix II). The patient may be weaned from the respirator when he or she is able to trigger his or her own inspirations, when inspiratory pressures required are 35 cm water or less, and when expirations shorten and wheezing becomes low-pitched and disappears after nebulized bronchodilators. At this point, muscle relaxants and sedatives are withheld entirely, and the patient is disconnected from the ventilator with the endotracheal tube remaining in place. An open, humidified "T" tube facilitates gradual increase, in time tolerated without ventilator support. If the patient has stable vital signs, normal blood gases in 30 to 40 per cent oxygen, inspiratory effort of -25 cm H_2O, vital capacity of ≥ 5 cc/kg after 4 or 6 hours on the "T" tube, extubation may be performed. Intermittent mandatory ventilation can be helpful in weaning some patients.[26] Mean total duration of controlled and assisted ventilation and weaning of patients managed in the preceding manner was about 57 hours in a recently reported series.[27]

Complications. Potential complications of mechanical ventilation include mechanical failure of the instrument or power source, improper warming or humidification of inspired air, oxygen toxicity, introduction of pathogens into the respiratory tract, atelectasis, pneumothorax (manifested by sudden increase in peak pressure developed by a volume-preset machine), pneumomediastinum, and subcutaneous emphysema.[23] Complications of endotracheal intubation include intubation of a bronchus, kinking of the tube, obstruction by mucous plug, accidental extubation, and nasal hemorrhage. Hoarseness may occur after extubation, and when intubation has been prolonged or the cuff overinflated, the formation of ulcers or granulomas, paralysis of small muscles of the larynx, and subglottic stenosis also may occur.[28] Hypertension, hypotension, and cardiac arrhythmias may be noted, usually in a temporal relationship with the administration of medications.

There is increasing interest in the use of intravenously administered isoproterenol in the presention of respiratory failure. It is said to prevent the need for mechanical ventilation[29, 30] and to cause fewer complications than mechanical ventilation. No prospective controlled studies of the use of intravenously administered isoproterenol in the prevention of respiratory failure have been conducted, and therefore general recommendations for its use in this condition cannot be made at the present time.

REFERENCES

1. Bierman, C. W., Pierson, W. E., and Shapiro, G. G.: The treatment of status asthmaticus in children. South. Med. J., 68:1556, 1975.
2. Bierman, C. W., and Pierson, W. E.: The pharmacologic management of status asthmaticus in children. Pediatrics, 54:245, 1974.
3. Franklin, William: Treatment of severe asthma. N. Engl. J. Med., 290:469, 1974.
4. Pierson, W. E., Bierman, C. W., Stamm, S. J., and Van Arsdel, P. P., Jr.: Double-blind trial of aminophylline in status asthmaticus. Pediatrics, 48:642, 1971.
5. Pierson, W. E., Bierman, C. W., and Kelley, V. C.: A double-blind trial of corticosteroid therapy in status asthmaticus. Pediatrics, 53:867, 1974.
6. Shapiro, G. G., Eggleston, P. A., Pierson, W. E., Ray, C. G., and Bierman, C. W.: Double-blind study of the effectiveness of a broad-spectrum antibiotic in status asthmaticus. Pediatrics, 54:282, 1974.
7. Shapiro, G. G., Simons, E., Garra, B., Pierson, W. E., and Bierman, C. W.: Double-blind evaluation of the effectiveness of nebulized metaproterenol and isoproterenol in childhood status asthmaticus. J. Allergy Clin. Immunol., 57:258, 1976.
8. Dabbous, S. A., Tkachyk, J. S., and Stamm, S. J.: Double-blind study of the effects of corticosteroids in the treatment of bronchiolitis. Pediatrics, 37:477, 1966.
9. Knowles, G. K., and Clark, P. J. H.: Pulsus paradoxus as a valuable sign indicating severity of asthma. Lancet, 2:1356, 1973.
10. Papilledema in chest disease (Editorial). Br. Med. J., 2:1486, 1963.
11. Eggleston, P. A., Ward, B. H., Pierson, W. E., and Bierman, C. W.: Radiographic abnormalities in acute asthma in children. Pediatrics, 54:442, 1974.
12. McFadden, E. R., Jr., and Lyons, H. A.: Arterial blood gas tension in asthma. N. Engl. J. Med., 278:1026, 1968.
13. Stamm, S. J.: Reliability of capillary blood for the measurement of Pa_{O_2} and oxygen saturation. Dis. Chest, 52:191, 1967.
14. Straub, P. W., Buhlmann, A. A., and Rossier, P. H.: Hypovolemia in status asthmaticus. Lancet, 2:923, 1969.
15. Simons, F. E. R., Pierson, W. E., and Bierman, C. W.: Current status of the use of theophylline in children. Pediatrics, 55:735, 1975.
16. Mitenko, P. A., and Ogilvie, R. I.: Rational intravenous doses of theophylline. N. Engl. J. Med., 289:600, 1973.
17. Logsdon, P. J., Middleton, E., Jr., and Coffey, R. G.: Stimulation of leukocyte adenylcyclase by hydrocortisone and isoproterenol in asthmatic and nonasthmatic subjects. J. Allergy Clin. Immunol., 50:45, 1970.
18. Ellul-Micallef, R., and Fenech, F. F.: Effect of intravenous prednisolone in asthmatics with diminished adrenergic responsiveness. Lancet, 2:1269, 1975.
19. Freedman, B. J., and Hill, G. B.: Comparative study of duration of action and cardiovascular effects of bronchodilator aerosols. Thorax, 26:46, 1971.
20. Bierman, C. W.: Pneumomediastinum and pneumothorax complicating asthma in children. Am. J. Dis. Child., 114:42, 1967.
21. McFadden, E. R., Jr., Kisser, R., and Degroot, W. J.: Acute bronchial asthma: Relations between clinical and physiological manifestations. N. Engl. J. Med., 288:221, 1973.
22. Downes, J. J., Wood, D. W., Striker, T. W., and Pittman, J. D.: Arterial blood-gas and acid-base disorders in infants and children with status asthmaticus. Pediatrics, 42:238, 1968.
23. Downes, J. J., Fulgencio, T., and Raphaely, R. C.: Acute respiratory failure in infants and children. Pediatr. Clin. North Am., 19:423, 1972.
24. Wood, D. W., Downes, J. J., and Lecks, H. I.: The management of respiratory failure in childhood status asthmaticus. Experience with 30 episodes and evolution of a technique. J. Allergy, 42:261, 1968.
25. Levin, N., and Dillon, J. B.: Status asthmaticus and pancuronium bromide. J.A.M.A., 222:1265, 1972.

26. Downs, J. B., Klein, E. F., Desautels, D., Modell, J. H., and Kirby, R. R.: Intermittent mandatory ventilation: A new approach to weaning patients from mechanical ventilators. Chest, *64*:331, 1973.
27. Simons, F. E. R., Pierson, W. E., and Bierman, C. W.: Respiratory failure in childhood status asthmaticus. Am. J. Dis. Child., in press.
28. The price of therapeutic artificial ventilation (Editorial). Lancet, *1*:1161, 1973.
29. Wood, D. W., Downes, J. J., Scheinkopf, H., and Lecks, H. I.: Intravenous isoproterenol in the mangement of respiratory failure in status asthmaticus. J. Allergy Clin. Immunol., *50*:75, 1972.
30. Cotton, E. K., and Parry, W.: Treatment of status asthmaticus and respiratory failure. Pediatr. Clin. North Am., *22*:163, 1975.

APPENDIX I: TREATMENT OF RESPIRATORY FAILURE IN STATUS ASTHMATICUS

Intubation

1. Nasogastric tube passed, gastric contents emptied.
2. Suction upper airway.
3. Ventilate with 100 per cent oxygen by bag and mask.
4. Medications:*

	Dose:
diazepam or	0.1 mg/kg–0.3 mg/kg
pentobarbital	2 mg/kg
atropine	0.01 mg/kg (maximum 0.5 mg)
succinylcholine	1–2 mg/kg

5. Tube, polyvinyl chloride:
   a. Low pressure cuff in patients > 20 kg, uncuffed tube in patients < 20 kg.
   b. Secure with tape and tincture of benzoin.
   c. Measure distance from external nares to proximal end of tube.
   d. Check tube position by radiograph.

Mechanical Ventilation: Volume-Preset Ventilator†

1. Tidal volume (corrected): 10–12 cc/kg.
2. Rate: 10–20/min.
3. Flow rate: 50–70 L/min.
4. Temperature of inspired air-oxygen mixture: 37°C; humidity: 80–100°.
5. Inspired oxygen concentration: minimum required for satisfactory oxygenation.
6. Medications:

	Dose:
d-tubocurarine	0.4–0.6 mg/kg
pancuronium bromide	0.05–0.8 mg/kg
diazepam	0.1–0.3 mg/kg
morphine	0.1–0.2 mg/kg
chloral hydrate	20–30 mg/kg

Criteria for Weaning

1. Disappearance of bronchospasm after nebulized isoproterenol (0.05 per cent) or other beta-adrenergic drug.
2. Normal arterial blood gases in 30 to 40 per cent oxygen.
3. Assist mode.
4. Pressure required: 30 to 35 cm H_2O or less.
5. Expiration-inspiration ratio <2:1.
6. Vital capacity ≥ 15 cc/kg.
7. Tidal volume ≥ 5 cc/kg.
8. Inspiratory effort: −25 cm H_2O.

---

*Use these drugs, particularly succinylcholine, with *extreme* caution in the hypoxic patient (see text).

†After initiation, modify ventilator settings as patient's clinical signs and blood gas measurements change. Change only one ventilator setting at a time. Model number MA-1: Bennett Respiration Products, Inc., Santa Monica, Calif. (patients > 10 kg). Model number LS-104-150: Bourns, Inc., Life Systems Operation, Riverside, Calif. (patients < 10 kg).

APPENDIX II: FLOW SHEET FOR MONITORING OF PATIENTS DURING MECHANICAL VENTILATION IN STATUS ASTHMATICUS

Date _____ Weight (kg) _____ Time (hr) _____

	0000	0100	0200	0300	0400	0500	0600	0700
Temperature (°C)								
Cardiovascular								
pulse*								
blood pressure†								
Respiratory‡								
rate/minute								
ausculation								
exhaled volume (cc)								
tidal volume (cc)								
peak inspiratory pressure (cm H_2O)								
flow rate (L/min)								
FI_{O_2} (%)								
temperature (°C)/humidity (%) of inspired air								
suction								
positioning								
chest physiotherapy								
Fluid Balance								
input: intravenous fluid cc/hr	/	/	/	/	/	/	/	/
output: urine output (cc),§ nasogastric tube drainage (cc)	/	/	/	/	/	/	/	/

Laboratory Tests
blood gases: Pa_{O_2} (mm Hg), Pa_{CO_2} (mm Hg),
pH
urine specific gravity
serum electrolytes (mEq): Na, Cl, HCO_3, K
chest roentgenogram
other

Medications
aminophylline
hydrocortisone
beta-adrenergic drug
muscle relaxant
sedative
other

---

*Continuous electrocardiographic monitoring.
†Indwelling radial artery catheter with strain gauge.
‡Continuous monitoring with low pressure alarm in inspiratory line (Bunn LT50 Pediatric Alarm System, John Bunn Co., 11035 Walden Avenue, Alden, NY 14004).
§All patients catheterized.

Chapter Fourteen

THE RESPIRATORY DISTRESS SYNDROME OF THE NEWBORN

GEORGE W. BRUMLEY, M.D.,
LILLIAN R. BLACKMON, M.D.

Adaptation from intra-uterine to extra-uterine life is a dramatic and complex event in which the lung undergoes transition from a fluid-filled dormant organ receiving about 10 per cent of fetal cardiac output[1] to an air-filled dynamic organ receiving almost all the cardiac output and responsible for oxygen uptake, carbon dioxide excretion, and indirectly acid-base stability.

When this transition is imperfect the result is either apnea or, more commonly, labored rapid breathing. The latter indicates a wide range of diagnostic possibilities to be considered for the proper choice of therapy. If congenital anomalies of the respiratory system, asphyxia, pneumonia, pneumothorax, aspiration (stomach contents, amniotic fluid, meconium, or blood), delayed resorption of alveolar fluid, and congestive heart failure are ruled out as diagnoses, there remains generalized atelectasis due to incomplete aeration of the lung at birth, to surfactant depletion,[2] or to both. Such labored or distressed breathing with pulmonary atelectasis persisting beyond the immediate newborn period, laboratory evidence of hypoxia, carbon dioxide retention, and metabolic acidosis represents the clinical entity once known as the idiopathic respiratory distress syndrome, and now by the last three words, or their initials, RDS. This is the clinical counterpart of the disease characterized by pathologists as hyaline membrane disease (HMD). Labored breathing from other causes will not be referred to as

From the Department of Pediatrics, Division of Perinatal Medicine, Duke University Medical Center, Durham, North Carolina.

194

RDS in this presentation. Respiratory failure will be used to indicate pulmonary functional inadequacy of any etiology resulting in the accumulation of carbon dioxide ($P_{CO_2} > 65$ mm Hg).

Numerous unproved therapeutic regimens[3] have been proposed for RDS and have confused the physician and often placed the marginally involved infant at greater risk. Current information suggests that such hazards at least can be surmounted, and that survivors not only may have normal lungs but may be comparable to their siblings in intelligence.[4, 5, 6] To achieve this outcome, management must be individualized. The following diagnostic and therapeutic approach is not curative, but attempts to rule out causes of distressed breathing other than RDS and provides compensation and stabilization until spontaneous recovery is possible.

DIAGNOSIS

History and Physical Examination

The majority of infants who develop RDS are less than 38 weeks' gestation and have experienced significant birth asphyxia, with Apgar scores below 7 at 1 and 5 minutes.[7, 8, 9, 10] High risk factors which are frequently noted in the pregnancy history are anemia, antepartum uterine bleeding, and delivery by cesarean section before the onset of labor.[11, 12] Other possible predisposing factors may be maternal diabetes,[13] an infant who is the second born of twins,[14] and a history of RDS in siblings.[15]

The signs and symptoms of increased respiratory work and decreased intrathoracic gas volume are usually apparent from birth and become more severe over the first 4 to 6 hours of life. The classical symptom complex includes tachypnea with respiratory rates of 80 to 100 per minute, intercostal, subcostal, and sub-xyphoid retractions, nasal flaring, sternal in-drawing, and an expiratory grunt. Auscultatory findings vary with age, with fine inspiratory rales and delayed alveolar air entry being characteristic early. Later, decreased and delayed alveolar air entry and progression to tubular breath sounds may occur, indicating more severe impairment of alveolar ventilation. Cyanosis in room air within 4 to 6 hours from birth almost always is seen. Systemic manifestations of the oxygenation deficit commonly are seen, and include temperature instability, hypotension or poor peripheral perfusion or both, decreased urinary output, edema, ileus with abdominal distention, and neurological depression. Without therapeutic intervention to improve oxygenation, these signs worsen and death frequently occurs within 72 hours.

Laboratory Assessment

The infant who persists with distressed breathing after a satisfactory airway and normal body temperature are established requires blood analysis for oxygen and acid-base status. If cyanosis is observed with the infant breathing room air, environmental oxygen sufficient to relieve the cyanosis is first instituted. A percutaneous peripheral arterial sample (either radial or temporal) is preferable. An arterialized capillary sample may be obtained from a warmed finger, heel, or ear lobe. If abnormal values, i.e., pH < 7.20, arterial CO_2 tension (Pa_{CO_2}) > 60 mm Hg, are obtained, or environmental oxygen supplementation is required beyond 2 to 4 hours of age, the umbilical artery is catheterized using an aseptic technique. An Argyle umbilical artery catheter (1980) of an appropriate size (5 French for infants larger than 1500 gm birth weight and 3½ French for infants smaller than 1500 gm birth weight) is inserted into the abdominal aorta to the level of the bifurcation (L4–5 interspace on abdominal x-ray). The appropriate length of catheter to insert is estimated by doubling the distance measured from the base of the umbilicus to an inguinal skin crease with the hips flexed and abducted. The proper placement is confirmed by abdominal x-ray. The umbilical artery catheter permits the frequent sampling required for adequate management of oxygen supplementation and ventilatory support. Though the known complications of an umbilical artery or vein catheter are of low incidence,[16, 17, 18, 19] because of their severity, the use of either solely for the routine administration of parenteral fluids is not justifiable. If the umbilical artery cannot be used, serial radial or temporal artery sampling is feasible; capillary samples may be quite satisfactory for acid-base evaluation, though poor peripheral perfusion of many RDS babies invalidates this source for reliable oxygen sampling. We do not use the femoral artery for blood sampling because of the inherent dangers of this approach.

A moderate degree of asphyxia from compromise in placental blood flow during the last stages of labor normally may produce a pH of 7.20 with respiratory acidosis and Pa_{CO_2} as great as 60 mm Hg. This falls rapidly with the onset of breathing and the pH approaches normal within a few hours. Unless intra-uterine hypoxia is prolonged, the infant at birth has a normal serum bicarbonate level of approximately 21 mEq/L. A bicarbonate level below 17 mEq/L is indicative of a significant reduction in buffering capacity and will result in an acidotic pH unless adequate respiratory compensation occurs. After the first 12 hours, carbon dioxide retention in excess of 45 mm Hg in arterial or arterialized capillary blood is considered abnormal though no therapeutic measures are necessary unless significant acidosis results (pH < 7.30).[20] Oxygen tension in arterial blood should reach 65 mm Hg by 1 hour of age.[21]

If pulmonary atelectasis worsens and ventilation-perfusion imbalance increases, retention of carbon dioxide results in a persistent respiratory acidosis and respiratory failure (Pa_{CO_2} >65 mm Hg) may develop. Larger degrees of atelectasis appear to be responsible for increasing right-left shunts through the parenchyma of the lung.[22] The clinically apparent cyanosis resulting from this admixture correlates well with the low arterial oxygen tension (Pa_{O_2}) found in the presence of added inspired oxygen. Neonatal arterial oxygen levels below 30 mm Hg probably do not provide for adequate tissue oxygenation so that significant amounts of lactic acid are produced from anaerobic glycolysis. The consumption of bicarbonate in buffering this added non-volatile acid produces a metabolic acidosis and compounds the respiratory acidosis already present. The acidosis may be complicated further by the inability of the neonatal kidney to excrete acid and effectively compensate the respiratory acidosis.[23]

Radiographic Examination

A chest x-ray should be obtained in all infants with respiratory distress and respiratory failure, provided the infant can tolerate the stress of the procedure. Irreducible risks of manipulation, hypothermia, and the disruption of oxygen and endotracheal tubes are acceptable, even in the most marginal infant, if a tension pneumothorax, diaphragmatic hernia, or misplaced endotracheal tube are suspected. In such instances, if portable x-ray equipment is not available, the physician should accompany the infant to the x-ray department and be prepared to minimize trauma and resuscitate the patient.

The radiographic differential diagnosis of respiratory distress of Capitano and Kirkpatrick[24] (Table 1) warrants a few added comments. In the immediate neonatal period, the appearance of amniotic fluid aspiration may not differ significantly from that of delayed resorption of alveolar fluid. Both show patchy to diffuse water densities scattered throughout all lung fields, but delayed resorption of alveolar fluid may be characterized further by increased vascular streaking, probably due to lymphatic engorgement of the perivascular spaces as the alveolar fluid is removed from the lung by the lymphatics.[25] Aspiration of meconium usually has been heralded by meconium in the posterior pharynx at birth and substantiated by the findings of perihilar streaking on x-ray and patchy densities suggesting areas of atelectasis. This is true particularly when the meconium in the upper airways was noted to be thick and adequate removal by direct tracheal suction was not accomplished. The hallmark of RDS, diffuse atelectasis, appears as "ground-glass" opacification of peripheral lung fields, upon which is superimposed an air bronchogram. Decreased lung volume may be present as evidenced by elevated diaphragms and narrowed rib spaces.

TABLE 1   **Radiographic Differential Diagnosis of**
Respiratory Distress in the Newborn Infant*

Primary Pulmonary	Non-pulmonary
Abnormalities associated with a shift of the mediastinum	
Cystic adenomatoid malformation	Diaphragmatic hernia or eventration
Agenesis	Hydrothorax
Atelectasis	Pneumothorax
Congenital lobar emphysema	Tumor
Abnormalities not associated with shift of the mediastinum	
Fetal aspiration syndrome	Abnormal thoracic cage
Hemorrhage	Airway obstruction
Hyaline membrane syndrome†	Cardiovascular abnormalities
Pneumonia	
Pulmonary dysmaturity	
Transient tachypnea of the newborn	

*From Capitano, M. A., and Kirkpatrick, J. A., Jr.: Roentgen examination in the evaluation of the newborn infant with respiratory distress. J. Pediatr., 75:896, 1969.
†Usually designated as RDS in this chapter.

The stronger infant with respiratory failure, however, may have an unimpressive x-ray at variance with the biochemical evidence of carbon dioxide retention. The better fixation of the thorax (in the larger infant) appears to permit the development of sufficient transpulmonary pressure to expand the atelectatic lung so that the radiographic evidence of atelectasis may be lacking at maximal inspiration. These findings need not negate other more basic evidence of respiratory failure in RDS.

Other conditions likely to produce parenchymal radiographic changes are pneumonia, marked congestive heart failure, and pulmonary hemorrhage. Although the onset of congestive heart failure in the immediate newborn period is unusual, when present it usually is accompanied by other evidence of cardiac disease. An exception to this is the often normal cardiac size of the infant with infradiaphragmatic total anomalous pulmonary venous drainage. In such instances the radiographic picture of pulmonary vascular engorgement and the evidence of marked right-sided hypertrophy on the electrocardiogram will be of help to properly identify cardiac disease as primary, though the attendant right heart failure also may cause secondary respiratory failure.

TREATMENT

The treatment of RDS is multifaceted and requires constant attention to all of the factors to be discussed. It is important that therapy does not become an iatrogenic source of further insult to the precariously balanced infant. For a detailed discussion of the historical background and recent advances which form the basis of our understanding and treatment of RDS, the reader is referred to a recent review by Farrell and Avery.[26] The current therapy of RDS is directed toward three goals: (1) the alleviation of the oxygenation deficiency, (2) the prevention of progressive atelectasis, and (3) the maintenance of homeostasis of all systems until recovery of normal lung function occurs.

Alleviation of Oyxgenation Deficiency

Tissue hypoxia results in anaerobic metabolism and a precipitous fall in pH as lactic acid is incompletely buffered. Therefore, the development of metabolic acidosis in the absence of other known causes—e.g., bicarbonate wasting in urine, ketoacidosis or exogenous hydrogen ion loading—is direct evidence of inadequate tissue oxygenation. Moreover, anaerobic glycolysis derives only approximately 20 per cent of the potential energy (adenosine triphosphate) from glucose oxidation and the significant quantity of waste heat ordinarily a byproduct of the Krebs cycle is no longer available for temperature maintenance.

Rudolph and Yuan[27] have shown, in newborn calves, that pulmonary vascular resistance increases markedly with a Pa_{O_2} below 50 to 60 mm Hg. This effect was enhanced by concomitant acidosis (pH less than 7.25). Thus, adequate oxygenation in the neonate is important to facilitate cardiopulmonary adaptation by reducing pulmonary arteriolar spasm and inducing closure of the patent ductus arteriosus. Scopes and Ahmed[28] found that the metabolic response to cold stress was blocked at a Pa_{O_2} lower than 50 mm Hg and as a result deep body temperature decreased markedly in the hypoxemic infant. Rigatto and Brady[29] have noted an increase in periodic breathing in otherwise asymptomatic growing preterm infants with a Pa_{O_2} below 60 mm Hg, suggesting a paradoxical depression of the respiratory center. The oxygenation deficiency that characterizes RDS and results from intrapulmonary shunting[22] must be alleviated to reduce the systemic manifestations of hypoxia and avoid death.

Oxygen therapy basically is oriented toward the prevention of anaerobic metabolism and the maintenance of a normal adult circulation. The exact arterial oxygen content that will accomplish these objectives without causing oxygen toxicity is unknown. Usher[30] has suggested that arterial oxygen tensions in excess of 55 mm Hg in infants with RDS cause more severe x-ray changes and right-to-left shunting. Nelson[31] has proposed limiting environmental oxygen to that necessary to maintain the Pa_{O_2} between 40 and 50 mm Hg unless the infant shows worsening systemic symptoms. We are not convinced that the primary pulmonary pathology of RDS results from oxygen toxicity and would prefer to have a larger margin of safety against central nervous system hypoxia. We therefore attempt to maintain the arterial oxygen tension (Pa_{O_2}) of infants under therapy for respiratory failure between 60 and 80 mm Hg.

We advocate the use of oxygen in the delivery room to facilitate cardiopulmonary adaptation for any distressed infant.[32] The continuation of such therapy for more than the immediate few hours postdelivery requires justification, since it is imperative that no infant be given supplemental oxygen indiscriminately, especially for non-pulmonary causes of RDS, e.g., intracranial hemorrhage, sepsis, or hypoglycemia.

Since cyanosis often presents the significant dilemma of cardiac versus pulmonary disease, Table 2, modified from Nelson,[31] may be of value in making this differential. As Nelson aptly points out, the pathology rarely is pure and most often involves mixed cardiopulmonary malfunction.

An important adjunct in supporting tissue oxygenation is the provision of adequate oxygen-carrying capacity. Increasing hemoglobin by 1 gm per 100 ml increases oxygen content by 1.34 ml as compared to increasing the Pa_{O_2} from 10 to 100 mm Hg, which increases the dissolved oxygen volume by only 0.2 ml. It is our practice to record the volume of blood removed for samples and either to replace whole blood on a volume for volume basis or to maintain a hemoglobin of 15 to 16 gm per 100 ml with repeated packed cell transfusions.

The widespread use of oxygen has brought an awareness of its significant potential ophthalmic and pulmonary toxicity. Arterial oxygen tension should be determined at intervals of 4 to 6 hours, or less if indicated, to avoid prolonged exposure to either hypoxia or hyperoxia. In the rare circumstance in which Pa_{O_2} determinations are not available,

TABLE 2   Differentiation of Causes of Hypoxemia*

Defect	Inspired Gas		Oxygen
	Air		
	Pa_{O_2}	Pa_{CO_2}	Pa_{O_2}
Hypoventilation	↓ ↓ ↓	↑ ↑ ↑	→
Diffusion	↓	↓	→
Venous admixture (Veno-arterial shunting)	↓ ↓ ↓	→	↓

*All indications are illustrative, approximate, and refer to pure (rare) rather than mixed (common) defects.
Pa_{O_2} = Arterial oxygen tension.
Pa_{CO_2} = Arterial carbon dioxide tension.
↑ , ↓ ,→ = increase, decrease or no change with respect to normal values.

the inspired oxygen concentrations can be reduced daily until clinical cyanosis is evident and the environmental oxygen then can be increased by 5 to 10 per cent. Oxygen therapy obviously should be terminated as early as possible, i.e., as soon as the Pa_{O_2} is greater than 60 mm Hg in room air or the infant is acyanotic in room air. The American Academy of Pediatrics has recommended that environmental oxygen concentrations be measured at least every 2 hours with an oxygen analyzer calibrated on a daily basis with room air and 100 per cent oxygen.[33]

The drying effect of dehydrated oxygen may be disastrous for the infant with RDS whose cough is often compromised and in whom even the largest airway is obstructed easily by inspissated secretions. Thus, oxygen should be administered fully hydrated at ambient temperature. Warming the hydrated oxygen has the advantage of reducing cold stress to the infant and decreasing free water requirements. There is some evidence to suggest that chilling of the "mask" area of the face leads to increased oxygen consumption,[34, 35] an effect that is undesirable in the infant who has difficulty maintaining adequate oxygen uptake. Overheating the inspired gas, however, may produce restlessness and hyperoxia in the mature infant, especially after the newborn period.

Prevention of Progressive Atelectasis

Studies by Gregory and others have indicated the therapeutic value of continuous positive airway pressure in the management of RDS.[36] Chernick and Vidyasagar[37, 38] showed that continuous negative pressure around the thorax had the same efficacious result with significant improvement in neonatal morbidity. The physiological effects of continuous distending pressure (CDP) have been documented by several workers.[39, 40] These include a prompt increase in oxygenation, an initial brief decrease followed by an increase in lung compliance and minimal change in Pa_{CO_2}. Two controlled studies[41, 42] have suggested that the early use of CDP, either positive or negative, may alter the progression of the disease and shorten the duration of oxygen therapy. However, an increased incidence of air leak with resultant pneumothorax has been reported in infants treated with CDP.[43]

The indications for the initiation of CDP vary with different centers. In general, we begin CDP using the nasal route (similar to the method described by Kattwinkel et al.[44]) when the Pa_{O_2} becomes less than 60 mm Hg in an $F_{I_{O_2}}$* of greater than 50 per cent. Holding the $F_{I_{O_2}}$ constant, a pressure of 6 to 8 cm H_2O is applied. As the oxygenation

---

*$F_{I_{O_2}}$ = Fractional concentration of inspired oxygen.

deficit may decrease precipitously with the addition of CDP, it is necessary to follow arterial oxygen tension closely. With improvement, the Fi_{O_2} is reduced in small increments until near room air and then pressure is decreased. If oxygenation is not improved, pressure is increased stepwise to a maximum of 10 to 12 cm H_2O, and if necessary the Fi_{O_2} is increased. A few patients may require endotracheal intubation for more direct application of the distending pressure to the lung. We prefer to begin mechanical ventilatory assistance at this point rather than increase pressure beyond the aforementioned limit.

The next level of commitment in the care of these infants is to provide ventilatory assistance, a form of therapy which appears to increase the rate of recovery significantly.[45] Responsibility for a ventilatory assistance program is demanding of staff, equipment, and time. The 24-hour availability of well-trained personnel who are familiar with the ventilator to be used and thoroughly aware of the complications of this mode of therapy is an indispensable requirement. Therefore, before initiating mechanical ventilatory assistance the physician must assess carefully the need for ventilatory assistance, and consider whether referral to a better equipped and staffed intensive care nursery is indicated.

The decision to embark upon ventilatory support is prompted by periods of sustained apnea, rising arterial carbon dioxide tension in excess of 65 mm Hg, falling arterial oxygen tension below 50 mm Hg in Fi_{O_2} of greater than 80 per cent, and/or persistent pH below 7.20. At times in marginal patients respirator therapy can be postponed by intermittent periods of manual ventilation with bag and mask or with the nasal prongs of the CDP apparatus. There appears to be no totally satisfactory infant ventilator at present but, in general, there is a preference for volume limitation. Moreover, it must be considered that most if not all present modes of ventilatory support impose some risk of morbidity upon the patient.

At the outset, the method for attaching the ventilator to the patient is critical. The nasal adaptor, face mask, naso- or orotracheal tube and tracheostomy each have virtues and vigorous proponents. We use oral or nasotracheal tubes for the full duration of ventilatory support, if possible, and change subsequently to a tracheostomy if there is evidence of serious trauma to the larynx. Certainly, the most significant problem with endotracheal tubes is their fixation to prevent extubation or inadvertent passage into one of the main stem bronchi with collapse of the contralateral lung. Since right bronchial intubation is the most frequent misplacement, decreased ventilation on auscultation of the left upper lobe or an acute rise in arterial carbon dioxide should alert one to this complication. Not only does this complication worsen respiratory failure, but it also exposes the ventilated lung to significant increased ventilatory pressures with the risk of lung rupture and pneumothorax. Therefore, the fixation of the endotracheal tube must be accomplished by taping, suturing, or whatever means necessary to guarantee its stability. There appears to be no justification for the use of cuffed endotracheal tubes in infants.[46] We have not had any experience with nasal adaptors or face masks, although these methods have received support in recent publications.[47, 48]

Though not suitable for infants weighing less than 1500 gm because of the buffeting imposed upon the patient, the negative pressure type respirator reportedly has been more successful than the positive pressure type in larger infants with respiratory failure. Reports by Stern[49] and Linsao[50] indicate that many infants can be ventilated in this way without intubation and that bacterial contamination of the upper respiratory tract by opportunistic organisms is greatly reduced. The effect of negative pressure ventilation upon intrathoracic structures appears to be significantly different from that of positive pressure ventilators in that it promotes venous return to the right heart. In addition, there is a significant reduction in lung parenchymal complications as compared with positive pressure respirators using similar oxygen concentrations. Beyond these observations, there are few hard data to support one type of ventilator over another. (See also Chapter 11.)

In the choice of a ventilator, the method of humidification also must be assessed. Hydration of the inspired gas frequently is limited by the small tidal volume in the immature infant with RDS. Heated humidification is preferable to nebulization because of the particulate water produced by the latter. Since high levels of water content are possible with nebulizers, care must be taken that condensation in the respirator tubing does not inadvertently drown the patient. Provisions also must be made to monitor and control possible bacterial contamination of such equipment to minimize the hazards of nosocomial infection. Recent reappraisals of the contribution of mist therapy to bronchial hydration suggest that systemic fluid maintenance is a more important variable in minimizing the increased viscosity of secretions than the ventilatory type of hydration unit or water particle size.[51]

Maintenance of Homeostasis

Thermal Environment. Almost all infants who weigh less than 2500 gm or are hypoxic require some method of supplemental temperature support to achieve thermal neutrality (i.e., environmental conditions in which endogenous heat production is minimal) when nursed unclothed. The actual temperature of the neutral thermal environment varies so greatly with weight, gestational age, and postnatal age that no arbitrary rules can be given. For most unclothed infants below 1500 gm (3 lb, 5 oz) birth weight, neutral thermal environment can be provided in an incubator with an air temperature between 90° and 94°

(32° and 35°C), some 20°F above that of delivery room or nursery.[52, 53, 54] Temperature supplement for the infant can be obtained either by convection, as in the usual incubator, or from a radiant heat source, either of which can be servocontrolled. Since provision of such support is rarely adequate in the delivery room, prompt wrapping and early removal to an adequately equipped nursery are important aspects of care. Hyperthermia, which is also a stress, may cause increased oxygen consumption and should be avoided.

Support of Circulation.   Hypotension is a frequent finding in infants with RDS.[55, 56] The pathogenesis may be related to intrapartum blood loss as with placenta previa, to severe asphyxia, or to decreased vascular volume from capillary leak or air block.[57] The Doppler ultrasound method for assessing arterial blood pressure has proved to be efficacious and reliable.[58, 59] We believe blood pressure should be monitored at least at hourly intervals until the infant is stable and at frequent intervals thereafter. The normal values reported by Usher,[60] Kitterman,[61] and Bucci[62] are used in our nursery. When acute blood loss is suspected from the labor history and the infant shows clinical evidence of hypotension, we transfuse blood, 10 to 20 ml per kg, drawn aseptically from the fetal vessels of the placenta into a heparinized syringe. If autotransfusion is not possible and the need for volume expansion appears acute, a solution of 5 per cent albumin in Ringer's lactate is administered, again at 10 to 20 ml per kg. This latter approach is recommended also when capillary leakage is felt to be the cause of the hypotension. Correction of acidosis as outlined further on and relief of air block by closed chest drainage are instituted as indicated. Hypotension is a very serious complicating factor in RDS. Its subtle and insidious influence often is unappreciated unless blood pressure is measured at frequent intervals.

Correction of Acidosis.   There are no specific or reliable clinical signs of acid-base derangements. The physician who treats the infant with RDS or any form of respiratory failure must have access to facilities to determine accurate blood pH, carbon dioxide, and oxygen measurements to permit the proper choice and control of therapy.

In the delivery room a decision must be made as to whether to treat the depressed infant immediately and empirically or to await laboratory results. Under such circumstances, the infant with persistent bradycardia (less than 100 beats per min), cardiac standstill, or unresponsiveness to adequate cardiopulmonary resuscitation can be treated empirically with 1 to 3 mEq of sodium bicarbonate per estimated kg of body weight diluted 1:1 with sterile water. The slow, 5 to 10 minute administration of this therapy into the umbilical vein avoids the delay of umbilical artery catheterization or peripheral vein localization. Such alkali therapy will reduce metabolic acidosis, but not excessively overtreat the infant who has no bicarbonate depletion. There is little evidence that mild metabolic alkalosis is harmful.

In the nursery, the acidosis encountered in the infant with RDS is most often of mixed metabolic and respiratory origin.[55] The focus of treatment is dual: to eliminate the cause and to provide rapid correction when the degree of acidosis is such as to cause compromise of cardiopulmonary function. The management of inadequate tissue oxygenation and perfusion and the resultant metabolic acidosis has been discussed previously, as has the employment of ventilatory assistance to enhance carbon dioxide excretion. Rapid correction of acidemia of a moderate to severe degree, pH less than 7.25, is indicated in the acute circumstance to avert further decompensation and particularly to avoid reflex increase in pulmonary vascular resistance with reversion to right-to-left shunting through fetal channels.[55]

The calculation of the dose of base, either sodium bicarbonate or tris(hydroxymethyl)aminomethane (THAM) is empirical, since only the base deficit of the blood is measurable and in the clinical setting there is seldom a steady state. The use of pH alone to interpret acid-base derangements is inadequate since the pH is the resultant of both pulmonary and renal function. Empirical therapy based upon pH without benefit of carbon dioxide and bicarbonate levels is, therefore, capricious and may seriously complicate subsequent appropriate therapy.

To calculate the bicarbonate dose required to effect base compensation when there is a significant metabolic component, one determines the baseline or "original" pH, Pa_{CO_2}, and serum bicarbonate as represented in Table 3. For the purposes of such calculations, it is assumed that the pulmonary excretion of carbon dioxide will not be altered acutely, and thus pH and bicarbonate are the only variables subject to change. Using the nomogram in Figure 1, the "compensated bicarbonate" is determined by extending a line from the Pa_{CO_2} value, which has remained unchanged, through the desired pH (> 7.30) to intersect with the HCO_3^- line. The difference between the "original" and the

TABLE 3 Derivation of the Total Correcting Dose of Bicarbonate from Data in Figure 1*

Bicarbonate	pH	Pa_{CO_2} mm Hg	HCO_3^- mEq/L
Original (---)	7.10	55	16
Compensated (. . .)	7.30	55	26

*Compensated – Original $\times$ 0.6 body wt (kg) = total correcting dose
bicarbonate   bicarbonate   bicarbonate

(26 mEq − 16 mEq) (0.6) (3.0 kg) = 18 mEq

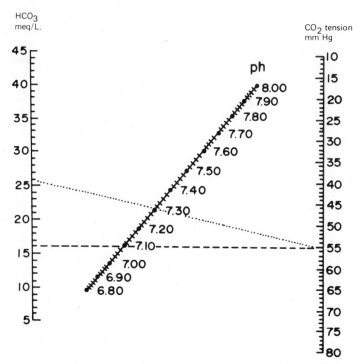

Figure 1. Nomogram derived from the Henderson-Hasselbalch equation. (Modified from McLean, F. C.: Physiol. Rev., *18*:511, 1938.)

"compensated" HCO_3^- is the bicarbonate required per liter total body water to repair or compensate the acidosis as indicated in the equation in Figure 1 for an infant weighing 3.0 kg.

In asphyxiated infants, the size of the bicarbonate space appears to be smaller than that in infants with more chronic types of acidosis, so that the newborn infant with metabolic acidosis of short duration is often overcorrected by formulas assuming the bicarbonate space to relate to body weight in kilograms by a factor of 0.6.[63] To obviate this possible overcorrection of such infants, we prefer to give one-half the correcting dose of alkali and repeat the acid-base measurements in 15 minutes, giving the remainder of the calculated dose if necessary to achieve a pH goal of 7.30 or higher. To diminish the osmotic effect of administering a hypertonic solution, the calculated dose is diluted 1:1 with sterile water and injected slowly over a period of 5 to 10 minutes.

The use of tris(hydroxymethyl)aminomethane (THAM) to correct metabolic acidosis or the mixed acidosis of respiratory distress is warranted in infants in whom prior treatment with sodium bicarbonate has caused hypernatremia. Reportedly, THAM also has the advantage of rapid intracellular penetration and the capacity to buffer non-volatile organic acids as well as carbon dioxide. However, carbon dioxide production renders any buffer ineffectual in the absence of adequate pulmonary function. When indicated, the formula: Body wt (kg) × negative B.E. = ml 0.3 M THAM, taken from Strauss,[64] may be used to calculate the dosage of iso-osmolar (0.3 M) THAM. This formula considers only metabolic acidosis since base excess (B.E.) is, by definition, the titratable base at normal pH, temperature 38°C, and Pa_{CO_2} 40 mm Hg. Therefore, alkalinization for hypercapnia with THAM must be executed in steps of treatment and acid-base assessment until the desired effect is obtained. Except in the presence of hypernatremia, THAM is used infrequently in our nursery and appears to have no significant advantage over bicarbonate.

An often neglected but important effect of such therapy is hyperosmolarity and its influence upon the capillary bed, blood pressure, and cerebrospinal fluid pressure. Recent articles by Finberg[65, 66] indicate the hazards of hyperosmolarity with specific reference to the use of bicarbonate, THAM, and hypertonic glucose so commonly used in resuscitation and the treatment of acid-base derangements. Since hypoxia, an important component of RDS, is certainly a capillary insult, the potential additive effect of hyperosmolarity must be considered and avoided. Simmons and Adcock[67] recently reported a relationship between hypernatremia resulting from repeated dosage with bicarbonate and intraventricular hemorrhage. In accordance with their experience, we attempt to limit the total amount of bicarbonate used in 24 hours to the recommended maximum of 8 mEq/kg. (See also Chapter 20 in this book.)

Fluids and Calories

All neonates require fluid and caloric support from the first hours of life, and the infant with RDS has increased requirements because of the excessive respiratory water losses and caloric consumption associated with the increased work of breathing. Depending on maturity and the degree of respiratory failure, during the first days of life we maintain the infant with more significant RDS on 10 per cent glucose in water at 75 to 100 ml per kg initially, increasing to 120 to 180 ml per kg beyond the third day.[68] This provides 60 or more calories per kilogram as a fat-sparing caloric provision,[69] which may be inadequate with the increased work of breathing. Such fluids, infused through an umbilical artery catheter or preferably a peripheral vein, usually are begun within four hours after birth. With the establishment of good renal function after the first day of life, sodium (20 mEq/L per day), potassium (20 mEq/L per day), and chloride (40 mEq/L per day) should be added to the infusate.[70] Infants who are nursed in open bassinets under radiant heaters have been shown to have marked insensible water losses, as much as 3 to 4 ml/kg/hr for the very small preterm infant.[71] Thus, in infants weighing less than 1500 gm, glucose solution at a rate of 100 to 150 ml per kg may be administered initially with an increase to 200 ml per kg later as dictated by body weight, urine output, and specific gravity.

Because glucose intolerance has been reported in the very immature,[72] a 5 per cent solution of glucose in water probably is preferable for these infants to avoid hypertonicity from hyperglycemia. However, individual glucose requirements are difficult to predict. Blood glucose measurements must be performed frequently and the glucose infusion modified accordingly to maintain a blood level of 50 to 100 mg per 100 ml. If the neonate is to be sustained intravenously for more than 4 days, a comprehensive evaluation of nutritional status must be performed and total intravenous nutrition be considered.[73]

Thoughtful deliberation is required before oral feedings are attempted in the infant with RDS. Not only may paralytic ileus be present as part of the infant's response to his or her attendant metabolic derangements, but also a predisposition for poorly coordinated swallowing and aspiration of stomach contents. Even the tachypnea of the infant with delayed resorption of alveolar fluid or low grade metabolic acidosis may compromise the use of the intestinal tract as a route for hydration and caloric intake. Once the evidence of ileus has subsided, oral feedings may be undertaken cautiously. We prefer to use constant slow infusion via oroduodenal tubes because of the protection this route provides against aspiration and sudden abdominal distention, which often occur with gastric feedings, as well as the marked advantage in achieving an adequate caloric intake. There are reported serious complications with this method of feeding,[74, 75] but these have been infrequent in our experience. In addition, by the use of oroduodenal tube feeding, parenteral alimentation with its inherent risks is avoided.

Monitoring

Many different kinds of equipment are now available for cardiorespiratory, temperature, blood pressure and inspired oxygen monitoring. In our experience, these adjuncts are important and of significant help to the nurse and physician in the provision of factual information and second-to-second assessment of the sick infant. Intradermal electrodes have been used in our nursery to provide low impedance signals for cardiorespiratory monitoring without troublesome skin problems or the false alarms characteristic of surface electrodes. Laboratory support also is required for the frequent micromeasurements of oxygen, acid-base parameters, and electrolytes. While an alert and sufficient staff can substitute for monitoring vital signs, there is no satisfactory replacement for biochemical determinations.

Personnel

When physicians must relinquish the care of the distressed infant to the nursing staff, the ability and number of that staff become a pivotal issue. It is imperative that the physician who is responsible for such infants be informed as to the competence of the personnel and the specific coverage to be provided for the infant in question. Lucey's assessment of the intensive care nursery as a place in which "people care intensely" epitomizes this consideration and appropriately relegates facilities and equipment to their proper, necessary, but subordinate role.[76]

Complications of RDS

Complications associated with RDS and its management are significant both in their number and their influence upon its course; they derive from every aspect of the disease and its treatment and from the prematurity of the patients. The following enumeration illustrates the breadth of these problems and directs the reader to more definitive discussion of each. Anticipation of their development and advance preparation for appropriate therapy are essential to minimize their impact on outcome.

Acute Complications. Acute complications are infection, particularly superimposed pneumonias,[7] intracranial hemorrhage,[77, 78] hyperbilirubinemia,[79] hypocalcemia,[80] air leak with pneumothorax,[81, 82] and acute deterioration due to failure or malfunction of mechanical support systems.[83] Less frequent in occurrence are necrotizing enterocolitis,[84] disseminated intravascular coagulation,[85] patent ductus arteriosus,[86, 87] and pulmonary hemorrhage.[88] The onset of any of these may be gradual or precipitous and the ultimate effect lethal or severely damaging. An essential aspect of the management of the infant with RDS is frequent and repeated assessment by physical examination and by biochemical determinations to detect complications early in their development. Early treatment is critical if a deleterious effect is to be avoided.

Chronic Complications. With the advent of mechanical ventilatory support and the increased survival rate of infants with severe RDS, a syndrome of chronic respiratory insufficiency has been seen with increasing frequency. Northway and others[89] first described the clinical and pathological picture, related the findings to exposure to high oxygen environments, and proposed the term "bronchopulmonary dysplasia" for the disorder. Subsequent reports[90, 91, 92] have confirmed their observations. There continues to be a debate on the relative importance of pulmonary maturity, high oxygen environment, and mechanical positive pressure ventilatory support in the development of this complication. Baro-injury has been most strongly implicated.

Other chronic complications of RDS that have been reported are injury to the larynx and trachea,[93, 94, 95] impairment of somatic growth,[4, 6] mental and neurological handicaps,[4, 6, 96, 97] and propensity to recurrent severe respiratory infections in infancy.[98] Residual abnormality in pulmonary function persisting into childhood has been documented in some survivors.[4, 98-101]

Other Proposed Modes of Therapy

While the treatment presented here admittedly is aimed only at supporting the patient without further insult until spontaneous recovery takes place, various theories of pathogenesis have led to other proposed therapies. To the reader considering such possibilities, we recommend the review of etiological theories and comprehensive bibliography collected by Nelson.[102] It is sufficient to say that results with specific therapies, e.g., aerosolized surfactant[55] and pulmonary vasodilators such as acetylcholine[55, 103] and tolazoline hydrochloride (Priscoline), have not been encouraging. Recovery, which appears to be dependent upon restoration of a normal oxygen and acid-base environment for the lung, adequate pulmonary perfusion, and the recovery of surfactant synthesis, cannot be hastened by known therapy. Pulmonary recovery is usually complete, although the persistent morbidity of some infants who have survived RDS suggests that the ischemic insult may have permanent anatomical effects.

Prediction of RDS

Gluck and associates[104] in 1971 reported the estimation of fetal pulmonary maturity by determining amniotic fluid ratio of lecithin to sphingomyelin. As sphingomyelin concentration remains relatively constant in the amniotic fluid, increase in saturated lecithin, a vital constituent of the pulmonary surfactant, becomes apparent over time by comparison. Previous investigators[105-110] had established phospholipids in amniotic fluid as probably derived from the fetal lung and increasing with gestational age. With the lecithin-sphingomyelin measurement it became possible to predict those fetuses who had achieved maturity and were, therefore, at decreased risk of developing RDS. Subsequently, Clements and co-workers[111] introduced the "shake test," which correlated surfactant concentration in amniotic fluid with the formation of a stable foam. These tests have been evaluated by other investigators and their reliability in predicting RDS confirmed.[112-115] With either method it is now possible to predict the likelihood that a given infant will develop RDS and to plan selective termination of high-risk pregnancy prior to term, but after pulmonary maturation has occurred.

Steroids

A considerable body of laboratory and subsequent clinical information indicates that treatment of the pre-34-week-old fetus with glucocorticoids induces maturation of the lung and reduces the incidence of RDS.[116-121] The application of this therapy prenatally appears to have few complications, and the advantages probably outweigh the potential and as yet unknown hazards. Such treatment, however, must be used only by expert obstetrical and neonatal personnel who can provide the subsequent support required by very immature neonates. Lack of attention to this requirement will negate whatever beneficial effect the fetus receives from steroid therapy.

Conclusion

It has become increasingly evident that the provision of care as outlined here is expensive and requires a highly organized team approach, particularly when mechanical ventilatory support is necessary. The improved outcome both in terms of increased survival and reduced neurological and mental handicap does, in our opinion, justify the tremendous outlay in resources to provide intensive care. Regionalization of facilities for perinatal intensive care provides both conservation of available resources and access of all needful neonates to intensive care. Early recognition of the at risk mother and of the infant in distress, attention to supportive care, and transfer of mother or infant to a perinatal center for management should further decrease the morbidity and mortality of RDS.

REFERENCES

1. Rudolph, A. M.: The changes in the circulation after birth: Their importance in congenital heart disease. Circulation, *41*:343, 1970.
2. Brumley, G. W., Hodson, W. A., and Avery, M. E.: Lung phospholipids and surface

tension correlations in infants with hyaline membrane disease, and in adults. Pediatrics, *40*:13, 1967.

3. Sinclair, J. C.: Prevention and treatment of the respiratory distress syndrome. Pediatr. Clin. North Am., *13*:711, 1966.

4. Stahlman, M., Hedvall, G., Dolanski, E., Foxelius, G., Burko, H., and Kirk, V.: A six-year follow-up of clinical hyaline membrane disease. Pediatr. Clin. North Am., *20*:433, 1973.

5. Stewart, A. L., and Reynolds, E. O. R.: Improved prognosis for infants of very low birth weight. Pediatrics, *54*:724, 1974.

6. Johnson, J. D., Malachowski, N. C., Grobstein, R., Welch, D., Daily, W. J. R., and Sunshine, P.: Prognosis of children surviving with the aid of mechanical ventilation in the newborn period. J. Pediatr., *84*:272, 1974.

7. Cohen, M. M., Weintraub, D. H., and Lilienfeld, A. M.: The relationship of pulmonary hyaline membranes to certain factors in pregnancy and delivery. Pediatrics, *26*:42, 1960.

8. Fisch, R. O., Gravem, H. J., and Engel, R. R.: Neurological status of survivors of neonatal respiratory distress syndrome. A preliminary report from the collaborative study. J. Pediatr., *73*:395, 1968.

9. James, L. S.: Physiology of respiration in newborn infants and in the respiratory distress syndrome. Pediatrics, *24*:1069, 1959.

10. Burns, P. D., Cooper, W. E., and Drose, V. E.: Maternal-fetal oxygen and acid-base studies and their relationship to hyaline membrane disease in the newborn infant. Am. J. Obstet. Gynecol., *82*:1079, 1961.

11. Fedrick, J., and Butler, N. R.: Certain causes of neonatal death. I. Hyaline membranes. Biol. Neonate, *15*:229, 1970.

12. Fedrick, J., and Butler, N. R.: Hyaline membrane disease. Lancet, *2*:768, 1972.

13. Robert, M. F., Neff, R. K., Hubbell, J. P., Taeusch, H. W., and Avery, M. E.: Association between maternal diabetes and the respiratory-distress syndrome in the newborn. N. Engl. J. Med., *294*:357, 1976.

14. Rokos, M. U., Vaeusorn, O., Nachman, R., and Avery, M. E.: Hyaline membrane disease in twins. Pediatrics, *42*:204, 1968.

15. Graven, S. N., and Misenheimer, H. R.: Respiratory distress syndrome and the high risk mother. Am. J. Dis. Child., *109*:489, 1965.

16. Wigger, H. J., Bransilver, B. R., and Blanc, W. A.: Thromboses due to catheterization in infants and children. J. Pediatr., *76*:1, 1970.

17. Egan, E. A., and Eitzman, D. V.: Umbilical vessel catheterization. Am. J. Dis. Child., *121*:213, 1971.

18. Balagtas, R. C., Bell, C. E., Edwards, L. D., and Levin, S.: Risk of local and systemic infections associated with umbilical vein catheterization: A prospective study in 86 newborn patients. Pediatrics, *48*:359, 1971.

19. Symansky, M. R., and Fox, H. A.: Umbilical vessel catheterization: Indications, management and evaluation of the technique. J. Pediatr., *80*:820, 1972.

20. Albert, M. S., and Winters, R. W.: Acid-base equilibrium of blood in normal infants. Pediatrics, *37*:728, 1966.

21. Oliver, T. K., Jr., Demis, A. J., and Bates, G. D.: Serial blood-gas tensions and acid-base balance during the first hour of life in human infants. Acta Paediatr., *50*:346, 1961.

22. Murdock, A. I., Kidd, B. S. L., Llewellyn, M. A., Reid, M. McC., and Swyer, P. R.: Intrapulmonary venous admixture in the respiratory distress syndrome. Biol. Neonate, *15*:1, 1970.

23. Edelmann, C. M., Jr., Soriano, J. R., Boichis, H., Gruskin, A. B., and Acosta, M. I.: Renal bicarbonate reabsorption and hydrogen ion excretion in normal infants. J. Clin. Invest., *46*:1309, 1967.

24. Capitano, M. A., and Kirkpatrick, J. A.: Roentgen examination in the evaluation of the newborn infant with respiratory distress. J. Pediatr., *75*:896, 1969.

25. Avery, M. E., Gatewood, O. B., and Brumley, G. W.: Transient tachypnea of newborn. Possible delayed resorption of fluid at birth. Am. J. Dis. Child., *111*:380, 1966.

26. Farrell, P. M., and Avery, M. E.: Hyaline membrane disease. Am. Rev. Resp. Dis., *111*:657, 1975.

27. Rudolph, A. M., and Yuan, S.: Response of the pulmonary vasculature to hypoxia and H$^+$ ion concentration changes. J. Clin. Invest., *45*:399, 1966.

28. Scopes, J. W., and Ahmed, I.: Indirect assessment of oxygen requirements in newborn babies by monitoring deep body temperature. Arch. Dis. Child., *41*:25, 1966.
29. Rigatto, Henrique, and Brady, June P.: Periodic breathing and apnea in preterm infants. II. Hypoxia as a primary event. Pediatrics, *50*:219, 1972.
30. Usher, R. H.: Liberal versus restricted indications for oxygen in RDS, a controlled trial (abst.). Combined Program and Abstracts, 80th Annual Meeting, American Pediatric Society and the 40th Annual Meeting, Society for Pediatric Research, Atlantic City, New Jersey, April 29–May 2, 1970, p. 83.
31. Nelson, N. M.: Compromised convalescence from hyaline membrane disease. Pediatics, *44*:158, 1969.
32. Klaus, M., and Meyer, B. P.: Oxygen therapy for the newborn. Pediatr. Clin. North Am., *13*:731, 1966.
33. American Academy of Pediatrics: Hospital Care of the Newborn. 5th ed., Evanston, Ill., 1971, pp. 92–94.
34. Mestýan, J., Járai, I., Bata, G., and Fekete, M.: The significance of facial skin temperature in the chemical heat regulation of premature infants. Biol. Neonate, 7:243, 1964.
35. Pribylova, H.: Effect of temperature of inspired air on the metabolic response of the newborn. Rev. Czech. Med., *17*:133, 1971.
36. Gregory, G. A., Kitterman, J. A., Phibbs, R. H., Tooley, W. H., and Hamilton, W. K.: Treatment of the idiopathic respiratory distress syndrome (IRDS) with continuous positive airway pressure (CPAP). N. Engl. J. Med., *284*:1334, 1971.
37. Chernick, V., and Vidyasagar, D.: Continuous negative chest wall pressure in hyaline membrane disease: One year experience. Pediatrics, *49*:753, 1972.
38. Chernick, V.: Continuous negative chest wall pressure therapy. Pediatr. Clin. North Am., *20*:407, 1973.
39. Bancalari, E., Garcia, O., and Jesse, M. J.: Effects of continuous negative pressure on lung mechanics in idiopathic respiratory distress syndrome. Pediatrics, *51*:485, 1973.
40. Wiebe, H., Brooks, J., and Gregory, G. A.: The effect of continuous positive airway pressure on lung function in infants with the respiratory distress syndrome. Pediatr. Res., *9*:402, 1975.
41. Fanaroff, A. A., Cha, C. C., Sosa, R., Crumrine, R. S., and Klaus, M. H.: A controlled trial of continuous negative external pressure in the treatment of severe respiratory distress syndrome. J. Pediatr., *82*:921, 1973.
42. Rhodes, P. G., and Hall, R. T.: Continuous positive airway pressure delivered by face mask in infants with the idiopathic respiratory distress syndrome: A controlled study. Pediatrics, *52*:1, 1973.
43. Chernick, V.: Mechanical ventilation. Iatrogenic Problems in Neonatal Intensive Care. 69th Ross Conference on Pediatric Research, Hilton Head Island. South Carolina, 1975, p. 68.
44. Kattwinkel, J., Fleming, D., Cha, C. C., Fanaroff, A. A., and Klaus, M. H.: A device for administration of continuous positive airway pressure by the nasal route. Pediatrics, *52*:131, 1973.
45. Minkowski, A., Monset-Conchard, M., and Amiel-Tison, C.: Symposium on artificial ventilation. Biol. Neonate, *16*:1, 1970.
46. Sinclair, J. C.: Problems associated with prolonged nasotracheal intubation. Problems of Neonatal Intensive Care Units. 59th Ross Conference on Pediatric Research, Columbus, Ohio, 1969, p. 69.
47. Gruber, H. S., and Klaus, M. H.: Intermittent mask and bag therapy: An alternate approach to respirator therapy for infants with severe respiratory distress syndrome. J. Pediatr., *76*:194, 1970.
48. Helmrath, T. A., Hodson, W. A., and Oliver, T. K., Jr.: Positive pressure ventilation in the newborn infant: The use of a face mask. J. Pediatr., *76*:202, 1970.
49. Stern, L., Ramos, A. D., Outerbridge, E. W., and Beaudry, O. P.: Negative pressure artificial respiration: Use in treatment of respiratory failure of the newborn. Can. Med. Assoc. J., *102*:595, 1970.
50. Linsao, L. S., Levinson, H., and Swyer, P. R.: Negative pressure artificial respiration: Use in treatment of respiratory distress syndrome of the newborn. Can. Med. Assoc. J., *102*:602, 1970.
51. Parks, C. R.: Mist therapy: Rationale and practice. J. Pediatr., *76*:305, 1970.

52. Oliver, T. K., Jr.: Temperature regulation and heat production in the newborn. Pediatr. Clin. North Am., *12*:765, 1965.
53. Scopes, J. W., and Ahmed, I.: Range of critical temperatures in sick and premature newborn babies. Arch. Dis. Child., *41*:417, 1966.
54. Hey, E. N., and Katz, G.: The optimum thermal environment for naked babies. Arch. Dis. Child., *45*:328, 1970.
55. Chu, J., Clements, J. A., Cotton, E. K., Klaus, M. H., Sweet, A. Y., and Tooley, W. H.: Neonatal pulmonary ischemia. Pediatrics (Suppl.), *40*:709, 1967.
56. Neligan, G. A., and Smith, C. A.: The blood pressure of newborn infants in asphyxial states and in hyaline membrane disease. Pediatrics, *26*:735, 1960.
57. Brazy, J. E., and Blackmon, L. R.: Hypotension and bradycardia: associated with airblock in the neonate. To be published.
58. Black, I., Kotrapa, N., and Massie, H.: Application of Doppler ultrasound to blood pressure measurement in small infants. J. Pediatr., *81*:933, 1972.
59. Gordon, L. S., Johnson, P. E., Penido, J. R., Printup, C. A., Dietrick, W. R., and Buggs, H.: Systolic and diastolic blood pressure measurements by transcutaneous Doppler ultrasound in premature infants in critical care nurseries and at closed-heart surgery. Anesth. Analg., *53*:914, 1974.
60. Usher, R.: *In* Silverman, W. A., ed.: Dunham's Premature Infants. New York, Paul B. Hoeber, Inc., 1961, p. 546.
61. Kitterman, J. A., Phibbs, R., and Tooley, W. H.: Aortic blood pressure in normal newborn infants during the first twelve hours of life. Pediatrics, *44*:959, 1969.
62. Bucci, G., Scalamandrè, A., Savignoni, P. G., Mendicini, M., Picece-Bucci, S., and Piccinato, L.: The systemic systolic blood pressure of newborns with low weight. A multiple regression analysis. Acta Paediatr. Scand. (Suppl.), 229, 1972.
63. Palmer, W. W., and Van Slyke, D. D.: Studies on acidosis. IX. Relationships between alkali retention and alkali reserve in normal and pathological individuals. J. Biol. Chem., *32*:499, 1917.
64. Strauss, J.: Tris (hydroxymethyl) amino-methane (Tham): A pediatric evaluation. Pediatrics, *41*:667, 1968.
65. Finberg, L.: Dangers to infants caused by changes in osmolal concentration. Pediatrics, *40*:1031, 1967.
66. Kravath, R. E., Aharon, A. S., Abal, G., and Finberg, L.: Clinically significant physiological changes from rapidly administered hypertonic solutions: acute osmol poisoning. Pediatrics, *46*:267, 1970.
67. Simmons, M. A., Adcock, E. W., III, Bard, H., and Battaglia, F. C.: Hypernatremia and intracranial hemorrhage in neonates. N. Engl. J. Med., *291*:6, 1974.
68. Roy, R. N., and Sinclair, J. C.: Hydration of the low birth-weight infant. Clin. Perinatol., *2*:393, 1975.
69. Krauss, A. N., and Auld, P. A. M.: Metabolic requirements of low-birth-weight infants. J. Pediatr., *75*:952, 1969.
70. Sinclair, J. C., Driscoll, J. M., Jr., Heird, W. C., and Winters, R. W.: Supportive management of the sick neonate: Parenteral calories, water and electrolytes. Pediatr. Clin. North Am., *17*:863, 1970.
71. Wu, P. Y. K., and Hodgman, J. E.: Insensible water loss in preterm infants: Changes with postnatal development and non-ionizing radiant energy. Pediatrics, *54*:704, 1974.
72. Dweck, H. S., and Cassady, G.: Hyperglycemia and very low birth weight. Pediatrics, *53*:189, 1974.
73. Heird, W. C., and Driscoll, J. M., Jr.: Newer methods of feeding low birth weight infants. Clin. Perinatol., *2*:309, 1975.
74. Boros, S. J., and Reynolds, J. W.: Duodenal perforation: A complication of neonatal transpyloric tube feeding. J. Pediatr., *85*:107, 1974.
75. Chen, J. W., and Wong, P. W. K.: Intestinal complications of nasojejunal feeding in low-birth-weight infants. J. Pediatr., *85*:109, 1974.
76. Lucey, J. F.: Closing remarks. Problems of Neonatal Intensive Care Units. 59th Ross Conference on Pediatric Research, Columbus, Ohio, 1969, p. 95.
77. Harrison, V. C., Hesse, H. deV., and Klein, M.: Intracranial hemorrhage associated with hyaline membrane disease. Arch. Dis. Child., *43*:116, 1968.
78. Fedrick, J., and Butler, N. R.: Certain causes of neonatal deaths. II. Intraventricular haemorrhage. Biol. Neonate, *15*:257, 1970.

79. Brown, A. K.: Variations in the management of neonatal hyperbilirubinemia: Impact on our understanding of fetal and neonatal physiology. *In* Bilirubin Metabolism in the Newborn. Birth Defects: Original Article Series, National Foundation—March of Dimes, 6:22, 1970.

80. Tsang, R. C., and Oh, W.: Neonatal hypocalcemia in low birth weight infants. Pediatrics, 45:773, 1970.

81. Kirshner, P. A., and Strauss, L.: Pulmonary interstitial emphysema in the newborn infant, precursors and sequelae: A clinical and pathologic study. Dis. Chest, 46:417, 1964.

82. Thibeault, D., Lachman, R., Laul, V., and Kwong, M.: Pulmonary interstitial emphysema, pneumomediastinum and pneumothorax. Am. J. Dis. Child., 126:611, 1973.

83. Iatrogenic Problems in Neonatal Intensive Care. 69th Ross Conference on Pediatric Research, Hilton Head Island, South Carolina, 1975.

84. Frantz, I. D., L'Heurex, P., Engel, R. R., and Hunt, C. E.: Necrotizing enterocolitis. J. Pediatr., 86:259, 1975.

85. Alstatt, L. B., Dennis, L. H., Sundell, H., Malan, A., Harrison, V., Hedvall, G., Eichelberger, J., Fogel, B., and Stahlman, M.: Disseminated intravascular coagulation and hyaline membrane disease. Biol. Neonate, 19:227, 1971.

86. Kitterman, J. A., Edmunds, L. H., Gregory, G. A., Heymann, M. A., Tooley, W. H., and Rudolph, A. M.: Patent ductus arteriosus in premature infants. Incidence, relation to pulmonary disease and management. N. Engl. J. Med., 287:473, 1972.

87. Thibeault, D. W., Emmanouilides, G. C., Nelson, R. J., Lackman, R. S., Rosengart, R. M., and Oh, W.: Patent ductus arteriosus complicating the respiratory distress syndrome in preterm infants. J. Pediatr., 86:120, 1975.

87a. Editorial: Prostaglandins and the ductus arteriosus. Lancet, 2:837, 1976.

88. Rowe, S., and Avery, M. E.: Massive pulmonary hemorrhage in the newborn. II. Clinical considerations. J. Pediatr., 69:12, 1966.

89. Northway, W. H., Jr., Rosan, R. C., and Porter, D. Y.: Pulmonary disease following respirator therapy of hyaline membrane disease: Bronchopulmonary dysplasia. N. Engl. J. Med., 276:357, 1967.

90. Banarjee, C. K., Girling, D. J., and Wigglesworth, J. S.: Pulmonary fibroplasia in newborn babies treated with oxygen and artificial ventilation. Arch. Dis. Child., 47:509, 1972.

91. Anderson, W. R., and Strickland, M. B.: Pulmonary complications of oxygen therapy in the neonate: Postmortem study of bronchopulmonary dysplasia with emphasis on fibroproliferative obliterative bronchitis and bronchiolitis. Arch. Pathol., 91:506, 1971.

92. Berg, T. J., Pagtakhan, R. D., Reed, M. H., Langston, C., and Chernick, V.: Broncho-pulmonary dysplasia and lung rupture in hyaline membrane disease: Influence of continuous distending pressure. Pediatrics, 55:51, 1975.

92a. Taghizadeh, A., and Reynolds, E. R.: Pathogenesis of bronchopulmonary dysplasia following hyaline membrane disease. Am. J. Pathol., 82:241, 1976.

93. Symchych, P. S., and Cadotte, M.: Squamous metaplasia and necrosis of the trachea complicating prolonged nasotracheal intubation of small newborn infants. J. Pediatr., 71:534, 1967.

94. Hatch, D. J.: Prolonged nasotracheal intubation in infants and children. Lancet, 1:1272, 1968.

95. Rasche, R., and Kuhns, L. R.: Histopathologic changes in airway mucosa of infants after endotracheal intubation. Pediatrics, 50:632, 1972.

96. Reynolds, E. O. R., and Taghizadeh, A.: Improved prognosis of infants mechanically ventilated for hyaline membrane disease. Arch. Dis. Child., 49:505, 1974.

97. Fitzhardinge, P. M.: Early growth and development in low-birthweight infants following treatment in an intensive care nursery. Pediatrics, 56:162, 1975.

98. Outerbridge, E. W., Nogrady, M. B., Beaudry, P. H., and Stern, L.: Idiopathic respiratory distress syndrome. Recurrent respiratory illness in survivors. Am. J. Dis. Child., 123:99, 1972.

99. Westgate, H. D., Fisch, R. O., Langer, L. O., and Staub, H. P.: Pulmonary and respiratory function changes in survivors of hyaline membrane disease. Dis. Chest, 55:465, 1969.

100. Lamarre, A., Linsao, L., Reilly, B. J., Swyer, P. R., and Levison, H.: Residual pulmonary abnormalities in survivors of idiopathic respiratory distress syndrome. Am. Rev. Resp. Dis., 108:56, 1973.

101. Bryan, M. H., Hardie, M. J., Reilly, B. J., and Swyer, P. R.: Pulmonary function studies during the first year of life in infants recovering from the respiratory distress syndrome. Pediatrics, 52:169, 1973.
102. Nelson, N. M.: On the etiology of hyaline membrane disease. Pediatr. Clin. North Am., 17:943, 1970.
103. Moss, A. J., Emmanouilides, G. C., Rettori, O., and Adams, F. H.: Acetylcholine in the treatment of idiopathic respiratory distress syndrome. J. Pediatr., 69:817, 1966.
104. Gluck, L., Kulovich, M., Borer, R., Brenner, P. H., Anderson, G. G., and Spellacy, W. N.: Diagnosis of the respiratory distress syndrome by amniocentesis. Am. J. Obstet. Gynecol., 109:440, 1971.
105. Helmy, F. M., and Hack, M. H.: Comparison of the lipids in maternal and cord blood and of human amniotic fluid. Proc. Soc. Exp. Biol. Med., 110:91, 1962.
106. Adams, F. H., Fujiwara, T., and Rowshan, G.: The nature and origin of the fluid in the fetal lamb lung. J. Pediatr., 63:881, 1963.
107. Adams, F. H., Moss, A. J., and Fagan, L.: The tracheal fluid in the fetal lamb. Biol. Neonate, 5:151, 1963.
108. Adams, F. H., Desilets, D. T., and Towers, B.: Physiology of the fetal larynx and lung. Ann. Otol. Rhinol. Laryngol., 76:735, 1967.
109. Biezenski, J. J., Pomerance, W., and Goodman, J.: Studies of the origin of amniotic fluid lipids. I. Normal composition. Am. J. Obstet. Gynecol., 102:853, 1968.
110. Graven, S. N.: Phospholipids in human and monkey amniotic fluid. Pediatr. Res., 2:318, 1968.
111. Clements, J. A., Platzker, A. C. G., Tierney, D. F., Hobel, C. J., Creasy, R. K., Margolis, A. J., Thibeault, D. W., Tooley, W. H., and Oh, W.: Assessment of the risk of the respiratory distress syndrome by a rapid test for surfactant in amniotic fluid. N. Engl. J. Med., 286:1077, 1972.
112. Bhagwanni, S. G., Fahmy, D., and Turnbull, A. C.: Bubble stability test compared with lecithin assay in prediction of respiratory distress syndrome. Br. Med. J., 1:697, 1973.
113. Boehm, F. H., Srisupundit, S., and Ishii, T.: Lecithin/sphingomyelin ratio and a rapid test for surfactant in amniotic fluid. A comparision. Obstet. Gynecol., 41:829, 1973.
114. Merola, J. C. L., Johnson, L. M., Bolognese, R. J., and Corson, S. L.: Determination of fetal pulmonary maturity by amniotic fluid lecithin/sphingomyelin ratio and rapid shake test. Am. J. Obstet. Gynecol., 119:243, 1974.
115. Mukherjee, T. K., Rajegowada, B. K., Glass, L. L., Auerbach, J., and Evans, H. E.: Amniotic fluid shake test versus lecithin/sphingomyelin ratio in the antenatal prediction of respiratory distress syndrome. Am. J. Obstet. Gynecol., 119:648, 1974.
116. DeLemos, R. A., Shermata, D. W., Knelson, J. H., Kotas, R., and Avery, M. E.: Acceleration of appearance of pulmonary surfactant in the fetal lamb by administration of corticosteroids. Am. R. Resp. Dis., 102:459, 1970.
117. Kotas, R. V., Fletcher, B. D., Torday, J., and Avery, M. E.: Evidence for independent regulators of organ maturation in fetal rabbits. Pediatrics, 47:57, 1971.
118. DeLemos, R. A., and McLaughlin, G. W.: Induction of the pulmonary surfactant in the fetal primate by intrauterine administration of corticosteroids. Pediatr. Res., 7:425, 1973.
119. Farrell, P. M., and Zachman, R. D.: Induction of choline phosphotransferase and lecithin synthesis in the fetal lung by corticosteroids. Science, 179:297, 1973.
120. Liggins, G. C., and Howie, R. N.: A controlled trial of antepartum glucocorticoid treatment for prevention of the respiratory distress syndrome in premature infants. Pediatrics, 50:515, 1972.
121. Lung Maturation and the Prevention of Hyaline Membrane Disease. 70th Ross Conference on Pediatric Research, Dorado Beach, Puerto Rico, 1975. In press.

Chapter Fifteen

THE BLEEDING NEONATE

BERTIL E. GLADER, PH.D., M.D.,
GEORGE R. BUCHANAN, M.D.

Serious and often life-threatening hemorrhages commonly occur in neonates, particularly in large intensive care nurseries which care for low birth weight infants. We describe here a practical clinical approach to the diagnosis and management of the varied and unique causes of neonatal bleeding. More detailed information regarding pathophysiology can be found in other currently available reviews.[1-5]

NORMAL NEONATAL HEMOSTASIS

Normal hemostasis depends on the cooperative interaction of platelets, which adhere to subendothelial surfaces and aggregate to form small plugs, and soluble plasma proteins, which react in an orderly sequence leading to the deposition of a fibrin clot (Fig. 1). Generalized bleeding may result whenever a qualitative or quantitative abnormality of platelets or clotting proteins is present. During the newborn period, developmental abnormalities in certain hemostatic components can be associated with an increased propensity to hemorrhage in infants. For example, the cord blood content of vitamin K–dependent clotting factors (II, VII, IX, and X) is reduced to between 30 and 70 per cent of the mean values in older children, and generally the activity of these factors is lower in prematures than in term infants. During the first few days of life the concentration of vitamin K–dependent factors decreases even further, although this postnatal decrease largely can be

From the Department of Pediatrics, Harvard Medical School, and the Division of Hematology, Children's Hospital Medical Center, Boston, Mass. 02115.

Research supported by the Medical Foundation, Inc., USPHS grant 5-T01-AM-05581, and the Children's Hospital Medical Center Clinical Research Center USPHS grant FR-00128. Dr. Glader is a recipient of a Research Career Development Award (AM-00156) from the National Institutes of Health.

217

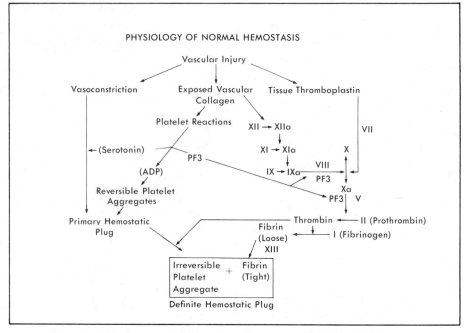

PHYSIOLOGY OF NORMAL HEMOSTASIS

Figure 1. This figure summarizes the role of platelets and clotting factors in the production of the hemostatic plug following vascular injury. Abbreviations: PF3 = platelet factor 3; ADP = adenosine diphosphate.

prevented by prophylactic vitamin K administration at birth. In premature infants, however, transient hepatic immaturity may cause a less than optimal response to vitamin K administration. The clotting factors not dependent on vitamin K for their "activation" are either normal (fibrinogen, V, VIII) or only mildly reduced (XI, XII, XIII). Platelet counts in term and premature newborns are the same as in older children (Table 1). Neonatal platelet function (measured *in vitro* by platelet aggregometry) may be transiently abnormal,[6, 7] but this impairment is of questionable clinical significance since the bleeding time (an *in vivo* measure of platelet function) is normal.[6]

APPROACH TO THE BLEEDING INFANT

History and Physical Examination. The pediatrician confronted with a bleeding infant must carefully assess the total clinical setting, since the history and physical examination can be as diagnostically useful as any laboratory test. Important historical information includes familial bleeding problems, maternal illnesses (especially infections), drug administration (maternal and neonatal), and documentation that vitamin K was given at birth. The general observation of whether an infant is "sick" or "well" at the onset of bleeding also is an important diagnostic key. Certain hemorrhagic disorders, such as disseminated intravascular coagulation (DIC), occur almost exclusively in "sick" infants (babies with sepsis, hypoxia, acidosis, hepatosplenomegaly, hypoglycemia, or problems related to prematurity). On the other hand, bleeding manifestations in otherwise "well" infants (normal birth weight, alert, vigorous, and without hepatosplenomegaly, hypoxia, or evidence of systemic disease) usually are due to immune-mediated thrombocytopenia, classic hemorrhagic disease of the newborn (vitamin K deficiency), or isolated clotting factor deficiencies. The physical examination further defines the nature of the bleeding disorder. Normal infants may have petechiae over presenting parts secondary to venous congestion and the trauma of delivery. These petechiae are seen shortly after birth, but they gradually disappear and are not associated with bleeding. On the other hand, generalized petechiae, small superficial ecchymoses, and mucosal bleeding suggest a platelet abnormality, most commonly thrombocytopenia. Larger ecchymoses, some forms of localized bleeding (cephalohematomas, umbilical cord bleeding, gastrointestinal hemorrhage) or diffuse bleeding from several sites (skin, mucous membranes, venipuncture sites) usually are associated with a generalized coagulation disturbance due to vitamin K deficiency, DIC, or liver disease.

Laboratory Evaluation.   The etiology of bleeding usually can be ascertained by simple diagnostic tests (Table 1). (1) *Platelet counts* are measured directly or estimated from the peripheral blood smear (platelet count = average number of platelets per oil immersion field × 15,000). Platelet counts are the most helpful of the simple laboratory tests available, since most neonates with serious bleeding problems are

TABLE 1   Normal Values for Screening Laboratory Tests in the Neonate

	Premature Infant	Term Infant	Child over 1–2 mo of Age
Platelet count (μl)	150,000–400,000	150,000–400,000	150,000–400,000
Platelets on peripheral blood smear	10–20 platelets per oil immersion field, including one or two small clumps	Same	Same
Prothrombin time (PT) (sec)*	14–22	13–20	12–14
Partial thromboplastin time (PTT) (sec)*	35–55	30–45	23–35
Fibrinogen (mg/100 ml)	150–300	150–300	150–300

*Normal values may vary from laboratory to laboratory, depending on the particular reagents employed.

In full term infants who have received vitamin K, PT and PTT values generally fall within the normal "adult" range by several days (PT) to several weeks (PTT) of age. Small premature infants (under 1500 gm) tend to have longer PT and PTT's than larger babies.

thrombocytopenic. Common causes of thrombocytopenia include increased destruction (DIC, infection, immune thrombocytopenia), sequestration in an enlarged spleen, and removal from the circulation following exchange transfusion (blood over several hours old has few platelets). Thrombocytopenia caused by decreased platelet production (aplastic anemia, leukemia) rarely is seen during the newborn period. Significant bleeding from decreased platelets generally is associated with platelet counts less than 30,000 per μl. (2) *Prothrombin time* (PT) is a test of the extrinsic clotting cascade (factors VII, X, V, II, and fibrinogen). (3) *Activated partial thromboplastin time* (PTT) is a measure of the intrinsic clotting system (factors XII, XI, IX, VIII, X, V, II, and fibrinogen). (4) *Fibrinogen* can be determined on the same plasma sample as the PT and PTT. Other laboratory tests, such as fibrin split products, specific factor assays, platelet aggregation, and bleeding time rarely are necessary for diagnosis and therapy in bleeding infants. Two important variables must be considered when collecting venous blood for neonatal coagulation studies. First, the ratio of blood to anticoagulant (3.8 per cent sodium citrate) should be 19:1.[8] The usual ratio (9:1) may give spurious results in neonates with hematocrits over 60 per cent. Secondly, blood should not be drawn from heparinized catheters since even minute amounts of this anticoagulant can prolong the PTT.

Blood Components Used in Therapy of Bleeding Infants

PLATELET TRANSFUSIONS. A unit of platelets is defined as that number of platelets obtained from 1 unit of blood. Platelets are suspended in plasma, approximately 1 unit of platelets in 15 to 30 ml plasma. The administration of 1 unit of platelets to a neonate generally elevates the platelet count to well over 100,000 per μl. Subsequently, the platelet count should decline slowly over 8 to 10 days. Failure of a neonate to sustain a platelet increase indicates increased platelet destruction (sepsis, DIC, antiplatelet antibody).

FRESH FROZEN PLASMA. Plasma which is frozen and stored immediately after separation contains adequate concentrations of all clotting factors. Fresh frozen plasma (10 to 15 ml/kg) given every 12 hours provides adequate hemostasis for most causes of bleeding due to lack of clotting factors. Whenever coagulation factors and platelets are given at the same time, the volume of platelet concentrate (largely plasma) needs to be included in calculating plasma therapy.

CLOTTING FACTOR CONCENTRATES. Patients with factor VIII deficiency (classical hemophilia) or factor IX deficiency (Christmas disease) require high factor levels in rare cases of severe bleeding. In order to avoid problems with fluid overload, concentrated factor preparations should be employed.

TABLE 2 Differential Diagnosis of Bleeding in the Neonate

Clinical Evaluation	Laboratory Studies			Likely Diagnosis
	Platelets	PT	PTT	
"Sick"	↓	↑	↑	DIC
	↓	N	N	Platelet consumption (infection, necrotizing enterocolitis, renal vein thrombosis)
	N	↑	↑	Liver disease
	N	N	N	Compromised vascular integrity (associated with hypoxia, prematurity, acidosis, hyperosmolality)
"Healthy"	↓	N	N	Immune thrombocytopenia Occult infection or thrombosis Bone marrow hyperplasia (rare)
	N	↑	↑	Hemorrhagic disease of newborn (vitamin K deficiency)
	N	N	↑	Hereditary clotting factor deficiencies
	N	N	N	Bleeding due to local factors (trauma, anatomical abnormalities) Qualitative platelet abnormalities (rare) Factor XIII deficiency (rare)

FRESH WHOLE BLOOD. This therapy is used for exchange transfusion as well as to replace volume losses associated with severe hemorrhage. Banked whole blood more than 12 hours old contains few platelets and decreased quantities of labile clotting factors (V and VIII); packed red blood cells are devoid of platelets as well as significant amounts of clotting proteins. Therefore, fresh whole blood should be used in conditions in which hemostasis, as well as RBC replacement, is a goal. Alternatively, packed RBC's, fresh plasma, and platelet concentrates can be given if fresh whole blood is not available.

A differential diagnosis of bleeding in newborn infants is presented in Table 2. This classification is based on clinical evaluation (sick or healthy infants) and simple laboratory tests (platelet counts, PT, PTT).

BLEEDING IN SICK NEONATES

Disseminated Intravascular Coagulation (DIC)

DIC, which probably occurs to some extent in all sick infants, represents an inappropriate activation of the clotting process.[9, 10] A number of "trigger" mechanisms (hypoxia, acidosis, tissue necrosis, infection, and endothelial injury) result in the utilization and consumption of clotting factors and platelets. This leads to a variety of clinical consequences, the most common of which is diffuse bleeding due to severe depletion of hemostatic elements. Thrombosis with necrosis, organ dysfunction, and microangiopathic hemolytic anemia also can be seen. Infants with DIC invariably are sick and symptoms of the underlying condition (shock, bacterial sepsis, asphyxia) often overshadow the bleeding manifestations. The diagnosis of clinically significant DIC is suggested by moderate to severe thrombocytopenia and a prolonged PT and PTT which are unresponsive to parenteral vitamin K. Decreased fibrinogen and the presence of fragmented red blood cells on the peripheral smear also may be seen. Specific measurement of fibrin split products or consumable factors usually is not needed in order to arrive at the diagnosis.

There is general agreement that successful management of infants with DIC depends on effective removal of conditions which "trigger" the coagulation process. The most important therapeutic considerations thus are directed at the control of infection, hypoxia, acidosis, and hypotension. Extremely ill infants who are actively bleeding from multiple sites and whose clotting study measurements become increasingly abnormal also should receive specific therapy for the hemorrhagic disorder. There is little consensus, however, regarding what form of specific therapy to employ.

Our approach is to administer fresh platelet concentrates (1 unit every 12 to 24 hours) and fresh frozen plasma (10 to 15 ml/kg body weight every 12 to 24 hours). In some infants receiving large volumes of these blood products it is necessary to adjust the volume of other administered fluids. It has been said that platelet and plasma transfusions without concomitant heparin may add "fuel to the fire" and accelerate thrombosis.[11] In our experience, however, this has not been the case, and frequently we see clinical improvement following this conservative approach. This occurs despite the fact that consumption of platelets and clotting factors continues unabated. The beneficial effects of these measures are only transient and transfusion support may be necessary for a number of days. The ultimate correction of DIC depends on rectifying the underlying process.

In those infants who continue to bleed after platelet and plasma transfusions, other forms of therapy such as exchange transfusion are considered. Exchange transfusion is a rational approach which provides clotting factors and platelets, and it may remove fibrin degradation products and some of the toxic factors causing DIC.[12] In addition, adult red blood cells have a lower oxygen affinity than neonatal RBC's, and this may reduce the tissue damage due to hypoxia. Heparin also is useful as a means of arresting the consumptive process, and isolated reports suggest that the response to heparin may be dramatic. In our experience, however, heparin dosage and effects are difficult to monitor and one is never certain whether persistent hemorrhage is due to excessive or insufficient heparinization. Furthermore, heparin does not prolong survival in experimental models of DIC,[13] and it has been demonstrated that heparin fails to improve survival[14] or even reduce hemorrhage[15] in older patients with DIC. We use heparin primarily in those infants with DIC characterized by marked thrombosis, such as gangrenous necrosis of the skin (purpura fulminans). In these cases, in which increased fibrin deposition is not associated with compensatory fibrinolysis, heparin is administered in doses of 10 to 15 units per kg body weight per hour as a continuous infusion. Once the infant is heparinized, plasma and platelet transfusions are continued until there is evidence of a beneficial response (i.e., cessation of thrombus formation). (See also Chapter 22 in this book.)

Hemorrhage Secondary to Platelet Consumption in Sick Neonates

Diffuse bleeding that is clinically indistinguishable from DIC occasionally is seen in sick thrombocytopenic infants in whom the PT and PTT are normal. Hemorrhage due to thrombocytopenia in these cases is secondary to increased destruction of circulating platelets. In contrast to immune thrombocytopenias, which also are characterized by rapid platelet consumption (see further on), infants in this category generally are very sick. Commonly the underlying pathology is thrombosis (renal vein thrombosis, necrotizing enterocolitis) or infection. Corrigan has demonstrated that bacterial septicemia may be associated with bleeding and thrombocytopenia in the absence of evidence for DIC.[16] Thrombocytopenia also is a common manifestation of intrauterine viral and protozoal infections, and, in these cases, decreased platelet production may combine with increased consumption to cause thrombocytopenia. As a general rule, occult infection should be suspected in any ill neonate with unexplained thrombocytopenia. Therapy for these infants obviously is directed at the underlying pathology. Platelet transfusions should be given if there is a definite bleeding tendency or if platelets are less than 10,000 per μl.

Bleeding Due to Liver Disease

The liver synthesizes nearly all clotting factors and thus it is not surprising that severe liver disease commonly is associated with a generalized hemorrhagic diathesis.[17] The PTT and PT are prolonged, but in contrast to hemorrhagic disease of the newborn (see further on), there is little or no response to vitamin K administration. Fibrinogen levels frequently are depressed and other evidence of liver disease usually is present (hepatomegaly, direct hyperbilirubinemia, elevated serum transaminase). Effective therapy in the presence of severe liver disease is difficult because the underlying diseases are serious, and DIC or splenic sequestration of platelets may contribute to the hemorrhagic tendency. Treatment consists of vitamin K and fresh whole blood or fresh frozen plasma.

Bleeding in Sick Neonates with Normal Platelets, PT, and PTT

Sick neonates, particularly prematures, often have serious pulmonary and central nervous system hemorrhage, the pathophysiology of which is not clearly defined. Frequently there is laboratory evidence of DIC, but in many cases no hemostatic abnormalities are detected.[3] Local factors such as hypoxia, acidosis, and hyperosmolality presumably compromise vascular integrity and lead to bleeding. In the absence of coagulation abnormalities, plasma and platelet transfusions are not useful, and therapy must be directed at the underlying pathological processes. These serious hemorrhages, however, generally are refractory to most forms of therapy.

BLEEDING IN APPARENTLY HEALTHY NEONATES

Immune Thrombocytopenias

These disorders are characterized by petechiae, ecchymoses, and mucosal bleeding in healthy, vigorous neonates within the first 48 hours of life. The PT and PTT are normal, but the platelet count is markedly reduced. Thrombocytopenia is secondary to transplacental passage of maternal IgG antibody which coats the infant's platelets and leads to their premature destruction by reticuloendothelial cells. Two general forms of immune-mediated platelet destruction are recognized: isoimmune thrombocytopenia and thrombocytopenia secondary to maternal disease.

Isoimmune Thrombocytopenia.   This is analogous to erythroblastosis due to ABO or Rh incompatibility in that the infant's platelets contain an antigen (inherited from father) which is lacking on maternal platelets.[18] During gestation, fetal platelets enter the maternal circulation and stimulate antiplatelet antibody production. The antibody in the majority of cases is directed against the PLA–1 antigen (infant positive, mother negative), while antibodies against various HL–A antigens are responsible for the remainder. It should be noted that *in vitro* diagnostic tests which specifically type platelet antigens are not readily available, and the diagnosis of this disorder usually must be based on clinical grounds and simple laboratory tests. The key diagnostic feature is isolated thrombocytopenia in a healthy neonate whose mother has a normal platelet count and a negative medical history and physical examination.

Most neonates with isoimmune thrombocytopenia have no major clinical problems.[19] Nevertheless, significant bleeding can occur within hours after birth, and serious intracranial hemorrhages have been seen. For this reason, we believe that infants with isoimmune thrombocytopenia should receive definitive treatment in the presence of significant thrombocytopenia (platelets less than 30,000 per μl). The most effective form of therapy is transfusion of platelets lacking the offending antigen (i.e., maternal platelets).[20] Following this, the platelet count generally increases (100,000 to 150,000 per μl), bleeding ceases, and transfused platelets survive normally (6 to 8 days). Administration of random donor platelets usually is not effective since 97 per cent of the general population have the platelet antigen (PLA–1 positive) to which maternal antibody is directed. Corticosteroid administration and exchange transfusions to remove antibody have been advocated in the past,[21] but now it generally is agreed that the most effective therapy consists of maternal plateletpheresis (a procedure which can be undertaken by most blood banks) and transfusion of these platelets into affected infants.[19] In most cases a single platelet transfusion is sufficient, although a second infusion occasionally is required to sustain a platelet increase. Following a good response to maternal platelet transfusions, thrombocytopenia may occur 5 to 7 days post-transfusion. Bleeding rarely is seen at this time and additional platelet transfusions usually are unnecessary. Platelet counts may remain depressed for 2 to 8 weeks until passively transferred antibody is catabolized.

In contrast to Rh sensitization, first-born infants frequently suffer from isoimmune thrombocytopenia. Furthermore, the recurrence rate in subsequent pregnancies is very high (up to 85 per cent). The currently available *in vitro* tests to detect whether a given fetus is affected unfortunately are of little prognostic value. Therefore, to prevent possible intracranial hemorrhage during delivery, we advocate elective cesarean section for mothers who previously have had infants with isoimmune thrombocytopenia.

Immune Thrombocytopenia Secondary to Maternal Disease. This differs from the isoimmune variety in that the offending antibody is directed against antigens common to all platelets. Invariably there is maternal thrombocytopenia, while the neonate is affected to the extent that antibody crosses the placenta and interacts with fetal platelets. The reasons for decreased platelets in the mother are as varied as the causes of adult immune thrombocytopenia (e.g., idiopathic, systemic lupus erythematosus). The likelihood of a child developing thrombocytopenia is determined in large part by the state of maternal disease.[22] If the mother had immune thrombocytopenia in the past, but now has a normal platelet count, there is a low probability that her infant will develop thrombocytopenia. On the other hand, a low maternal platelet count increases the likelihood of neonatal thrombocytopenia. The clinical features of infants with this disorder are virtually identical to those with isoimmune thrombocytopenia. The prognosis usually is good, and significant bleeding beyond the first few days of life is most unusual.[19] Steroids (prednisone 2 mg/kg/day) are given to infants with platelet counts less than 10,000, or those who show any evidence of bleeding. Therapy should be limited to the first 2 weeks of life, since this is the period of greatest risk for severe hemorrhage. In contrast to isoimmune thrombocytopenia, platelet transfusions have little role in the management of these patients since the antiplatelet antibody usually is directed against a "public antigen" present on all platelets. Nevertheless, in the presence of life-threatening hemorrhage, platelet transfusions or exchange transfusion followed by administration of platelets, should be attempted.

Hemorrhage Due to Nonimmune Thrombocytopenia in Healthy Neonates

Some of the same causes of thrombocytopenia responsible for bleeding in sick infants also apply to apparently healthy neonates. In particular, occult infection or localized thrombosis should be considered. Rarely, thrombocytopenia due to bone marrow hypoplasia (leukemia, aplastic anemia) or hereditary defects in platelet production can cause bleeding in the newborn period. Despite earlier reports to the contrary, thiazides probably do not cause neonatal thrombocytopenia.

Hemorrhagic Disease of the Newborn

Newborn infants lack vitamin K stores, and unless the vitamin is given at birth, a marked deficiency of factors II, VII, IX, and X may ensue within the first few days of life. Premature infants, particularly, are prone to develop factor deficiency because of transient hepatic immaturity. Hemorrhagic disease of the newborn classically occurs at 2 to 4 days of age and is manifested by cutaneous, umbilical, gastrointestinal or central nervous system hemorrhage. Unless there is massive blood loss or shock, however, these babies appear well. The prolonged PT and PTT reflects defects in both intrinsic and extrinsic clotting systems. Treatment consists of a single dose of intravenous vitamin K (Aquamephyton, 1.0 mg). The response to therapy is a dramatic cessation of bleeding and correction of laboratory abnormalities within 4 to 6 hours. Transfusion with fresh frozen plasma or vitamin K-dependent factor concentrates (Proplex or Konyne) can be used for life-threatening hemorrhages, but this form of therapy rarely is necessary.

Bleeding due to vitamin K deficiency is generally preventable by prophylactic intramuscular administration of the vitamin at birth. The most common cause of neonatal hemorrhagic disease is inadvertent failure to administer the vitamin. For this reason, bleeding infants who meet the clinical and laboratory criteria of this disorder should be given intravenous vitamin K, even if the vitamin reportedly was given earlier. Infants born to mothers receiving medication known to impair vitamin K function (coumarin anticoagulants, hydantoin anticonvulsants) also may hemorrhage, even at the time of birth. In addition, neonates (especially prematures) receiving total parenteral alimentation without vitamin K supplementation can bleed, but this can be prevented by prophylactic administration of vitamin K (0.5 mg intramuscularly each week).

Hereditary Clotting Factor Deficiencies

Hemophilia A (deficiency of factor VIII coagulant activity), hemophilia B or Christmas disease (deficiency of factor IX), and von Willebrand's disease (deficiency of factor VIII protein and coagulant activity) constitute over 99 per cent of all hereditary clotting factor deficiencies. Neonatal bleeding due to von Willebrand's disease is extremely rare, if it occurs at all. Furthermore, as Baehner and Strauss have observed,[23] bleeding in the neonatal period is unusual in classical hemophilia and Christmas disease. The well-known muscle and joint hemorrhages characteristic of older hemophiliacs do not begin until infants start to crawl and walk. Nevertheless, hereditary clotting factor deficiencies must be considered when bleeding occurs in healthy-appearing neonates, usually male, in whom a prolonged PTT is the only coagulation abnormality. Definitive diagnosis ultimately requires a specific assay of coagulation factors. Both factors VIII and IX can be evaluated in the newborn period since maternal clotting factors do not cross the placenta. Factor IX activity in neonates is transiently depressed, but this minimal decrease usually does not obscure the diagnosis of Christmas disease in the infant who has received supplemental vitamin K. Significant bleeding in the newborn period most commonly presents following circumcision. For minimal bleeding, fresh frozen plasma and local measures (pressure, topical thrombin) usually are sufficient while appropriate factor concentrates should be employed in those rare cases of severe life-threatening hemorrhages. The desired level of plasma factor activity depends on the severity of the clinical condition (for details see Donaldson and Kisker, and Abildgaard).[24, 25]

Bleeding in Healthy Neonates with Normal Platelets, PT, and PTT

The most common hemorrhages seen in healthy neonates are due to local vascular factors and are not associated with detectable hemostatic abnormalities. For example, birth trauma commonly causes bruises and petechiae in healthy infants with no underlying coagulation defect. Also the extensive blood loss seen with gastrointestinal hemorrhages usually is due to local anatomical factors or swallowed maternal blood as detected by the Apt test.[26] This simple procedure distinguishes gastrointestinal blood loss due to neonatal hemorrhage or swallowed maternal blood:

1. Mix 1 volume of stool or vomitus with 5 volumes of water.
2. Centrifuge mixture, and separate clear pink supernatant (hemolysate).
3. Add 1 ml 1 per cent NaOH to 4 ml hemolysate. Mix and observe color change after 2 minutes. Hemoglobin A changes from pink to yellow-brown color (this indicates maternal blood). Hemoglobin F resists denaturation and remains pink (this indicates fetal blood).

Gastrointestinal bleeding seldom (10 to 15 per cent of cases) is associated with platelet or coagulation abnormalities.[27]

A few rare coagulation disorders also must be considered in this group of infants. (1) Hereditary deficiency of factor XIII (fibrin-stabilizing factor) does not cause abnormal screening tests, but rarely may produce clinically significant hemorrhage due to the presence of a friable clot. Characteristically, the umbilical stump begins to ooze at 24 to 48 hours of age, after a period of apparently adequate hemostasis. The definitive diagnosis, which requires a specialized coagulation laboratory, is made by demonstrating that the infant's fibrin clot is soluble in 5 M urea.[28] In suspected cases of factor XIII deficiency, local measures are employed for mild bleeding while fresh frozen plasma is used for more severe hemorrhage. (2) Qualitative platelet defects (due to drugs or intrinsic platelet disorders) are rare causes of neonatal bleeding. The diagnosis of these entities is suggested by a prolonged bleeding time in the presence of an adequate number of platelets. *In vitro* platelet aggregation studies, if available, also are abnormal. Bleeding due to qualitative platelet abnormalities generally responds to platelet transfusions.

SUMMARY

Serious bleeding episodes in newborn infants usually can be diagnosed following careful clinical assessment and a few simple laboratory tests. Certain conditions are found almost exclusively in "sick" infants, whereas other coagulation abnormalities occur in otherwise "healthy" neonates. Successful management of hemorrhage necessitates a correct diagnosis which thereby dictates appropriate therapy. In some cases, such as in DIC, successful outcome ultimately depends on correction of the underlying pathophysiology which triggered the coagulation disturbance.

REFERENCES

1. Oski, F. A., and Naiman, J. L.: Hematologic Problems in the Newborn. Philadelphia, W. B. Saunders Co., 1972.
2. Hathaway, W. E.: The bleeding newborn. Semin. Hematol., *12*:175, 1975.
3. Chessells, J. M., and Hardisty, R. M.: Bleeding problems in the newborn infant. Progr. Hemostasis Thromb., *2*:333, 1974.
4. Glader, B. E.: Bleeding disorders in the newborn infant. *In* Shaffer, A. J., and Avery. M. E., eds.: Diseases of the Newborn. 4th ed., Philadelphia, W. B. Saunders Co., 1977.
5. Bleyer, W. A., Hakami, N., and Shepart, T. H.: The development of hemostasis in the human fetus and newborn infant. J. Pediatr., *69*:838, 1971.
6. Mull, M. M., and Hathaway, W. E.: Altered platelet function in newborns. Pediatr. Res., *4*:229, 1970.
7. Corby, D. G., and Schulman, I.: The effects of antenatal drug administration on aggregation of platelets of newborn infants. J. Pediatr., *79*:307, 1971.
8. Koepke, J. A., Rodgers, J. L., and Ollivier, M. J.: Pre-instrumental variables in coagulation testing. Am. J. Clin. Pathol., *64*:591, 1975.
9. Hathaway, W. E., Mull, M. M., and Pechet, G. S.: Disseminated intravascular coagulation in the newborn. Pediatrics, *43*:233, 1969.
10. Whaun, J. M., and Oski, F. A.: Experience with disseminated intravascular coagulation in a children's hospital. Can. Med. Assoc. J., *107*:963, 1972.
11. Deykin, D.: The clinical challenge of disseminated intravascular coagulation. N. Engl. J. Med., *283*:636, 1970.
12. Gross, S., and Melhorn, D. K.: Exchange transfusion with citrated whole blood for disseminated intravascular coagulation. J. Pediatr., *78*:415, 1971.
13. Corrigan, J. J., and Kiernat, J. F.: Effect of heparin in experimental gram-negative septicemia. J. Infect. Dis., *131*:138, 1975.
14. Corrigan, J. J., and Jordan, C. M.: Heparin therapy in septicemia with disseminated intravascular coagulation. N. Engl. J. Med., *282*:778, 1970.
15. Al-Mondhiry, H.: Disseminated intravascular coagulation: Experience in a major cancer center. Thromb. Diath. Haemorrh., *34*:181, 1975.
16. Corrigan, J. J.: Thrombocytopenia: A laboratory sign of septicemia in infants and children. J. Pediatr., *85*:219, 1974.
17. Roberts, H. R., and Cedarbaum, A. I.: The liver and blood coagulation: Physiology and pathology. Gastroenterology, *63*:297, 1972.
18. Shulman, N. R., Marder, V. J., Hiller, M. C., and Collier, E. M.: Platelet and leukocyte isoantigens and their antibodies: Serologic, physiologic and clinical studies. Progr. Hematol., *4*:222, 1964.
19. Anthony, B., and Krivit, W.: Neonatal thrombocytopenic purpura. Pediatrics, *30*:776, 1962.
20. McIntosh, S., O'Brien, R. T., Schwartz, A. D., and Pearson, H. A.: Neonatal isoimmune purpura: Response to platelet infusions. J. Pediatr., *82*:1020, 1973.
21. Pearson, H. A., Shulman, N. R., Marder, V. J., and Cone, T. E., Jr.: Isoimmune neonatal thrombocytopenia purpura. Clinical and therapeutic considerations. Blood, *23*:154, 1964.
22. Laros, R. K., and Sweet, R. L.: Management of idiopathic thrombocytopenic purpura during pregnancy. Am. J. Obstet. Gynecol., *122*:182, 1975.
23. Baehner, R. L., and Strauss, H. S.: Hemophilia in the first year of life. N. Engl. J. Med., *275*:524, 1966.
24. Donaldson, V. H., and Kisker, C. T.: Blood coagulation in hemostasis. *In* Nathan, D. G., and Oski, F. A., eds.: Hematology of Infancy and Childhood. Philadelphia, W. B. Saunders Co., 1974, p. 561.
25. Abildgaard, C. F.: Current concepts in the management of hemophilia. Semin. Hematol., *12*:223, 1975.
26. Apt, L., and Downey, W. S.: Melena neonatorum: The swallowed blood syndrome. J. Pediatr., *47*:6, 1955.
27. Sherman, N. J., and Clatworthy, H. W., Jr.: Gastro-intestinal bleeding in neonates: A study of 94 cases. Surgery, *62*:614, 1967.
28. Britten, A. F. H.: Congenital deficiency of factor XIII (fibrin-stabilizing factor). Am. J. Med., *43*:751, 1967.

Chapter Sixteen

DIABETIC KETOACIDOSIS AND COMA

ROBERT SCHWARTZ, M.D.

Diabetic acidosis, even with coma, may not be so alarming in its implications as are some other problems discussed in this book. Yet it certainly belongs among the critical illnesses, demanding as it does prompt action to restore a delicate physiological balance. Because the therapeutic response is very sensitive to precise management, improper therapy may be all the more dangerous. Management of diabetic coma therefore confronts the pediatrician with a more dramatic challenge than either the early recognition of diabetes in the previously normal child or the prevention of ketoacidosis in those with known diabetes, both of which should be more common problems. The mortality in diabetic acidosis and coma is admittedly very low. It should be non-existent.

The frequency of presentation with ketoacidosis in children with diabetes mellitus has been variously reported as low as 18 per cent by Danowski[1] and as high as 52 per cent by Jackson.[2] Knowles indicated that 45 per cent of diabetic children had serum carbon dioxide concentrations of less than 20 mM/L at the initial episode of diabetes.[3] In his observations, recurrence of attacks varied widely; no subsequent acidosis occurred in 46 per cent of the children, whereas 13 per cent had 10 attacks or more each to account for almost half of all attacks tabulated. Knowles found acidosis most prevalent in the first 5 years of known diabetes, regardless of age at diagnosis, and in the teen years, regardless of duration.[3] Severe ketoacidosis (serum $CO_2 < 10$ mM/L and coma) occurs in less than 20 per cent of initial admissions.[1]

While the fundamental common biochemical basis for hereditary

From the Section on Reproductive and Developmental Medicine, Brown University Program in Medicine and the Department of Pediatrics, Rhode Island Hospital, Providence, Rhode Island.

juvenile diabetes mellitus remains to be elucidated, the non-vascular metabolic derangements in large measure can be attributed to defective insulin secretion.

The metabolic derangements that result concern: (1) volume depletion, both extracellular and intracellular; (2) osmotic alterations between volume compartments; (3) acid-base disequilibrium with acidosis and buffer depletion; (4) alterations in erythrocyte control of oxygen dissociation from hemoglobin; and (5) caloric deficiency, i.e., "metabolic starvation."

Immunoreactive insulin measurements indicate low normal values in plasma which fail to rise in response to several stimuli (glucose, arginine, tolbutamide).[4] Although a physiological recovery may occur after initial treatment, permanent deficiency of insulin secretion follows within weeks to months after onset. The several resultant physiological disturbances are well shown by the two diagrams (Figs. 1 and 2), reproduced by courtesy of Dr. Rachmiel Levine. These diagrams, however, do not indicate the important role of relative or absolute hyperglucagonemia as emphasized by Unger.

Insulin deprivation (Fig. 1) is associated with impairment of peripheral utilization of carbohydrates, caused in part by defective glucose uptake in insulin-sensitive tissues, especially muscle and adipose tissue. In addition, decreased synthesis of glycogen in the liver and increased synthesis of glucose from amino acids (gluconeogenesis) raise the hepatic glucose output. These two factors, coupled with a continuing and sometimes increased dietary intake of carbohydrate, result in hyperglycemia. Since glucose contributes to the effective osmotic pressure of the extracellular fluid, hyperglycemia is associated with cellular dehydration as cell water shifts to the extracellular compartment. In the kidney the hyperglycemia results in a filtered glucose load exceeding the reabsorptive mechanism of tubular transport, thus producing an "osmotic" or "solute" diuresis. This in turn obligates both water and electrolyte (sodium and chloride) loss and results in extracellular fluid depletion when there is also a failure of intake. As the derangement progresses, additional solute for excretion is derived from protein catabolism (urea) and the ketoacidosis (organic acids), both of which require water and cation loss.

In the peripheral adipose tissue cells (Fig. 2) decreased lipogenesis and increased lipolysis occur. The latter produces an excess of non-esterified or free fatty acids (FFA or NEFA) which, bound to albumin, are transported in the plasma to the liver and other tissues for further metabolism. In the liver, increased degradation of fatty acids to two carbon fragments (acetyl-coenzyme A) is associated with increased formation of organic acids, especially "ketone acids" (β-hydroxybutyric and acetoacetic acids). The latter, as relatively strong organic acids (pK's approximately 4.7), interact with cellular and extracellular

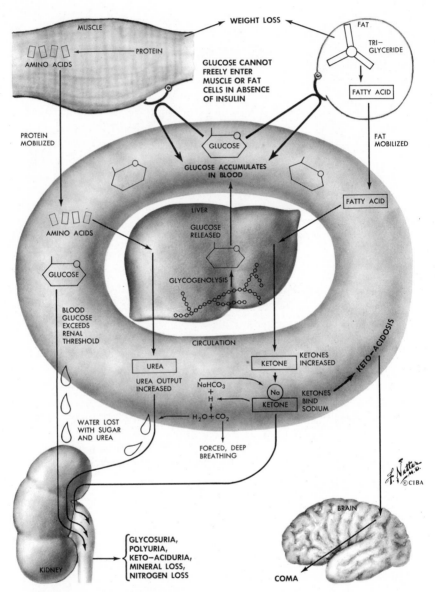

Figure 1. Pathophysiological effects of insulin deprivation. Not shown is the production of hydrogen ions due to organic acids (including "ketones"). Ketones do not "bind sodium" but are associated with cation at physiological pH, and to a large extent appear in the urine in this form. (© Copyright 1965, CIBA Pharmaceutical Company, Division of CIBA-Geigy Corporation. Reproduced with permission from The CIBA Collection of Medical Illustrations, by Frank H. Netter, M.D. All rights reserved.)

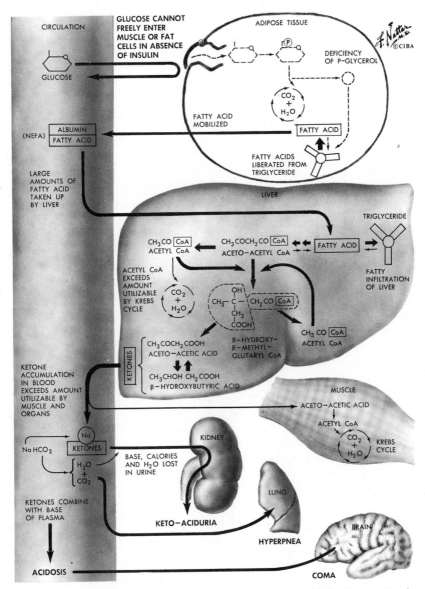

Figure 2. Ketoacidosis in diabetes. Substitution of ketone acids for "ketones" and cation for "base" would clarify terminology concepts. NEFA = FFA. (© Copyright 1965, CIBA Pharmaceutical Company, Division of CIBA-Geigy Corporation. Reproduced with permission from The CIBA Collection of Medical Illustrations, by Frank H. Netter, M.D. All rights reserved.)

buffers and, at physiological pH's, exist principally in ionized form rather than as free organic acid.

The magnitude of systemic metabolic acidosis is dependent upon the rate of organic acid synthesis and metabolism coupled with renal compensatory mechanisms for excreting hydrogen ion. Three factors — urinary pH gradient, titratable acidity (determined by concentration of organic acids and phosphate), and ammonium production particularly — affect the rate at which systemic buffers are depleted. When hydrogen ion production exceeds the total of these three limiting mechanisms, acidosis proceeds inexorably toward an unphysiological state no longer compatible with cellular function.

Buffer depletion in metabolic acidosis is evident in part in the measured bicarbonate concentration of plasma. The so-called plasma anion gap is an approximation of organic acid accumulation in the plasma. This is derived by determining the difference in the sum of measured cations and anions. The measured cations are sodium and potassium, while the anions are chloride, bicarbonate, and protein. Protein equivalents are equal to 2.43 times the serum protein concentration in grams per 100 ml.

$$\Sigma \text{ cations} - \Sigma \text{ anions} =$$
$$\Sigma\,([Na]_p + [K]_p) - \Sigma\,([Cl]_p + [HCO_3^-]_p + 2.43[Pr]_p)$$

The total buffer deficit of the body is the resultant of two major components. One, represented by the loss of volume including osmolar (Na, K, Cl) and buffer (HCO_3^-) components, requires replacement from exogenous sources; the other, represented by organic "ketone" acids within the body, is a measure of potential buffer. When lipogenesis is increased and lipolysis decreased by administration of insulin and glucose, not only is organic acid (hydrogen ion) production diminished, but also the "ketone acids" in peripheral tissues are metabolized to CO_2 and H_2O, and the regeneration of some buffer occurs. However, the initial bicarbonate concentration alone cannot be relied upon to predict quantitatively the buffer regeneration with therapy.

While the principal alterations expressed here relate primarily to extracellular volume depletion and metabolic acidosis, hypertonicity and loss of cellular volume are accompanied by depletion of potassium and phosphate. Though such depletion is frequent and significant, it may not be reflected in the initial serum potassium and phosphate concentrations, which may even be elevated.

Although Guest and Rapoport first described alterations in red cell organic phosphates in 1939, their physiological significance was not appreciated sufficiently until the role of 2,3-diphosphoglycerate (DPG) in hemoglobin affinity was discovered. There is now definitive evidence that diabetic ketoacidosis in the insulin-dependent subject is associated with decreased DPG as well as with an elevation of the glycohemoglobin (HbA_{Ic}) which has an increased affinity for oxygen. Furthermore, during therapy in the absence of exogenous phosphate, there is a decline in plasma inorganic phosphate which is important to restoration of erythrocyte DPG. Ditzel and Standl[5] have demonstrated that the low DPG and inorganic phosphate are associated with a shift of the oxygen dissociation curve to the left and with a significantly decreased $P_{50}O_2$ (in vivo) in adults.

Electrolyte deficits previously measured by balance techniques in children[6] and adults[7, 8, 9] with severe diabetic acidosis were summarized by Darrow[10] as (per kilogram body weight):

H_2O	Na	Cl	K
100 gm	8 mEq	6 mEq	6–10 mEq

To these may be added, from the work of Martin and co-workers[11] a

fourth electrolyte:

$$P$$
$$1.0 \text{ mM}$$

CLINICAL AND LABORATORY FINDINGS

The onset of symptoms associated with juvenile diabetes mellitus itself may vary in duration from 1 to 2 days to as long as several months before the appearance of clinically significant ketoacidosis, although in most instances the duration is less than 1 month. Polyuria and polydipsia are, of course, the most common symptoms; polyphagia, nocturia, and weight loss may be somewhat less evident. Infections and emotional upsets may be contributing factors. The rapidity of progression from carbohydrate intolerance to ketoacidosis is so unpredictable that continuous medical surveillance is recommended once the diagnosis of diabetes mellitus is suspected, with laboratory studies initially not only to establish the diagnosis but also to assess the degree of metabolic derangements, especially in those aspects that require emergency therapy. The diagnosis of diabetes mellitus is confirmed by the identification of glucosuria and ketonuria in the presence of a blood sugar (glucose) above 150 mg per 100 ml.

Vomiting, with the attendant absence of fluid and calorie intake, is an ominous symptom which signals rapid deterioration and progression to serious acidosis and coma. The early phases of acidosis may produce no gross changes in the character of respiration; however, by the time moderate acidosis (serum $CO_2 < 15$ mM/L) supervenes definite increases in depth and rate are apparent. With severe acidosis (serum $CO_2 < 10$ mM/L), the characteristic Kussmaul acidotic breathing is grossly and alarmingly obvious.

Acid-base derangement is evident in a serum pH which may be as low as 6.85 to 7.00 and a decreased carbon dioxide content reaching 2.5 to 10 mM/L in severe acidosis.* Under these circumstances, there is marked depression of the actual bicarbonate concentration, while the tension of carbon dioxide also is depressed (values of 10 to 20 mm Hg) in the presence of compensatory hyperventilation. Plasma ketones are elevated and approximate the bicarbonate depression. A rapid bedside test has been described by Lee and Duncan[12] which quantifies plasma ketone levels by serial dilution of plasma (1:1, 1:2, 1:4, 1:8, and so forth) and reaction with nitroprusside reagent. Since the latter does not react with β-hydroxybutyrate (which may account for 35 to 50 per cent of plasma ketones), the test is semiquantitative at best, but serves as a useful guide to adequacy of therapy. Diminution of the concentration of plasma ketones usually is reflected in a lessening of the metabolic acidosis and an improvement in the bicarbonate concentration.

In diabetic ketoacidosis, hyperglycemia may vary from 150 to as high as 2000 mg glucose/100 ml. Most frequently, a range of values from 250 to 600 mg/100 ml is observed. While the concentration of sodium in plasma is usually normal or slightly decreased, marked elevations of blood glucose are associated with a reciprocal decrease in sodium concentration. The value of chloride tends to parallel that of sodium. As already noted, plasma potassium initially is normal or even slightly elevated (5.5 to 6.0 mEq/L) in association with dehydration and metabolic acidosis. In the rare case of abnormally decreased plasma potassium, particular attention to early therapy with potassium is indicated.

Signs of dehydration (decreased skin turgor, softened eyeballs, dry mucous membranes) are not obvious until acute weight loss of at least 5 per cent has occurred. In diabetic acidosis occurring a month or more after the onset of unsuspected diabetes, signs of undernutrition predominate and weight loss alone is not a valid measure of fluid deficit. When dehydration is severe (15 per cent body weight loss), signs of circulatory insufficiency with hypotension and tachycardia may be present. Azotemia may reflect circulatory inadequacy and decreased renal perfusion as well as the additional urea production from increased protein catabolism.

Hyperlipidemia, including hypercholesterolemia, may be very marked (15 to 25 gm total lipids per 100 ml plasma), especially in patients with prolonged onset. Lactescence (milky plasma) should be recognized when drawing the initial blood sample or suspected by finding lipemia retinalis on physical examination. Hyperlipemia not only

---

*For those laboratories using the micro pH electrodes and the Astrup technique, familiarity with terminology and concepts such as buffer base (excess or deficit) and standard bicarbonate is indicated.

interferes with spectrophotometric analysis of hemoglobin, but also results in falsely low laboratory measurements of electrolytes and other aqueous phase substances because of volume displacement.[13] Thus markedly but deceptively low serum sodium values ($\pm$ 100 mEq/L) may be reported in the presence of very high blood glucose levels associated with hyperlipemia.

The state of consciousness may be as varied as other signs; however, in advanced ketoacidosis, semicoma or coma is evident. Differential diagnosis is seldom a problem. In rare instances, similar findings may occur following a head injury or in salicylate intoxication in young children, and the change in respiratory character sometimes is mistaken for a sign of primary respiratory disease such as pneumonia in young children. But once diabetes mellitus is thought of, the only possible diagnostic problem may arise from the occasional abdominal pain of acidosis and the question of appendicitis in a known diabetic.

THERAPY

Treatment of the child with diabetic acidosis is always urgent, perhaps more so than in some of the other "critical illnesses" discussed in this book, but the degree of urgency must be determined from clinical and laboratory assessment at admission, with particular emphasis on circulatory sufficiency and the extent of metabolic acidosis. Once the diagnosis has been confirmed (rapid blood glucose assessment may be made at the bedside with Dextrostix*), initial fluids, given primarily to expand circulatory volume, should consist of isotonic sodium in a balanced anion solution ($Cl + HCO_3$ at a ratio of 2:1) at a rapid rate of 20 ml per kg of body weight in the first 30 to 60 minutes.

If severe acidosis is present (pH < 7.15 and/or carbon dioxide content, combining power, or actual bicarbonate concentration less than 8 mM/L), sodium bicarbonate should then be given in a dose of 2 mEq/kg of body weight. This is easily accomplished with the 7.5 per cent sodium bicarbonate solution which contains 44.6 mEq in 50 ml (approximately 1 mEq/ml). Direct administration of this solution, with its osmolar load of 892×2 mOs/L, may raise the effective osmotic pressure of extracellular fluid enough to dehydrate brain cells and other cells further. Therefore dilution with distilled water is recommended: 50 ml of 7.5 per cent sodium bicarbonate to 250 ml distilled water results in a solution of 149 mEq/L (isotonic sodium bicarbonate). Initial therapy should avoid glucose administration, especially if marked hyperglycemia (> 300 mg per 100 ml) is present.

---

*Ames Company, Elkhart, Ind. 46514.

Correction of the ketoacidosis and hyperglycemia is dependent upon reversal of the pathophysiological mechanisms by insulin administration, which is given simultaneously with therapy for circulatory insufficiency and severe acidosis. This begins with an empirical administration of crystalline or regular insulin in a dosage of 3 to 4 units per kilogram of body weight for patients with severe acidosis and coma; lesser doses to 1 unit/kg are administered to patients less critically ill. Initial insulin is given by two routes: approximately half intravenously, the remainder subcutaneously. There have been recent recommendations for insulin in low (0.1 unit/kg/hr)[14] or high (1.0 unit/kg/hr)[15] dosage by continuous infusion after a prime injection. These techniques have not yet been established firmly. While this offers some advantage by virtue of continuous delivery of insulin by a constant infusion pump during the critical early phase of therapy, there is no substitute for continuous clinical and laboratory monitoring of the patient. For those who prefer this route, the technique of Genuth[15] is recommended. Regular insulin is given as an initial prime injection of 1.0 unit/kg intravenously, followed by continuous infusion of an equal amount, 1.0 unit/kg, throughout each succeeding hour. The infusion should be made up with 2.5 ml 25 per cent human albumin in 250 ml 5 per cent glucose and water plus 2.5 ml regular U100 insulin, resulting in 1 unit/ml in 250 mg per cent albumin. This therapy is maintained until plasma acetone is a trace or absent and glucose is 250 mg per 100 ml or less. If improvement is not evident in 4 hours, the rate of insulin infusion should be increased, i.e., doubled. Insulin resistance should be suspected. Note that insulin is administered independent of the intravenous fluids so that they may be varied separately as necessary.

Urgency in attention to circulatory insufficiency and acidosis should not lead to neglect of requirements for free water necessary in the presence of hyperosmolality and for correction of the significant negative water balance from hyperventilation and renal excretion. Such water may be provided by dilution of the electrolyte solution.

A program of therapy must be devised once initial emergency treatment has commenced. A detailed flow chart or data sheet containing critical clinical observations (especially body weight, blood pressure, pulse, respiration) and laboratory data (pH, CO_2, blood glucose, ketones, Na, K, phosphate, BUN, Hb) is essential to management. The frequency of observations depends upon the degree of critical concern; thus, while circulatory insufficiency is present or potential, blood pressure, pulse, and respiration are observed at least every 10 to 15 minutes. While acidosis is present, respiration is observed every 15 minutes and pH, CO_2 and ketones observed every 3 hours until significant improvement, whereupon the interval is increased. Blood sugar may be followed at 1- to 3-hour intervals at the bedside until stabilization at normoglycemia is assured. Body weight, Hb, and BUN need not be observed more frequently than every 12 hours. The recording of fluid balance must be meticulous and initially includes only intravenous fluids and urine; other volumes must be recorded subsequently. In addition, a balance of electrolytes, sodium, potassium, bicarbonate, phosphate, and glucose should be ascertained every 6 hours. Urine volumes may be collected separately, but cumulative periods of 6 hours are more practical. After the initial 24 hours of therapy, daily cumulative balances suffice.

The details of therapy are similar to those for other derangements of electrolyte physiology and are calculated from (1) previous deficit, (2) maintenance needs, and (3) continuing abnormal losses.

Previous Deficit. Since rapid restoration of the cellular deficit is not possible because of limitations of potassium administration, initial treatment is directed toward extracellular fluid restoration. According to the data of Darrow,[10] approximately half the estimated previous deficit may be restored as isotonic solution of sodium salts in the initial 24 hours.

Maintenance Needs. Specific maintenance requirements may be determined by a variety of techniques (based on surface area, calories metabolized, weight, or age), with an approximately similar range of values. Each physician must recognize the virtues and limitations of that system which he or she prefers. They may be summarized to include (a) 1500 to 1800 ml/M^2/24 hours; or (b) 150 ml/100 kcal metabolized/24 hours; or (c) insensible water losses, 10 to 50 ml/kg/24 hours + urine losses 10 to 50 ml/kg/24 hours, with a total of 20 to 100 ml/kg/24 hours; (d) 100−3X (X = age in years) ml/kg/24 hours. Maintenance fluids preferably contain one-fifth volume of isotonic solution of sodium salts and four-fifths free water (as 5 to 10 per cent glucose solution). Potassium in a concentration of 20 to 30 mEq/L also is included.

Continuing Abnormal Water Losses. Such losses due to hyperventilation and urinary output are highly variable and best assessed by acute changes in body weight relative to fluid balance.

The preceding recommendations may be summarized in an example for a 30 kg (1 M^2) child in severe ketoacidosis (Table 1). This results for the first 24 hours of therapy (when no glucose is to be given)

TABLE 1 Water and Sodium Requirements for First 24 Hours of Therapy

Data	Volume (ml/day)	Isotonic Na Solution (ml/day)	Na (mEq/day)	Electrolyte Free Water (ml/day)
Maintenance	1500	300	45.0	1200
Abnormal losses up to 50 per cent maintenance	750	150	22.5	600
ECF deficit 50 ml/kg	1500	1500	225.0	0
Total	3750	1950	292.5	1800

TABLE 2   Initial Emergency Therapy

Data	Volume (ml)	Isotonic Na Solution (ml)	Na (mEq)	Electrolyte Free Water (ml)
Isotonic NaCl 20 ml/kg and/or	600	600	90	0
NaHCO₃ 2 mEq/kg	400	400	60	0
Total	1000	1000	150	0

in a solution which is approximately half isotonic sodium solution plus supplemental potassium. Practically, the initial hour of therapy must be subtracted from the above to determine the remaining requirements. Thus, assuming the patient just discussed had circulatory insufficiency and severe acidosis and was treated promptly and adequately, see Table 2 for the amounts he or she would have received in the first hour.

Under these circumstances, and to avoid acute fluid overloads, the volume of isotonic sodium chloride should be reduced to 10 ml/kg and should be replaced in part by the isotonic sodium bicarbonate solution. If the total volumes (maximal) are as just noted, then the fluids to be given by the end of the first 24 hours will include those already administered plus the remainder in Table 3.

The remainder now represents approximately one-third isotonic sodium and two-thirds water instead of the half isotonic sodium for the total first 24 hours of therapy. The second phase of therapy (1 to 6 hours postadmission) is directed primarily toward expansion of extracellular volume and correction of acidosis (insulin and sodium bicarbonate).

Total fluids for the first day of therapy must be planned so that one-half to two-thirds of the remainder are administered in the initial 12 hours and the rest in the second half day. Thus in the example given 1375 ml total fluid remain for the first 12 hours (including 475 ml isotonic sodium solution). In the initial 6 hours (excluding the first) the amount would be: 688 ml fluid, 238 ml isotonic sodium solution.

TABLE 3   Continuing Therapy after Emergency Phase

Data	Volume (ml/day)	Isotonic Na Solution (ml/day)	Na (mEq/day)	Electrolyte Free Water (ml/day)
First 24 hours, total	3750	1950	292.5	1800
Minus first hour	1000	1000	150.0	0
Remainder	2750	950	142.5	1800

The remaining solution must contain some additional solute; otherwise it is dangerously hypotonic. Since glucose is not recommended in the presence of very high glucose concentrations, this may be achieved with 5 per cent fructose (450 ml). If not, an exception must be made to the 24-hour requirements given earlier and only 238 ml (an equal volume) of free water administered; the requisite additional free water administration is deferred until a later phase of therapy when glucose solution may be provided.

Once blood glucose concentration has fallen to 300 mg/100 ml or less (initially hourly determinations are suggested), then the appropriate vehicle is glucose as 5 or 10 per cent solution in place of either fructose or free water alone, with appropriate electrolyte.

Serial electrocardiograms are checked every 2 hours for (1) depression of the ST segment and lowering, flattening, or inversion of the T wave; (2) prolongation of the Q-T interval; (3) presence of an elevated, broad, or diphasic U wave which may be responsible for the impression of a prolonged Q-T interval; (4) occasional prolongation of the P-R interval, as indication of hypokalemia. Since potassium therapy usually is not recommended for the first 4 to 6 hours of treatment because of initial hyperkalemia, at approximately 4 hours post therapy, potassium phosphate is added in a concentration of 30 to 40 mEq/L. Potassium at 2 to 4 mM/kg/day and buffered phosphate at 2 to 3 mM/kg/day are recommended during the second phase of treatment. If symptoms of hypokalemia (muscle weakness or ileus) or very low serum values are observed (< 3.0 mEq/L), higher concentrations of potassium may be indicated. If concentrations exceeding 40 mEq/L are administered, careful monitoring of plasma potassium concentration is necessary, in addition to the electrocardiograms taken every two hours, to avoid cardiotoxicity.

Hypophosphatemia may be evident by 12 to 24 hours and should be treated by increasing the amount of phosphate in the infusate. If the plasma potassium level precludes use of buffered potassium phosphate, then buffer sodium phosphate should be used. Note that the addition of 3 mM/kg of potassium and 2 mM/kg of phosphate in the example of the 30 kg child reduces free water further. Thus, in Table 3 90 mM potassium and 60 mM phosphate for a total 150 mOsm would be equivalent to 500 ml water, thereby reducing total free water to 1300 ml for the first 24 hours of treatment. Additional free water may be provided either by increasing the total volume or by deferring sodium equivalent to potassium until the next 24-hour phase.

Regular insulin must be administered subcutaneously, unless given by continuous infusion, at least every 3 hours in a decreasing amount until ketosis is cleared, which may require 12 to 24 hours. When presenting findings are severe, the initial dose may be repeated once and then decreased by 50 per cent each subsequent period. At low levels of insulin (<5 U), a small 3 to 6 hourly dosage should still be maintained to avoid rebound ketonuria. A decrease in blood glucose is not sufficient reason alone for discontinuing insulin administration; rather, the amount of glucose administered parenterally should be increased from 5 to 10 per cent or greater solution. Monitoring of blood glucose at the bedside will serve to anticipate and correct hypoglycemia with glucose therapy.

Parenteral fluids are continued until the patient is free of ketones and aglycosuric. Even in the absence of vomiting, oral fluids should not be begun in the initial 12 hours, or even then if the sensorium is uncleared. Once consciousness is fully restored, fluids containing potassium may be introduced by mouth. Orange juice contains 40 mEq/L potassium and 10 per cent carbohydrate. Amounts of fluids and dosages of insulin during the second 24-hour period are dependent upon rate of repair of the estimated deficit and continuing losses. By this time, the extracellular deficit is usually minimal and beginning repair of cellular deficit through oral introduction of higher calories and protein may proceed. Regular insulin is preferred for an additional 24-hour period at regular intervals preceding oral intake. Periods exceeding 6 hours' duration without insulin are to be avoided. By the third day, a planned dietary regimen may be introduced with long-acting insulin. Further management is dependent upon many factors other than those just considered—especially upon the education and adjustment of the patient and family. Nevertheless, the efficiency and skill with which the preceding more critical illness has been managed will remain significant factors in the subsequent course and care of the patient.

REFERENCES

1. Danowski, T. S.: Diabetes Mellitus, with Emphasis on Children and Young Adults. Baltimore, Williams & Wilkins, 1957, p. 128.
2. Jackson, R. L., Hardin, R. C., Walker, G. L., Hendricks, A. B., and Kelly, H. G.: Degenerative changes in young diabetics in relation to level of control. Proc. Am. Diabetes Assoc., 9:307, 1949.
3. Knowles, H. C., Jr., Guest, G. M., Lampe, J., Kessler, M., and Skillman, T. G.: The course of juvenile diabetes treated with unmeasured diet. Diabetes, 14:239, 1965.
4. Parker, M. L., Pildes, R. S., Chao, K. L., Cornblath, M., and Kipnis, D. M.: Juvenile diabetes mellitus, a deficiency of insulin. Diabetes, 17:27, 1968.
5. Ditzel, J., and Standl, E.: The oxygen transport system of red blood cells during diabetic ketoacidosis and recovery. Diabetologia, 11:255, 1975.
6. Darrow, D. C., and Pratt, E. L.: Retention of water and electrolyte during recovery in a patient with diabetic acidosis. J. Pediatr., 4:688, 1942.
7. Butler, A. M., Talbot, N. B., Barnett, C. H., Stanbury, J. B., and MacLachlan, E. A.: Metabolic studies in diabetic coma. Trans. Assoc. Am. Physicians, 60:102, 1947.
8. Atchley, D. W., Loeb, R. F., Richards, D. W., Jr., Benedict, E. M., and Driscoll, M. E.: On diabetic acidosis: A detailed study of electrolyte balances following the withdrawal and re-establishment of insulin therapy. J. Clin. Invest., 12:297, 1933.
9. Nabarro, J. D. N., Spencer, A. G., and Stowers, J. M.: Metabolic studies in severe diabetic ketosis. Quart. J. Med., N. S., 21:225, 1952.

10. Darrow, D. C.: A Guide to Learning Fluid Therapy. Springfield, Ill., Charles C Thomas, 1964.
11. Martin, H. E., Smith, K., and Wilson, M. L.: The fluid and electrolyte therapy of severe diabetic acidosis and ketosis. Am. J. Med., 24:376, 1958.
12. Lee, C. T., and Duncan, G. G.: Diabetic coma: The value of a simple test for acetone in the plasma; an aid to diagnosis and treatment. Metabolism, 5:144, 1956.
13. Albrink, M. J., Hald, P. M., Man, E. B., and Peters, J. P.: The displacement of serum water by lipids of hyperlipemic serum. A new method for the rapid determination of serum water. J. Clin. Invest., 34:1483, 1955.
14. Page, M. McB., Alberti, K. G. M. M., Greenwood, R., Gumaa, K. A., Hockaday, T. D. R., Lowry, C., Nabarro, J. D. N., Pyke, D. A., Sonksen, P. H., Watkins, P. J., and West, T. E. T.: Treatment of diabetic coma with continuous low-dose infusion of insulin. Br. Med. J., 2:687, 1974.
15. Genuth, S.: Constant intravenous insulin infusion in diabetic ketoacidosis. J.A.M.A., 223:1348, 1973.

Chapter Seventeen

HYPOGLYCEMIA

ROBERT E. GREENBERG, M.D.,
ROBERT O. CHRISTIANSEN, M.D.

Hypoglycemia represents a significant emergency situation in pediatrics. Although recent studies indicate that cerebral tissue can utilize substrates other than glucose, especially in the newborn period and during prolonged fasting,[1] no substrate can successfully correct the neurophysiological sequelae of glucose deprivation on the central nervous system. Since permanent neurological effects of hypoglycemia correlate with the duration of time that cerebral tissue is deprived of glucose, early recognition and treatment of hypoglycemia are essential.

The diagnosis of hypoglycemia obviously depends on demonstration of a significant reduction in blood glucose concentration. Diagnostic criteria, similar to those developed by Cornblath and Schwartz,[2] have been widely accepted: two or more blood glucose values of less than 30 mg/100 ml in full-term infants; concentration of blood glucose less than 20 mg/100 ml in the neonate weighing less than 2500 gm; blood glucose values of less than 40 mg/100 ml in the older infant and child. Since hypoglycemia is defined in terms of the concentration of blood glucose, it is essential to utilize analytic methods that are specific for glucose. The most common method utilizes glucose oxidase, although other methods provide appropriate specificity. A rapid modification of the glucose oxidase method is represented by Dextrostix,* although accurate application of this diagnostic aid to hypoglycemia requires considerable training and experience.[3] Recently, a modifica-

From the Department of Pediatrics, University of New Mexico School of Medicine, Albuquerque, New Mexico, and Kaiser Foundation Hospital, South San Francisco, California.

Supported in part by Grants HD 03150 and HD 02147 from the National Institutes of Health and 2K3HD-7263 from the Career Development Review Branch (R.E.G.), National Institutes of Health.

*Ames Co., Inc., Elkhart, Ind. 46514.

244

tion of the Dextrostix method has been reported, enabling reproducible measurement of values in the range of 20 to 40 mg/100 ml.[4] Confirmation of results obtained by Dextrostix with reliable laboratory methods should be effected upon recognition of hypoglycemia.

Focusing on practical approaches to the infant or child with hypoglycemia, this discussion will consider the following areas: hypoglycemia in the newborn infant; hypoglycemia in the older infant and child; mechanisms underlying hypoglycemia, and approach to diagnosis; and therapy of the severely affected.

NEONATAL HYPOGLYCEMIA

The neonatal period presents a particularly difficult problem with respect to the regulation of blood glucose. Under normal conditions, the concentration of blood glucose declines during the first 24 hours after birth. Symptoms of hypoglycemia are often vague, nonspecific, and subtle. The incidence of asymptomatic hypoglycemia remains ill defined; equally obscure is the question of permanent sequelae, if any, of transient neonatal hypoglycemia, with or without attendant symptoms. Accordingly, careful attention to the symptomatology of neonatal hypoglycemia and to newborn infants at risk is essential.

Although irritability and convulsions were the first signs of hypoglycemia to be recognized, it is now well known that a myriad of other clinical findings should lead the clinician to suspect hypoglycemia. Such signs include tremor, cyanosis, apnea, listlessness, poor feeding, rotating eye motions, change in muscle tone, shrill cry, and instability of temperature regulation. Hypoglycemia may occur without clinical manifestations, a fact which has led some investigators to question the correlation between clinical signs and documented reductions in blood glucose concentration;[5] presence of clinical signs or symptoms has been found to correlate, however, with the duration of hypoglycemia.[6]

It has been possible, in recent years, to define a high risk population of newborn infants. Two major predisposing factors are apparent: (1) placental dysfunction, and (2) postnatal illness. Neonates predisposed to hypoglycemia as a consequence of intrauterine events often present as dysmature (small for dates) infants,[7] the smaller of discordant twins, and infants born of mothers with toxemia. Newborn infants with neonatal asphyxia, respiratory distress, hypothermia, or erythroblastosis fetalis exhibit an increased frequency of hypoglycemia. In addition, infants of diabetic mothers often develop hypoglycemia during the first 6 hours after birth. Severe and prolonged hypoglycemia has also been reported in infants of mothers treated with oral hypoglycemic agents.[8] Recognition of hypoglycemia in the neonate can be enhanced by routine determination of blood glucose concentration in high risk infants, and by prompt attention to previously described signs and symptoms.

Prompt and effective treatment should accompany recognition of hypoglycemia, regardless of the associated clinical findings. Recommended initial therapy consists of rapid intravenous infusion of 1 gm glucose/kg (2 ml/kg of 50 per cent glucose), followed by a constant infusion of glucose at a rate of 10 mg/kg/minute (75 ml/kg/24 hours of 20 per cent glucose). It must be remembered that this represents only approximate dosage; it is imprudent to assume that therapy is successful in maintaining a blood glucose concentration above 50 mg/100 ml without immediate and repetitive monitoring. Although neonatal hypoglycemia is usually transient, intravenous glucose administration should be maintained for at least 24 hours after the blood glucose concentration has been stabilized. Subsequently, the glucose infusion should be slowly decreased in conjunction with increasing oral feedings, since abrupt cessation of intravenous glucose may be associated with a recurrence of hypoglycemia. Prolonged infusion of concentrated glucose solutions may be complicated by thrombotic phenomena and excessive fluid administration; accordingly, the dangers of concentrated glucose solutions must be related to the ability of the newborn to handle fluid loads in an attempt to titrate therapy. The availability of infusion pumps applicable to intravenous therapy has markedly improved establishment of stabilized blood glucose concentrations.

If hypoglycemia cannot be successfully controlled by glucose infusion, empirical use of hydrocortisone in divided doses of 5 mg/kg/24 hr has been recommended by many investigators. Glucagon has recently been demonstrated to be capable of precociously inducing an increase in activity of phosphoenolpyruvate carboxykinase, an enzyme unique to the gluconeogenic pathway, in fetal, premature, and newborn rats.[9] Since neonatal hypoglycemia probably is related, in many instances, to relative inability to effect appropriate hepatic glucose output, utilization of intramuscular glucagon injections, 50 mcg/kg every 4 hours, is, at least, based on a rational theoretical framework. As previously indicated, all therapy is empirical and the concentration of blood glucose must be closely monitored.

HYPOGLYCEMIA IN THE OLDER INFANT AND CHILD

Permanent neurological sequelae result with greater frequency when repetitive episodes of hypoglycemia occur prior to 6 months of age. Fortunately, recognition of hypoglycemia in the older infant and child is easier than in the newborn infant. The signs and symptoms of hypoglycemia are a function of the rate of fall in blood glucose and the neurological sequelae of prolonged glucose deprivation. Pallor, sweating, and tremulousness accompany the adrenergic response to a rapid reduction in blood glucose concentration. The development of marked and persistent reductions in blood glucose results in listlessness, apathy, irritability, headache, visual disturbances, mental confusion, bizarre behavior, and, finally, convulsions and coma. Delineation of the relationship between symptoms and previous ingestion of food, time of day, and ingestion or administration of drugs aids in the detection of hypoglycemia. Hypoglycemia in the older infant and child may be defined by a concentration of blood glucose less than 40 mg/100 ml associated with suggestive signs and symptoms which disappear following restoration of normal blood glucose values. Signs and symptoms accompanying prolonged hypoglycemia, however, may not be obviated immediately by intravenous glucose administration.

Treatment of the severe, acute episode involves rapid intravenous administration of 2 ml/kg of 50 per cent glucose, followed by a constant infusion of glucose at a rate of 5 to 10 mg glucose/kg/minute, sufficient to maintain a blood glucose level above 50 mg/100 ml. After the concentration of blood glucose has been stabilized for 6 hours or longer, the rate of infusion can be progressively reduced unless the child is incapable of oral alimentation. Subsequent therapy depends on the severity and frequency of hypoglycemia and the nature of causative mechanisms.

MECHANISMS UNDERLYING HYPOGLYCEMIA, AND APPROACH TO DIAGNOSIS

The concentration of blood glucose is, essentially, a resultant of two interacting processes: peripheral glucose utilization and hepatic glucose production. Application of diagnostic methods to the study of the etiology of hypoglycemia in an affected child should attempt to estimate rates of these processes in as direct and rapid a fashion as possible. A distinction should be made between procedures utilized in the investigation of physiological mechanisms and those that may lead to specific therapy. Hypoglycemia in infancy and childhood almost always occurs under conditions of fasting, in contrast to the greater frequency of postprandial hypoglycemia in adults. A classification of etiological factors associated with hypoglycemia is outlined in Table 1. Utilizing the framework of this classification, the history can serve as an extremely important component in diagnosis.

Our approach to diagnosis emphasizes several concepts: diagnostic procedures should be used that lead to specific therapy with least danger to the patient; procedures that facilitate inclusion of the patient in clinical classifications which, in turn, are not indicative of specific

TABLE 1 Causes of Hypoglycemia in Childhood

I. Lack of available glucose or its precursors
   Malnutrition, severe
   Impaired absorption
      chronic diarrhea
      intestinal disaccharidase deficiency
      malabsorption of unknown etiology
      "dumping syndrome"

II. Increased peripheral glucose utilization
   Hyperinsulinism
      pancreatic tumors
      pancreatic hyperplasia
      nescidioblastosis
      "prediabetic" syndrome
      excessive exogenous insulin
      infants with erythroblastosis
   Tumors of mesothelial origin
   Defects in hormonal regulation
      growth hormone deficiency

III. Defects in glycogenolysis
   Glucose 6-phosphatase deficiency hepatorenal glycogenosis
   Hepatophosphorylase deficiency glycogenosis
   Amylo-1,6-glucosidase (debrancher) deficiency glycogenosis

IV. Defects in hepatic glucose formation and release
   Enzymatic defects in hepatic intermediary metabolism
      hereditary fructose intolerance
      galactosemia
      pyruvate carboxylase deficiency
      fructose-1,6-diphosphatase deficiency
      phosphoenolpyruvate carboxykinase deficiency
   Hepatic disease
      hepatitis
      cirrhosis
      malignant growth
   Defects in hormonal regulation
      adrenocortical insufficiency
         idiopathic adrenocortical atrophy
         destructive lesions
         enzymatic defects in hydrocortisone biosynthesis
         unresponsiveness of adrenal to ACTH
      hypopituitarism (selective or multiple defects in ACTH, TSH production)
      hypothyroidism
      glucagon deficiency
      adrenomedullary insufficiency (?)
   Defects in integrative function of the central nervous system
      congenital abnormalities, tumors, hemorrhage, injury, infection
   Pharmacological or toxic alterations in glucose homeostasis
      salicylates, biguanides, sulfonylureas, antihistamines, ethanol
   Limitation of gluconeogenic
      substrate
      ketotic hypoglycemia

V. Unknown etiology
   Leucine-induced hypoglycemia
   Idiopathic hypoglycemia of childhood
   Neonatal hypoglycemia
      infants of mothers with toxemia of pregnancy
      "small for dates" infants
      infants with neonatal asphyxia or respiratory distress syndrome

pathophysiological mechanisms are of little practical value; diagnostic procedures should be based on an understanding of the physiology of prolonged fasting; and the extent of diagnostic procedures must be determined, in part, by the severity and rate of recurrence of hypoglycemia and the age of the patient.

Recent studies have clarified the specific changes that accompany fasting, and provide insight into the changing pattern of hormonal control.[10, 11] In the absence of dietary carbohydrate, endogenous glucose production must increase in order to provide sufficient glucose to maintain a normal concentration of glucose in blood and, in turn, cerebral function. While enhancement of gluconeogenesis is appreciable, a marked reduction in the rate of glucose utilization occurs in prolonged fasting, such that very little glucose is utilized by any tissues except the formed elements of blood and brain. Protein catabolism is largely obviated by a marked increase in hydrolysis of triglycerides, with resultant release of free fatty acids and glycerol into the circulation. While overall glucose utilization is sharply reduced, the brain continues to consume glucose.

As a corollary to these events, the concentration of insulin falls to low but persistent levels in blood, while that of glucagon increases. Markedly enhanced rates of lipolysis lead to increased ketone body formation, so that absence of ketonuria during a prolonged fast may be regarded as an abnormal finding.

The capacity of the liver to produce new glucose is not saturated even if precursors, such as lactate and amino acids, are supplied at concentrations much higher than normally found in plasma. When an adult is fasted, glucose is produced from the following precursors: 50 per cent from amino acids, 10 per cent from glycerol (derived from lipolysis), and 30 per cent from lactate (derived from anaerobic glycolysis). Of the gluconeogenic amino acids, alanine is of principal importance.[12] Deficiencies in release of alanine by muscle appear to result in hypoglycemia.[13]

Based on these considerations, an approach to the diagnosis of the cause(s) of hypoglycemia might proceed as follows.

Response to Prolonged Fasting

Under careful observation, the child should be studied while fasting, with regular measurements of blood glucose, free fatty acids and/or glycerol, plasma insulin, and urinary ketone bodies. If one uses Dextrostix, when hypoglycemia occurs the fast can be discontinued without endangering the child.

This study gives evidence regarding: the rapidity of development of hypoglycemia; whether insulin secretion appropriately decreases as hypoglycemia develops; and whether enhanced rates of lipolysis accompany development of hypoglycemia.

In our experience, this single approach is most helpful in defining abnormalities in the control of insulin secretion. If the child fails to develop hypoglycemia after an 18- to 24-hour fast, no further studies are probably indicated since, regardless of etiology, the process is likely to be mild, although quite possibly recurrent.

Response to Consecutive Glucose Infusions

If hypoglycemia does occur, further information can be obtained by infusing glucose for 60 to 90 minutes at successive rates of 4, 8, and 12 mg/kg/minute and measuring the concentration of blood glucose during the last 15 minutes of each infusion period. Adam and co-workers[14] have developed a useful infusion protocol which allows one to make inferences regarding the magnitude of glucose utilization. For example, if excessive rates of glucose must be infused to maintain a blood glucose concentration in the low normal range, a rapid rate of peripheral glucose utilization may be inferred. On the other hand, maintenance of euglycemia with low rates of glucose infusion in a child who develops hypoglycemia during fasting suggests that the defect is inadequate hepatic glucose production.

Utilization of Specific Diagnostic Procedures

Specific procedures should be utilized based on information derived from the history and physical examination. For example, the child with marked hepatomegaly should be considered as possibly having glycogen storage disease or some form of intrahepatic pathology. Further, the child who develops postprandial hypoglycemia after taking a meal containing fructose should then be challenged with a fructose load.

Assessment of Hormonal Regulation

In the child with fasting hypoglycemia, the causative mechanism may reside in deficient secretion of hormones which are antagonistic to the action of insulin. Accordingly, appropriate techniques for measurement of growth hormone, thyroxine, and adrenal glucocorticoids should be employed.

MAINTENANCE THERAPY

Whenever possible, therapy should be directed toward causative mechanisms. In our hands, a specific diagnosis of the cause of infantile hypoglycemia is not possible in three-quarters of affected patients. If excessive or inappropriate insulin secretion is demonstrated, direct surgical intervention is advisable. In the usual situation, recurrent but infrequent episodes of hypoglycemia during fasting should be managed by frequent feedings, especially during the night. In spite of numerous assertions, there is little evidence that the composition of such frequent feeding is of major importance. In severely affected infants, use of adjunct therapy with epinephrine-like agents or adrenal glucocorticoids may assist in stabilizing blood glucose concentration. An antihypertensive, hyperglycemic sulfonamide (diazoxide) has been used extensively in the management of hypoglycemia. Since its principal mechanism of action depends on a diminution of insulin secretion in response to various physiological stimuli, effective control of hypoglycemia may not occur under conditions of prolonged fasting, when insulin secretion is already reduced. Hypertrichosis, edema, and hyperuricemia have been encountered as side effects of diazoxide administration.[15, 16]

REFERENCES

1. Owen, O. E., Morgan, A. P., Kemp, H. G., Sullivan, J. M., Herrera, M. G., and Cahill, G. F., Jr.: Brain metabolism during fasting. J. Clin. Invest., 46:1589, 1967.
2. Cornblath, M., and Schwartz, R.: Disorders of Carbohydrate Metabolism in Infancy. 2nd ed., Philadelphia, W. B. Saunders, 1976.
3. Chantler, C., Baum, J. D., and Norman, D. A.: Dextrostix in the diagnosis of neonatal hypoglycemia. Lancet, 2:1395, 1967.
4. Swiatek, K. R., Luebben, G., and Cornblath, M.: Screening method for determining glucose in blood and cerebrospinal fluid. Am. J. Dis. Child., 117:672, 1969.
5. Griffiths, A. D.: Association of hypoglycemia with symptoms in the newborn. Arch. Dis. Child., 43:688, 1968.
6. Raivio, K. O.: Factors affecting the development of symptoms in neonatal hypoglycemia. Ann. Paediatr. Fenn., 14:105, 1969.
7. Lubchenco, L. O., and Bard, H.: Incidence of hypoglycemia in newborn infants classified by birth weight and gestational age. Pediatrics, 47:831, 1971.
8. Zucker, P., and Simon, G.: Prolonged symptomatic neonatal hypoglycemia associated with maternal chlorpropamide therapy. Pediatrics, 42:824, 1968.
9. Yueng, D., and Oliver, I. T.: Factors affecting the premature induction of phosphopyruvate carboxylase in neonatal rat liver. Biochem. J., 108:325, 1968.
10. Cahill, G. F., Jr., Herrera, M. G., Morgan, A. P., Soeldner, J. S., Steinke, J., Levy, P. L., Reichard, G. A., Jr., and Kipnis, D. M.: Hormone-fuel interrelationships during fasting. J. Clin. Invest., 45:1751, 1966.
11. Cahill, G. F., Jr., and Owen, O. E.: Some observations on carbohydrate metabolism in man. In Dickens, F., Randle, P. J., and Whelan, W. J., eds.: Carbohydrate Metabolism and Its Disorders. New York, Academic Press, 1968, p. 497.

12. Felig, P., Pozefsky, T., Marliss, E., and Cahill, G. F., Jr.: Alanine: Key role in gluconeo-
    genesis. Science, *167*:1003, 1970.
13. Pagliara, A. S., Karl, I. E., Haymond, M., and Kipnis, D. M.: Hypoglycemia in infancy
    and childhood. Parts I and II. J. Pediatr., *82*:365 and 558, 1975.
14. Adam, P. A., Jr., King, K., and Schwartz, R.: Model for the investigation of intracta-
    ble hypoglycemia: Insulin-glucose interrelationships during steady state infu-
    sions. Pediatrics, *41*:91, 1968.
15. Baker, L., Kaye, R., Root, A. W., and Prasad, A. L. N.: Diazoxide treatment of idio-
    pathic hypoglycemia of infancy. J. Pediatr., *71*:494, 1967.
16. Koblenzer, P. J., and Baker, L.: Hypertrichosis lanuginosa associated with diazoxide
    therapy in prepubertal children: A clinicopathologic study. Ann. N.Y. Acad. Sci.,
    150:373, 1968.

Chapter Eighteen

ACUTE METABOLIC DISEASE IN INFANCY AND EARLY CHILDHOOD

DONOUGH O'BRIEN, M.D., F.R.C.P.
STEPHEN I. GOODMAN, M.D.

The infant or young child who becomes acutely and seriously ill with or without a preliminary period of "failure to thrive" and who shows marked and sometimes intractable metabolic acidosis with anorexia, lethargy, convulsions, and perhaps coma represents an infrequent but important problem. It has become increasingly apparent that a significant proportion of patients with this clinical picture are accounted for by inborn errors of intermediary metabolism; but from the standpoint of the practicing pediatrician, these still remain a group of rare and complex conditions, much discussed and rarely seen. In certain cases, more definitive physical signs offer some specific clue to diagnosis. For example, severe neonatal edema with hypoproteinemia may suggest cystic fibrosis; an odd smell may suggest branched-chain ketoaciduria; a large heart and macroglossia may suggest acid maltase deficiency (Pompe's disease); an electrolyte disturbance in the male may suggest the adrenogenital syndrome; and jaundice and hepatomegaly may suggest galactosemia.

The special purpose of this article is to call attention to that group of inborn errors that may be associated with sudden, severe, and perhaps fatal illness in early life. Individually rare but collectively worth recognition, many times they often can be promptly, accurately,

From the B. F. Stolinsky Research Laboratories, Department of Pediatrics, University of Colorado Medical Center, Denver, Colorado.

and inexpensively diagnosed and, as important, can be treated successfully. Furthermore, specific diagnosis then allows genetic counseling and the possibility of antenatal diagnosis in later pregnancies. Some typical case histories are presented as illustrations, together with a table of currently recognized diseases in this category and a second table listing some screening tests useful in diagnosis. The whole is intended as an *aide-mémoire* for the pediatrician, to assist him or her with the practicalities of diagnosis and initial management in this field.

CASE HISTORIES

Branched-Chain Ketoaciduria

D. D. was the product of an uncomplicated pregnancy and delivery. He appeared normal at birth and was discharged from the hospital at 3 days of age. At 5 days of age he became listless and began to feed poorly and was admitted to hospital 2 days later. A previous male sibling had died at 13 days of age with what was described as aspiration pneumonia.

Physical examination was completely normal except for moderate flaccidity, poor Moro and tonic neck reflexes, and a slight increase of deep tendon reflexes.

A hemogram and routine urinalysis were normal. The cerebrospinal fluid was normal and sterile; blood and urine cultures were negative. Serum pH, Pco_2, CO_2, Na, Cl, K, BUN, and glucose measurements were all normal. Chest x-ray revealed minimal bronchopneumonia at the right base.

On the second hospital day observation of a sweetish urinary odor led to an examination of serum amino acids, and the increased concentrations of leucine, isoleucine, and valine characteristic of branched-chain ketoaciduria were observed. Treatment with a diet low in branched-chain amino acids was promptly instituted. Now at the age of 7 years, the child is developmentally normal. This outcome is in sharp contrast to the prognosis for the untreated case, in which there is usually progressive neurological deterioration followed by death within the first 2 months of life.

Methylmalonic Aciduria

D. O., also a male, was discharged from the hospital at 3 days of age, following an uncomplicated term delivery. On the fourth day of life, he developed feeding difficulties, somnolence, and respiratory grunting, which prompted his hospitalization. Family history was non-contributory. On admission he was mildly jaundiced and his respirations were labored. Other positive physical findings were a slightly bulging anterior fontanelle with no neck stiffness, extreme lethargy, no Moro, suck, or grasp reflexes, and hypoactive deep tendon reflexes. His clinical condition steadily deteriorated until assisted ventilation was required.

Hemogram and routine urinalysis were normal. Biochemical measurements included a pH of 6.99, total CO_2 of 8 mEq/L, Na of 145 mEq/L, K of 4.8 mEq, BUN of 14 mg/100 ml, and a blood sugar of 3 mg/100 ml. The spinal fluid was clear, contained no cells, 210 mg/100 ml protein, and no detectable glucose. Cultures of blood, CSF, and urine were sterile. Chest x-ray showed diffuse infiltration, compatible with either infection or aspiration. Paper chromatography of amino acids in blood and urine were normal.

Severe metabolic acidemia suggested either renal tubular acidosis or organic acidemia. Gas chromatography of urinary organic acids revealed a large amount of methylmalonic acid characteristic of methylmalonic acidemia. A low protein diet and parenteral vitamin B_{12} in large doses, which might have been effective if given earlier, were instituted on the seventh day of life. They had no clinical effect and he died the next day.

Galactosemia

S. A., born in a small country hospital after a normal pregnancy and delivery, weighed 6 lbs, 6 oz at birth and was discharged on the fifth day of life. On the eighth day he was noted to be moderately jaundiced, and this increased up to the twelfth day when he was first seen by a pediatrician, at which time the serum total bilirubin measured 16.8 mg/100 ml. The liver edge was palpated 4 cm below the costal margin. There was also some pyuria and an umbilical discharge containing coagulase-positive staphylococci. Understandably, these observations led to a diagnosis of septicemia and treatment with antibiotics; his general condition then improved and the jaundice disappeared. On the twenty-eighth day the infant was seen again by the pediatrician. At this time, neonatal hepatitis was considered to be the most probable diagnosis. One week later the child had deteriorated clinically. A spinal fluid sugar at that time was 400 mg/100 ml and a blood sugar 300 mg/100 ml by a method that measured total reducing substances. Galactosemia was tentatively diagnosed and the infant placed on a galactose-free regimen. UDP galactose transferase activity was found to be < 8 ImU/gHb but treatment was ineffectual, and the infant died on the thirty-third day of life. Earlier sensitivity to the possibility of metabolic disease would almost certainly have saved his life.

DISCUSSION

Children's physicians already are accustomed to the idea of screening for inborn errors of metabolism in certain specified circumstances: for hyperphenylalaninemia and perhaps hypertyrosinemia in the newborn; for Wilson's disease in patients with liver disease; and for a more extended array of conditions in the mentally retarded. The idea that in certain cases sudden acute serious illnesses in infancy and early childhood also may be caused by inborn errors of metabolism is only now gaining widespread acceptance. The purpose of this article is to call attention to these conditions and to provide an introduction to and reference source for their diagnosis and initial management.

Table 1 is a compilation of some of the disorders that fall in this category. It is not all-inclusive in that certain well-known conditions such as cystic fibrosis have been omitted. The list is intended primarily to include those states in which there are non-specific signs, usually neurological, which may or may not be accompanied by severe acidosis. Distinguishing features such as special odors, in so far as they exist, are

Text continued on page 262

TABLE 1   Rare Inborn Errors of Metabolism Associated with Severe Clinical Disease in Infancy and Early Childhood[1,2,3]

Disorder	Biochemical Defect	Associated Clinical Findings	Lab Test (See Table 2)	Diagnosis	Treatment
In amino acid metabolism Hyperammonemia	a. Carbamyl phosphate synthetase[4,5]	Variable: from death in infancy to episodic vomiting and lethargy exacerbated by protein intake	1	Hyperammonemia	Protein restriction, α-keto acids
	b. Ornithine trans-carbamylase[6]	As above, but X-linked inheritance; males die in first week of life and females have variable and usually less severe course	1,2	Hyperammonemia, orotic aciduria	Protein restriction, α-keto acids
Citrullinemia[7]	Argininosuccinic acid synthetase	Variable: from neonatal lethargy, coma, and death to periodic vomiting, seizures, and mental retardation	1,3a,3b	Hyperammonemia, increased citrulline in blood and urine	Low protein diet
Argininosuccinic-aciduria[8]	Argininosuccinic acid lyase	Variable: from neonatal lethargy, coma, and death to mental retardation, periodic coma, ataxia, and trichorrhexis nodosa	1,3a,3b	Hyperammonemia, argininosuccinic acid in urine	Low protein diet
Hypervalinemia[9]	Valine α-ketoglutarate transaminase	Neonatal vomiting, lethargy, and failure to thrive	3a,3b	Increased valine in blood and urine	Low protein diet
Maple syrup urine disease, classical form[10]	Branched-chain keto-acid decarboxylase	Neonatal acidemia, lethargy, and feeding difficulty. Maple syrup-like odor to urine	3a,3b,4, 6,8	Increased branched-chain amino acids in blood and urine, increased branched-chain keto and hydroxy acids in urine	Diet low in branched-chain amino acids[10]

Disease	Enzyme defect	Clinical features		Biochemical findings	Treatment
Isovaleric acidemia[11]	Isovaleryl-CoA dehydrogenase	Metabolic acidemia, lethargy, and neurological symptoms. Odor of "sweaty feet"	6,8	Isovaleric acid, isovaleryl-glycine, and β-hydroxyisovaleric acid in urine	Low leucine diet[11]
β-Methylcrotonylglycinuria[12,13]	β-Methylcrotonyl-CoA carboxylase	Metabolic acidemia, vomiting, and irritability. Odor of "cat's urine"	6,8	β-Methylcrotonyl-glycine and β-hydroxyisovaleric acid in urine	Low protein diet. Some patients respond to large doses of biotin[13]
α-Methyl-β-Hydroxybutyric aciduria[14,15]	α-Methylacetoacetyl-CoA β-Ketothiolase	Variable: may present in infancy with metabolic acidemia, vomiting, and failure to thrive	6	α-Methylacetoacetic acid, α-methyl-β-hydroxybutyric acid, and tiglylglycine in urine	Low protein diet
Propionic acidemia[16,17]	Propionyl-CoA carboxylase	Metabolic acidemia, vomiting, and failure to thrive	6,3a,3b	Propionic acid, β-hydroxypropionic acid, methylcitric acid, and propionylglycine in urine; hyperglycinemia and hyperglycinuria	Low protein diet; some patients respond to biotin in large doses[17]
Methylmalonic aciduria[18,19,20]	a. Methylmalonyl-CoA racemase b. Methylmalonyl-CoA isomerase c. Defects in deoxyadenosyl-B_{12} synthesis	Metabolic acidemia, vomiting, and failure to thrive	5,6,3a,3b	Methylmalonic acid in blood and urine; hyperglycinemia and hyperglycinuria; (c) may have associated homocystinuria	Low protein diet; some of (b) and most of (c) respond to hydroxy- or cyano-B_{12} in large doses
Non-ketotic hyperglycinemia[21]	Glycine cleavage enzyme in brain	Seizures, microcephaly, mental retardation	3a,3b	Increased glycine in blood, urine, and cerebrospinal fluid	None

Table continued on following page

TABLE 1 Rare Inborn Errors of Metabolism Associated with Severe Clinical Disease in Infancy and Early Childhood[1,2,3] *(Continued)*

Disorder	Biochemical Defect	Associated Clinical Findings	Lab Test (See Table 2)	Diagnosis	Treatment
Hyper-β-alaninemia	β-Alanine-α-keto-glutarate transaminase (?)	Neonatal lethargy, seizures	3a,3b	Increased β-alanine in serum, β-alanine taurine, GABA, and β-AIB in urine	None
Sulfite oxidase deficiency[23]	Sulfite oxidase	Neonatal pyramidal signs, blindness, lens dislocations	7	Increased urine sulfite, thiosulfate, and S-sulfo-L-cysteine	None
Glutaric aciduria[24]	Glutaryl-CoA dehydrogenase	Intermittent metabolic acidemia, vomiting, choreoathetosis	6	Glutaric, glutaconic, and β-hydroxyglutaric acids in urine	Low protein diet
Pyroglutamic aciduria[25]	Glutathione synthetase	Neonatal metabolic acidemia with hemolytic anemia	6	Pyroglutamic acid in urine	Alkali therapy
Hereditary tyrosinemia[26]	Unknown: many cases due to fructose-1-phosphate aldolase deficiency (hereditary fructose intolerance)	Severe parenchymal liver disease progressing to cirrhosis, renal Fanconi syndrome with hypophosphatemic rickets	3a,3b,6	Increased serum methionine and tyrosine, generalized aminoaciduria, hypophosphatemia. Increased p-hydroxyphenyl-lactic acid and N-acetyltyrosine in urine	Diet low in tyrosine and phenylalanine, ? diet low in fructose
Pyridoxine-dependent seizures[27]	? neuronal glutamic acid decarboxylase	Neonatal seizures, irritability		Prompt response to pyridoxine	25 mg pyridoxine parenterally

In carbohydrate metabolism

Disease	Defect	Clinical features	Ref.	Laboratory findings	Treatment
Congenital lactic acidosis[28,29]	Pyruvate dehydrogenase complex, pyruvate carboxylase	Neonatal metabolic acidemia	3a,3b,6,11	Increased lactic and pyruvic acids in serum and urine, increased serum alanine	Low carbohydrate diet
Galactosemia, classical form[1]	UDP-galactose transferase	Vomiting, growth retardation, jaundice, hepatomegaly, lens opacities	10,9	Increased urine galactose, demonstration of enzyme defect in erythrocytes	Galactose restricted diet
Hereditary fructose intolerance[30,31]	Fructose-1-phosphate aldolase	Variable: may present in neonate with hypoglycemia, severe liver disease, and renal Fanconi syndrome with hypophosphatemic rickets	9,6,3a,3b	Same as "hereditary tyrosinemia" plus hypoglycemic response to oral fructose load (0.6 gm/kg)	Exclusion of cane sugar from diet
Fructose-1,6-diphosphatase deficiency[32]	Fructose-1,6-diphosphatase	Same as above	9,6,3a,3b	As above, specific enzyme assay	
Glucose-galactose malabsorption[33]	Enteric and renal transport of glucose and galactose	Diarrhea, vomiting, dehydration, failure to thrive	9	Glucose and galactose in stools	Galactose and glucose restricted diet

In metal metabolism

Disease	Defect	Clinical features	Ref.	Laboratory findings	Treatment
Familial hypomagnesemia[34]	Intestinal transport of magnesium	Seizures and tetany, responsive to Mg++ and not Ca++ therapy, progressive neurological deterioration	12	Hypocalcemia and serum magnesium less than 1.4 mEq/L	Mg++ IV (1 mEq/kg/day), then 4-5 mEq/kg/day PO until serum normal
Menkes' syndrome[35,36]	Intestinal transport of copper	Seizures, failure to thrive, pili torti, progressive neurological deterioration, X-linked recessive inheritance	13	Low serum copper and ceruloplasmin	None
Acrodermatitis enteropathica[37]	Intestinal transport zinc	Diarrhea, dermatitis, and alopecia on cow's milk formula	14	Serum zinc less than 60 mcg/100 ml	Zinc sulfate PO, diiodohydroxyquin (Diodoquin) PO

TABLE 2 Screening and Confirmatory Tests For Inborn Errors of Metabolism Causing Severe Clinical Disease In Infancy

Test	Availability*	Conditions Detected
1. Ammonia in plasma	B	Carbamyl-phosphate synthetase deficiency,[4,5] ornithine transcarbamylase deficiency,[6] citrullinemia,[7] argininosuccinic aciduria[8]
2. Orotacaciduria and screening test	A	Ornithine transcarbamylase deficiency[6]
3. Amino acid chromatography (a) paper	A	Citrullinemia,[7] argininosuccinic aciduria,[8] maple syrup urine disease,[10] hypervalinemia,[9] hyper-β-alaninemia,[22] non-ketotic hyperglycinemia,[21] hereditary tyrosinemia, propionic acidemia,[16,17] methylmalonic acidemia,[18,19,20] congenital lactic acidosis,[28,29] hereditary fructose intolerance,[30,31] fructose-1,6-diphosphatase deficiency[32]
(b) ion-exchange	C	Confirmation of above; request if any possibility of abnormality on paper chromatography
4. Dinitrophenylhydrazine test for keto acids in urine	A	Maple syrup urine disease, not specific[10]
5. Methylmalonic acid, urinary screening	A	Methylmalonic acidemia.[18,19,20] The test is erratically negative in the acute case and organic acid chromatography should always be carried out as well

6. Organic acids by combined gas chromatography-mass spectroscopy of urine extracts	C	Maple syrup urine disease,[10] isovaleric acidemia,[11] β-methylcrotonylglycinuria,[12,13] α-methyl-β-hydroxybutyric aciduria,[14,15] propionic acidemia,[16,17] methylmalonic acidemia,[18,19,20] glutaric aciduria,[24] pyroglutamic aciduria,[25] hereditary tyrosinemia, hereditary fructose intolerance,[30,31] fructose-1,6-diphosphatase deficiency,[32] congenital lactic acidosis[28,29]
7. Sulfite and thiosulfate in urine	A	Sulfite oxidase deficiency[23]
8. Unusual odor in sweat, breath, or urine		Maple syrup urine disease,[10] isovaleric acidemia,[11] β-methylcrotonylglycinuria[12,13]
9. Urine sugar chromatography	B	Hereditary fructose intolerance,[30,31] galactosemia,[1] glucose-galactose malabsorption[33]
10. Red cell screen for galactosemia	B	Galactosemia[1]
11. Serum lactic and pyruvic acids	B	Congenital lactic acidosis[28,29]
12. Serum magnesium	A	Familial hypomagnesemia[34]
13. Serum copper	A	Menkes' syndrome[35,36]
14. Serum zinc	C	Acrodermatitis enteropathica[37]

*A – could be carried out by any clinical laboratory.
B – likely available only in a major medical center.
C – probably available through specialized laboratories.

Serum or heparinized plasma samples should be separated from red cells and dispatched to the laboratory by the quickest route. Urine should be brought to <pH 3.0 for amino acids and pH 7.6 for organic acids. Except for ammonic, lactic, and pyruvic acid assays, which should be processed immediately, other tests can be carried out on mailed samples of 0.5 ml serum or 2 to 3 ml of a random urine sample.

listed; but in general, identification will depend on the laboratory. Few of these conditions are well described in standard pediatric texts.

The appropriate biochemical determinations are given in Table 2, in which tests have been divided into three categories: those that can be completed in any hospital clinical laboratory; those like one-dimensional amino acid chromatography that should be available in a group hospital clinical chemistry laboratory; and others, including organic acid chromatography, that need to be carried out in special centers. It is usually wise not to presume that a laboratory can carry out these tests and to check in advance its preparedness for a given test.

Sample collection and delivery is another consideration. Ideally, urine samples should be aliquots of a known 24-hour volume. Such accuracy is not always possible, and random specimens that have been stored frozen at a pH of 3 or lower for amino acids or pH 7 for organic acids are satisfactory. Five-milliliter samples can be sent air express in standard containers. Blood samples are sometimes hard to obtain from small infants except by heel prick. Thus, whole blood in heparinized capillaries, which can be protected in the mail by insertion into the folds of corrugated paper, is quite adequate, although plasma alone is always preferable.

REFERENCES

1. Stanbury, J. B., Wyngaarden, J. B., and Fredrickson, D. S.: The Metabolic Basis of Inherited Disease. 3rd ed., New York, McGraw-Hill, 1972.
2. Scriver, C. R., and Rosenberg, L. E.: Amino Acid Metabolism and Its Disorders. Philadelphia, W. B. Saunders Co., 1973.
3. Nyhan, W. L.: Heritable Disorders of Amino Acid Metabolism: Patterns of Clinical Expression and Genetic Variation. New York, John Wiley & Sons, 1974.
4. Gelehrter, T. D., and Snodgrass, P. J.: Lethal neonatal deficiency of carbamylphosphate synthetase. N. Engl. J. Med., 290:430, 1974.
5. Short, E. M., Conn, H. O., Snodgrass, P. J., Campbell, A. G. M., and Rosenberg, L. E.: Evidence for X-linked dominant inheritance of ornithine transcarbamylase deficiency. N. Engl. J. Med., 288:7, 1973.
6. Campbell, A. G. M., Rosenberg, L. E., Snodgrass, P. J., and Nuzum, C. T.: Ornithine transcarbamylase deficiency: A cause of lethal neonatal hyperammonemia in males. N. Engl. J. Med., 288:1, 1973.
7. Van der Zee, S. P. M., Trijbels, J. M. F., Monnens, L. A. H., Hommes, F. A., and Schretlen, E. D. A.: Citrullinemia with rapidly fatal neonatal course. Arch. Dis. Child., 46:847, 1971.
8. Carton, D., de Schrijver, F., Kiut, J., Van Durme, J., and Hooft, C.: Argininosuccinic aciduria: Neonatal varient with rapid fatal course. Acta Paediatr. Scand., 58:528, 1969.
9. Dancis, J., Hutzler, J., Tada, K., Waday, Y., Morikawa, T., and Arakawa, T.: Hypervalinemia. Pediatrics, 39:813, 1967.
10. Goodman, S. I., Pollak, S., Miles, B., and O'Brien, D.: The treatment of maple syrup urine disease. J. Pediatr., 75:485, 1969.
11. Levy, H. L., Erickson, A. M., Lott, I. T., and Kurtz, D. J.: Isovaleric acidemia: Results of family study and dietary treatment. Pediatrics, 52:83, 1973.

12. Stokke, O., Eldjarn, L., Jellum, E., Pande, H., and Waaler, P. E.: Beta-methylcro-
    tonyl-CoA carboxylase deficiency: a new metabolic error in leucine degradation.
    Pediatrics, 49:726, 1972.
13. Gompertz, D., Bartlett, K., Blair, D., and Stern, C. M. M.: Child with a defect in
    leucine metabolism associated with β-methylcrotonylglycinuria. Arch. Dis.
    Child., 48:975, 1973.
14. Keating, J. P., Feigin, R. D., Tenenbaum, S. M., and Hillman, R. E.: Hyperglycine-
    mia with ketosis due to a defect in isoleucine metabolism: a preliminary report.
    Pediatrics, 50:890, 1972.
15. Hillman, R. E., and Keating, J. P.: Beta-ketothiolase deficiency as a cause of the "ke-
    totic hyperglycinemia syndrome." Pediatrics, 53:221, 1974.
16. Hommes, F. A., Kuipes, J. R. G., Elema, J. D., Jansen, J. F., and Jonxis, J. H. P.:
    Propionicacidemia. Pediatr. Res., 2:519, 1968.
17. Barnes, N. D., Hull, D., Balgobin, L., and Gompertz, D.: Biotin-responsive propionic-
    acidemia, Lancet, 2:244, 1970.
18. Kang, E. S., Snodgrass, P. J., and Gerald, P. S.: Methylmalonyl coenzyme A racemase
    defect: another cause of methylmalonic aciduria. Pediatr. Res., 6:875, 1972.
19. Morrow, G. III, Barness, L. A., Cardinale, G. J., Abeles, R. H., and Flaks, J. G.: Con-
    genital methylmalonic acidemia: enzymatic evidence for two forms of the
    disease. Proc. Natl. Acad. Sci. (U.S.A.), 63:191, 1969.
20. Mahoney, M. J., Hart, A. C., Steen, V. D., and Rosenburg, L. E.: Methylmalonicaci-
    demia: biochemical heterogeneity in defects of 5'-deoxyadenosyl-cobalmin syn-
    thesis. Proc. Natl. Acad. Sci. (U.S.A.), 72:2799, 1975.
21. Perry, T. L., Urquhart, N., MacLean, J., Evans, M. E., Hansen, S., Davidson, A. G.
    F., Applegarth, D. A., MacLeod, P. J., and Lock, J. E.: Nonketotic hyperglycine-
    mia: glycine accumulation due to absence of glycine cleavage in brain. N. Engl. J.
    Med., 292:1269, 1975.
22. Scriver, C. R., Pueschel, S., and Danes, E.: Hyper-β-alaninemia associated with β-
    amino aciduria and γ-aminobutyric aciduria, somnolence and seizures. N. Engl.
    J. Med., 274:635, 1966.
23. Irreverre, F., Mudd, S. H., Heizer, W. D., and Laster, L.: Sulfite oxidase deficiency:
    studies of a patient with mental retardation, dislocated ocular lenses and abnor-
    mal urinary excretion of S-sulfo-L-cysteine, sulfite and thiosulfate. Biochem.
    Med., 1:187, 1967.
24. Goodman, S. I., Markey, S. P., Moe, P. G., Miles, B. S., and Teng, C. C.: Glutaric
    aciduria: a "new" disorder of amino acid metabolism. Biochem. Med., 12:12,
    1975.
25. Larsson, A., Zetterström, R., Hagenfeldt, L., Andersson, R., Dreborg, S., and Hör-
    nell, H.: Pyroglutamic aciduria (5-oxoprolinuria), an inborn error in glutathione
    metabolism. Pediatr. Res., 8:852, 1974.
26. Scriver, C. R., Partington, M., and Sass-Kortsak, A.: Conference on hereditary
    tyrosinemia. Can. Med. Assoc. J., 97:1045, 1967.
27. Rosenberg, L. E.: Inherited aminoacidopathies demonstrating vitamin dependency.
    N. Engl. J. Med., 281:145, 1969.
28. Farrell, D. F., Clark, A. F., Scott, C. R., and Wennberg, R. P.: Absence of pyruvate
    decarboxylase activity in man: a cause of congenital lactic acidosis. Science,
    187:1082, 1975.
29. Brunette, M. G., Delvin, E., Hacel, B., and Scriver, C. R.: Thiamine-responsive lactic
    acidosis in a patient with deficient low-K_m pyruvate carboxylase activity in liver.
    Pediatrics, 50:702, 1972.
30. Lindemann, R., Gjessing, L. R., Merton, B., Loken, A. C., and Halvorsen, S.: Amino
    acid metabolism in hereditary fructosemia. Acta Paediatr. Scand., 59:141, 1970.
31. Hulsmann, W. C., and Fernandes, J.: A child with lactacidemia and fructose
    diphosphatase deficiency in the liver. Pediatr. Res., 5:633, 1971.
32. Bakker, H. D., De Bfee, P. K., Ketting, D., Van Sprang, F. J., and Wadman, S. K.:
    Fructose-1, 6-diphosphatase deficiency: another enzyme defect which can pre-
    sent itself with the clinical features of "tyrosinosis." Clin. Chim. Acta., 55:41, 1975.
33. Meeuwisse, G. W., and Melin, K.: Studies in glucose-galactose malabsorption. Acta
    Paediatr. Scand. Suppl., 188:1, 1969.
34. Stromme, J. H., Nesbakken, R., Normann, T., Skjorten, F., Skyberg, D., and Johan-

nessen, B.: Familial hypomagnesemia. Biochemical, histological and hereditary aspects studied in two brothers. Acta Paediatr. Scand., *58*:433, 1969.

35. Danks, D. M., Stevens, B. J., Campbell, P. E., Gillespie, J. M., Walker-Smith, J., Blomfield, J., and Turner, B.: Menkes' kinky-hair syndrome. Lancet, *1*:1100, 1972.

36. Danks, D. M., Campbell, P. E., Stevens, B. J., Mayne, V., and Cartwright, E.: Menkes' kinky-hair syndrome: an inherited defect in copper absorption with widespread effects. Pediatrics, *50*:188, 1972.

37. Neldner, K. H., and Hambidge, K. M.: Zinc therapy of acrodermatitis enteropathica. N. Engl. J. Med., *292*:879, 1975.

Chapter Nineteen

SALICYLATE INTOXICATION

WILLIAM E. SEGAR, M.D.

Salicylate is a potent pharmacological agent, and the rational therapy for salicylate intoxication must be based on an understanding of its pharmacological actions and consequent pathophysiological effects.[1] Because it acts to uncouple oxidative phosphorylation in a manner analogous to that of 2,4-dinitrophenol, salicylate is, first of all, a general metabolic stimulant.[2] Oxygen consumption, carbon dioxide formation, and heat production are increased by its action; consequently, oxygen requirement, blood CO_2 concentration, and the need to eliminate heat also are increased. Respiration, heart rate, and cardiac output must increase to satisfy the demands imposed by the acceleration of metabolic processes. Increased heat production causes an increase in evaporated water losses from skin surfaces. Sweating usually occurs.

Second, salicylate interferes in a complex manner with the normal metabolism of carbohydrate.[3] Many factors seem to be involved, some tending to decrease and others to increase the blood glucose concentration, and clinically, either hyperglycemia or hypoglycemia may be observed. Hyperglycemia may be explained partially by the release of epinephrine due to activation of hypothalamic sympathetic centers. However, large doses of salicylate also decrease aerobic metabolism and increase glucose-6-phosphatase activity, effects which tend to increase the blood glucose level. Hypoglycemia, on the other hand, may be caused by an increased utilization of glucose by peripheral tissues or by interference with gluconeogenesis by salicylates. Recent studies suggest that brain glucose concentration may be decreased despite minimal alterations in blood glucose level.[4]

From the Department of Pediatrics, University of Wisconsin Medical Center, Madison, Wisconsin.

265

As a result of these salicylate-induced alterations in carbohydrate metabolism, organic acids, particularly lactic, pyruvic, and acetoacetic, accumulate.[5] Infants appear to be particularly susceptible to the toxic effects of salicylate on carbohydrate metabolism and are more likely to have disturbances in blood glucose concentration and severe metabolic acidosis than are older children.

Salicylate also is a known stimulant of the respiratory center of the central nervous system, and increased salicylate levels produce an increase in ventilation.[6] This effect, which occurs promptly after the ingestion of a toxic amount of salicylate, results in a net decrease in Pco_2 and a respiratory alkalosis, despite the fact the hypermetabolic action of salicylate would increase Pco_2. In turn, the renal excretion of sodium, potassium, and bicarbonate is increased, a known response to respiratory alkalosis. The excretion of potassium may be very great, since salicylate at toxic levels may increase potassium excretion to a rate that exceeds the creatinine clearance, by a mechanism unrelated to the accompanying metabolic alkalosis.[7] As a result of the loss of sodium and potassium bicarbonate, the patient's ability to compensate for the metabolic acidosis, which, in severely intoxicated children, is superimposed on the pre-existing respiratory alkalosis, is significantly compromised.

Dehydration, particularly in the infant or in the child with chronic salicylate intoxication, is an important and, often, an inevitable consequence of the pathophysiological processes noted. Both hyperventilation and sweating result in increased water and electrolyte expenditure. Vomiting and diarrhea occur frequently and contribute to the development of dehydration. Initially, the volume of urine will be increased by the increased solute load characteristic of any state of hypermetabolism and ketosis. It might be noted that once body water stores are depleted, salicylate no longer can induce effective sweating, and the hyperpyretic action of the drug no longer is balanced by effective defenses. Thus, hyperpyrexia accelerates dehydration, and dehydration potentiates hyperpyrexia. The magnitude of the water losses cannot be quantitated precisely. To our knowledge no balance studies have been performed on children recovering from salicylate intoxication. However, one might assume that the water losses are comparable to those observed in diabetic acidosis.[8-10] and would, in the severely intoxicated child, approximate 80 to 120 ml per kg of body weight.

DIAGNOSIS AND TREATMENT

The symptoms and clinical findings exhibited by the child with salicylate intoxication will vary depending on the age of the child, the amount of salicylate consumed, and whether the poisoning is a result of accidental ingestion or therapeutic overdosage. The severity of the illness often correlates poorly with the blood salicylate level and may be more severe than predicted from the salicylate concentration alone, particularly in infants and in children poisoned by therapeutic overdosage.

Mild Intoxication

Hyperventilation is frequently the only symptom of mild intoxication in a child 2 years old or older. Respiratory alkalosis is usually present. After emptying the child's stomach by the use of syrup of ipecac or by mechanical means, the physician need only be sure that the the child receives an adequate fluid intake, either orally or parenterally. The type of fluid given is of little importance because these children recover uneventfully.

Moderate Intoxication

The infant with salicylate intoxication, the child poisoned by therapeutic overdosage, or the older child with any disturbance in sensorium or hydration probably should be hospitalized and given parenteral fluid therapy. These moderately ill patients are not, by definition, significantly hypernatremic or hyperthermic. Recovery will be complete if the child is given adequate fluid therapy. Assuming that no significant dehydration exists, these children require maintenance therapy plus replacement of the concurrent abnormal losses that are the result of hyperventilation and diaphoresis. This additional fluid requirement can be provided by increasing maintenance therapy by 30 to 50 per cent. Because large amounts of potassium are lost in the urine as a response to the respiratory alkalosis, adequate potassium, usually at a concentration of 40 mEq/L, should be included in the intravenous fluids.

Severe Intoxication

The child with severe salicylate intoxication presents a major therapeutic challenge. Many are small infants who have received chronic overdosage and, despite plasma salicylate levels as low as 15 mg/100 ml, are gravely ill. Severe hyperthermia is common in this group and is an important cause of death. It is a result of the increase in heat production coupled with decreased efficiency of cooling mechanisms.

Severe hyperthermia cannot develop unless the normal heat-regulating mechanisms are impaired. Since these mechanisms depend, in part, upon the evaporation of water from the skin and lungs, as well as the loss of body heat by radiation and convection, they are compromised by dehydration. When the environmental temperature and humidity remain constant, an increase in the heat production must be compensated for by an increase in the evaporation of water or hyperthermia results. In circumstances in which normal body temperature cannot be maintained, sweat is formed, and its evaporation augments the cooling processes. This regulation of body heat requires a delicate balance between heat production and heat loss.

The central nervous system, especially the hypothalamic nuclei, plays an essential part in regulating the peripheral mechanisms concerned with the conservation or loss of body heat. Because of this action the hypothalamus has been termed the "thermostat" of the body. In fever the balance between heat production and heat loss persists, except that the "thermostat" is set at a higher level. Salicylate acts to reset the "thermostat" at a normal temperature. Heat production is not inhibited by salicylates; rather, it is, as noted earlier, increased. However, heat dissipation also is increased by means of increased insensible expenditure of water, as well as by the expenditure of large quantities of sweat. Salicylate, then, can reduce body temperature, but only through the loss of sizable quantities of water. This ability of salicylate to reduce body temperature to normal is undoubtedly due to its action on the central nervous system, for it can be prevented by the experimental production of hypothalamic lesions.[11] In any event, this combination of events can rapidly lead to lethal hyperpyrexia.

Moderate to severe dehydration usually is noted in the child who is seriously ill with salicylate intoxication. Shock and, rarely, acute renal failure may occur. The large respiratory and cutaneous water losses represent loss of water without equivalent loss of electrolyte. Hypernatremia occurs when the child's ability to excrete electrolyte, particularly sodium, is impaired by dehydration or when the renal transport of sodium is affected by the toxic action of salicylate. Significant hypernatremia is not infrequent, occurring in 5 of 25 severely intoxicated children reported by Segar and Holliday.[1] Severe hyperpyrexia and convulsions were observed in the same patients.

The infant with severe salicylate intoxication may be hypoglycemic or hyperglycemic. Glucosuria and ketonuria are present in the latter, and the clinical picture may be confused easily with that of diabetic acidosis. A history of salicylate ingestion and a blood salicylate determination are needed to establish the proper diagnosis. Hypoglycemia may be a more important physiological disturbance than hyperglycemia, since seizures and damage to the central nervous system are possible consequences. A blood sugar determination should be performed on all children with salicylate intoxication and if hypoglycemia exists, prompt therapy with a glucose-containing solution is essential. Indeed, all children with severe salicylate intoxication should receive intravenous glucose since, as noted earlier, the concentration of glucose in cerebrospinal fluid may be low despite normal concentrations in the blood.[7]

Finally, the child with severe salicylate intoxication may display alarming evidence of central nervous system dysfunction, including stupor, coma, convulsions (either focal or generalized), and, rarely, paralysis. The central nervous system symptoms can usually, but not always, be attributed to hyperpyrexia, disturbances in carbohydrate metabolism, hypernatremia, or severe acidosis and ketosis. Hill[12] has demonstrated that in experimental acute salicylate intoxication death occurs when a critical brain salicylate level is reached. Since these animals died in coma, usually after one or more convulsions, it appears that salicylate has a direct deleterious effect on the central nervous system.

Metabolic acidosis may be a serious and life-threatening complication of salicylate intoxication. Although the abnormalities in the chemical composition of the plasma can be corrected readily, the symptomatic recovery of the patient is, in our experience, less rapid than that of the child with diabetic acidosis of comparable severity.

The acidosis of salicylate intoxication is the end result of several pathological processes. Initially, during the stage of hyperventilation, respiratory alkalosis occurs as a result of the increased pulmonary excretion of carbonic acid. This decrease in plasma carbon dioxide tension produces, in turn, a decreased renal reabsorption of bicarbonate and increased excretion of both sodium and potassium bicarbonate.[13, 14] The loss of carbonic acid and of sodium bicarbonate diminishes the buffer capacity of the extracellular fluid to a measurable degree. Loss of potassium similarly leads to a decreased buffer capacity of intracellular fluid. Therefore, pH may change in either direction more readily than before.

The primary cause of the acidosis of salicylate intoxication, however, is the derangement of carbohydrate metabolism. Fat is mobilized and converted in the liver to ketone bodies, which are then utilized by cells for energy purposes. Since the ketone bodies are produced in excess of the capacities of tissue utilization and renal excretion, they accumulate as unmeasured anions in the body fluids. The bicarbonate and other buffer anions are reduced further by this accumulation of organic anions. The concentrations of lactic and pyruvic acids also increase in the body fluids as a result of faulty aerobic carbohydrate metabolism. Salicylate itself is an acid, and its ingestion will increase fixed cation excretion and, because it may displace some bicarbonate in plasma (2 or 3 mEq/L), will increase acidosis. Finally, impairment of renal function may augment the development of acidosis.

The metabolic acidosis of salicylate intoxication is therefore the result of the increased production of various organic acids in an organism whose defenses against acidosis are impaired by a pre-existing depletion of buffering capacity and are compromised further by inadequate renal function. Laboratory evidence of the metabolic acidosis includes a lower serum pH and total Pco_2 content. The child will exhibit Kussmaul respirations and, indeed, hyperventilation is needed for survival. If respiratory rate decreases, the Pco_2 increases and the blood pH, which is already low, may decrease to a level incompatible with life. Finally, myocardial performance may be inadequate—impaired as a result of acidosis, potassium deficiency, hyperthermia, and inefficient myocardial metabolism—and thus may lead to congestive heart failure.

Although adequate intravenous administration of fluids is the *sine qua non* of effective therapy, other important aspects of treatment should not be overlooked.

Hyperpyrexia must be attacked intelligently. Sponging the patient with tepid water is usually adequate. Ice-water sponging should be used judiciously, if at all, because this procedure may cause cutaneous vasoconstriction and interfere with heat loss, or cause shivering and thereby increase heat production. Convulsions may be treated with short-acting barbiturates. Intravenous injection of calcium gluconate is sometimes beneficial.

Care must be taken to avoid procedures and medications that depress respiration since, as noted, hyperventilation is required to increase CO_2 elimination and to prevent a further decrease of blood pH. Oxygen should be used only if the child is cyanotic or in heart failure. If respiratory depression occurs, artificial ventilation is needed and the pattern of hyperventilation must be maintained. Measurements of pH and Pco_2 should be made frequently to guide the rate and depth of artificial ventilation.

Tetany, should it occur, usually can be controlled by decreasing the amount of alkali administered and by the intravenous administration of calcium gluconate. Congestive heart failure also merits an attempt to correct the serum pH rapidly by the judicious administration of alkali because myocardial function may not improve until the serum pH exceeds 7.20.

Intravenous fluid therapy must (1) provide the child with his or her daily maintenance requirements of water and electrolytes, (2) correct pre-existing body fluid deficits, and (3) allow extra water to meet the abnormally great insensible water losses. The usual maintenance requirements are 100 ml of water, 3 mEq of sodium, 2 mEq of potassium, and 2 mEq of chloride per 100 kcal of caloric expenditure per day[15] (or 1500 ml of water, 45 mEq of sodium, 30 mEq of potassium, and 30 mEq of chloride per m^2/day). These amounts should be increased by 25 to 50 per cent to meet the increased requirements for water and electrolytes caused by hyperventilation and sweating.

The additional amount of intravenous fluids required to correct the pre-existing deficit in body fluids is determined by the degree of dehydration. If severe, 100 ml of water, 9 mEq of sodium, 6 mEq of potassium, and 6 mEq of chloride should be given per kilogram of body weight. If dehydration is not severe, proportionately lesser amounts of fluid are needed. As is always the case, deficit fluid therapy should be given in addition to that required for maintenance therapy and for the replacement of ongoing losses. An example of the recommended therapy per 24 hours for a child weighing 10 kg with severe dehydration due to salicylate intoxication is shown in Table 1.

If the serum sodium concentration is higher than 155 mEq/liter, the amount of sodium and chloride given as deficit therapy should be reduced by 25 to 50 per cent. Potassium is added to the intravenous fluids as soon as urine flow is established, and all intravenous fluids should contain 5 gm of glucose per 100 ml.

Perhaps not all physicians will wish to use the system of parenteral fluid therapy described here, although it and similar systems provide a degree of flexibility not otherwise available. However, if the use of polyionic solutions is preferred, those containing approximately 50 mEq of sodium and 40 mEq of potassium and chloride per liter are appropriate. The amount needed will vary from 150 to 250 ml/kg (2250 to 4000 ml/m^2), depending on the severity of the dehydration.

If the child is in shock, the initial therapy should consist of the rapid administration of Ringer's lactate solution, 20 to 40 ml/kg, given in a period of 20 to 30 minutes. Should anuria or severe oliguria persist once the child is adequately hydrated, hemodialysis or intermittent peritoneal dialysis should be instituted. The latter procedure is usually more easily accomplished and can be made more efficient by the addition of 5 per cent human serum albumin solution to the dialysis fluid.[16] However, if urinary output is satisfactory, dialytic procedures are seldom necessary.

It is well established that the renal excretion of salicylate is in-

TABLE 1 Recommended Intravenous Therapy for Child Weighing 10 Kilograms with Severe Dehydration Due to Salicylate Intoxication

Therapy	Amounts per 24 Hours			
	H$_2$O (ml)	Na (mEq)	K (mEq)	Cl (mEq)
Maintenance	1000	30	20	20
Deficit	1000	90	60	60
Replacement of abnormal losses	500	15	10	10
Total	2500	135	90	90

creased manyfold if the urine can be made alkaline. Sodium bicarbonate administration[17, 18] and the use of acetazolamide[19] or tris buffer have been recommended, and each, given properly, will increase the rate of salicylate excretion. However, both acetazolamide and tris buffer have major undesirable side effects which preclude their use except in carefully controlled experimental circumstances.[20, 21] Acetazolamide may be particularly dangerous because it produces an alkaline urine at the expense of increasing the systemic acidosis which, in turn, facilitates the entry of salicylate into the brain.[12] Alkalinization of the urine by the administration of sodium bicarbonate is less dangerous. However, as noted here, the child with mild or moderately severe salicylate intoxication will recover uneventfully if he or she receives an adequate fluid intake, irrespective of the rapidity of salicylate excretion. The use in these children of sodium bicarbonate or of other alkalinizing agents is, therefore, unnecessary.

The severely ill child, on the other hand, undoubtedly would be helped by the more rapid elimination of salicylate and by a prompt restoration of a more normal serum pH. Hill[12, 21] has shown that in experimental salicylate poisoning rapid alkalinization causes a decrease in muscle, brain, and liver salicylate concentrations. Since, as noted, salicylate probably has a direct toxic effect on the central nervous system as well as on the kidney, and one might assume that the more rapid removal of salicylate from tissue is advantageous, the temptation to use sodium bicarbonate therapy in the treatment of these children is strong. However, the large amounts of sodium bicarbonate needed to alkalinize the urine of the child with severe metabolic acidosis may increase the serum sodium concentration rapidly and significantly, thereby incurring the risk of central nervous system damage.[22] Furthermore, tetany occurs fairly frequently after the administration of alkali. In fact, the consequences of rapid alkalinization on the salicylate concentration in brain tissue of children with severe salicylate intoxication are uncertain despite Hill's studies. It has been shown that when alkali is administered to patients with diabetic ketoacidosis the pH of cerebrospinal fluid falls,[23] an effect that may adversely affect central nervous system functions and, quite possibly, increase the penetration of salicylate into the brain. Until these issues are examined thoroughly and resolved in the laboratory, it is the author's opinion that the dangers of giving large amounts of bicarbonate to produce alkalinization of the urine outweigh the admitted benefits and, therefore, sodium bicarbonate is not recommended for this purpose.

On the other hand, if an immediate increase in serum pH is required, as it might be if the patient were in myocardial failure or had profound coma or respiratory depression due to severe metabolic acidosis (serum pH < 7.20), the intravenous administration of sodium bicarbonate would be the treatment of choice, and 3 to 5 mEq/kg should be given rapidly. These recommendations concerning the use of sodium bicarbonate represent the author's opinion, based solely on his experience; statistical data utilizing survival rates and absence of neurological sequelae as the criteria of successful therapy are not available.

REFERENCES

1. Segar, W. E., and Holliday, M. A.: Physiological abnormalities of salicylate intoxication. N. Engl. J. Med., *259*:1191, 1958.
2. Smith, M. J. H.: Salicylates and metabolism. J. Pharm. Pharmacol., *11*:705, 1959.
3. Goodman, L. S., and Gilman, A.: The Pharmacological Basis of Therapeutics. 5th ed., New York, Macmillan, 1975.
4. Thurston, J. H., Pollock, P. G., Warren, S. K., and Jones, E. M.: Reduced brain glucose with normal plasma glucose in salicylate poisoning. J. Clin. Invest., *49*: 2139, 1970.
5. Schwartz, R., and Landy, G.: Organic acid excretion in salicylate intoxication. J. Pediatr., *66*:658, 1965.
6. Winters, R. W., White, J. S., Hughes, M. C., and Ordway, N. K.: Disturbances of acid-base equilibrium in salicylate intoxication. Pediatrics, *23*:260, 1959.
7. Quintanilla, A., and Kessler, R. H.: Direct effects of salicylate on renal function in the dog. J. Clin. Invest., *52*:3143, 1973.
8. Darrow, D. C., and Pratt, E. L.: Retention of water and electrolyte during recovery in patient with diabetic acidosis. J. Pediatr., *41*:688, 1952.
9. Atchley, D. W., Loeb, R. F., Richards, D. W., Jr., Benedict, E. M., and Driscoll, M. E.: On diabetic acidosis: detailed study of electrolyte balances following withdrawal and reestablishment of insulin therapy. J. Clin. Invest., *12*:297, 1933.
10. Nabarro, J. D. N., Spencer, A. G., and Stowers, J. M.: Metabolic studies in severe diabetic ketosis. Quart. J. Med., *21*:225, 1952.
11. Guerra (Perez-Carral), F., and Brobeck, R.: Hypothalamic control of aspirin antipyresis in monkey. J. Pharm. Exp. Ther., *80*:209, 1944.
12. Hill, J. B., Jr.: Salicylate intoxication. N. Engl. J. Med., *288*:1110, 1973.
13. Barker, E. S., Singer, R. B., Elkinton, J. R., and Clark, J. K.: Renal response in man to acute experimental respiratory alkalosis and acidosis. J. Clin. Invest., *36*:515, 1957.
14. Stanbury, S. W., and Thomson, A. E.: Renal response to respiratory alkalosis. Clin. Sci., *11*:357, 1952.
15. Holliday, M. A., and Segar, W. E.: The maintenance need for water in parenteral fluid therapy. Pediatrics, *19*:823, 1957.
16. Etteldorf, J. N., Dobbins, W. T., Summitt, R. L., Rainwater, W. T., and Fischer, R. L.: Intermittent peritoneal dialysis using 5 per cent albumin in the treatment of salicylate intoxication in children. J. Pediatr., *58*:226, 1961.
17. Oliver, T. K., Jr., and Dyer, M. E.: The prompt treatment of salicylism with sodium bicarbonate. Am. J. Dis. Child., *99*:553, 1960.
18. Whitten, C. F., Kesaree, N. M., and Goodwin, J. F.: Managing salicylate poisoning in children. Am. J. Dis. Child., *101*:178, 1961.
19. Schwartz, R., Fellers, F. X., Knapp, J., and Yaffe, S.: The renal response to administration of acetazolamide (Diamox) during salicylate intoxication. Pediatrics, *23*:1103, 1959.
20. Kaplan, S. A., and del Carmen, F. T.: Experimental salicylate poisoning: observations on the effects of carbonic anhydrase inhibitor and bicarbonate. Pediatrics, *21*: 762, 1958.
21. Hill, J. B.: Experimental salicylate poisoning: observations on the effects of altering blood pH on tissue and plasma salicylate concentrations. Pediatrics, *47*:658, 1971.
22. Kravath, R. E., Aharon, A. S., and Finberg, L.: Effect of hypertonic saline infusions on blood and cerebrospinal fluid. Pediatr. Res., *3*:352, 1969.
23. Ohman, J. L., Jr., Marliss, E. B., Aoki, T. T., Munichoodappa, C. S., Khanna, V. V., and Kozak, G. P.: The cerebrospinal fluid in diabetic ketoacidosis. N. Engl. J. Med., *284*:283, 1971.

Chapter Twenty

DEHYDRATION SECONDARY TO DIARRHEA

LAURENCE FINBERG, M.D.

Diarrhea, a symptom of a variety of disorders affecting infants, often leads to marked physiological disturbances. Vomiting, a common accompanying symptom, adds to and modifies the disturbances produced by diarrheal diseases. Enteric infections cause these symptoms more often than all other diseases combined, but non-infectious causes occasionally may also occur. The discussion here will deliberately limit consideration of the management of diarrhea to the physiological disturbances that accompany excessive loss of water and salts from the gastrointestinal tract. Etiological considerations, however important they may be, will not be pursued further. This emphasis is appropriate since survival following critical dehydration depends far more upon the correction of the physiological disturbance than upon the removal of the cause.

A critical stage in diarrheal disease may be defined as that which occurs when a volume of fluid equal in mass to about 10 per cent of the body weight has been lost over a period of a day or two. Clinically this usually occurs shortly after the illness has precluded oral intake through anorexia or vomiting. At this stage of illness parenteral fluid therapy should be employed. Oral intake should be curtailed during the early hours of therapy. The use of milk or other foods high in calories and solute markedly increases stool water losses and thus complicates management. Even if severe undernutrition coexists with the diarrhea, the first few hours nonetheless should be a period of brief starvation; the parenteral glucose will provide emergency calories.

From the Department of Pediatrics, Montefiore Hospital and Medical Center and the Department of Pediatrics of the Albert Einstein College of Medicine, Bronx, New York.

Although such routes of administration as intragastric drip and subcutaneous infusion have been employed successfully, their usage should be restricted to places where a deficiency of supplies or trained personnel interdicts the preferred parenteral route—continuous intravenous infusion. With modern equipment, skilled house officers and pediatricians should be able to use venipuncture technique with only rare recourse to venesection (cutdown).

CLINICAL EVALUATION

The plan for therapy begins with clinical assessment of the patient. When available, laboratory analyses add valuable complementary assistance. Even if chemical analyses cannot be performed for many hours, an initial blood sample to be analyzed for urea, N, Na^+, CO_2 content, Cl^-, and K^+ should be obtained. If enough blood and a sufficiently versatile laboratory are available, tests for Ca^{++}, pH, and Pco_2 are also of interest. The role of each of these determinations will be discussed as the areas of assessment are further delineated. Since weight of the patient (accurately determined and repeated at intervals) constitutes the most important and useful measurement, as much attention should be paid to the technique of weighing as to the laboratory procedures.

Clinical evaluation may be divided into five points of appraisal, in decreasing order of immediate importance: volume, osmolality, hydrogen ion status, intracellular ion deficits, and calcium ion homeostasis (Table 1). Each of these may be discussed profitably in terms of the method of clinical evaluation, usefulness of laboratory measurements, and calculation for physiological correction during each of the three phases of critical therapy; emergency, initial repletion, and early recovery. First, a 24-hour period of therapy will be considered: this will be followed by a breakdown for the first hour, the next 6 to 8 hours, and the remaining hours of the first 24. For the more seriously ill infants, a plan for the second day will be outlined, thus completing the critical therapy of dehydration.

Volume

Water volume repletion and maintenance constitute the most important facets of the care of dehydration.* The therapeutic volume needs are threefold: (1) the deficit, (2) the ongoing usual requirements for normal maintenance, and (3) continuing abnormal losses.

---

*Dehydration to the physiologist and clinician ordinarily means loss of water plus solute rather than the literal meaning of loss of water alone usually intended in other usages of the word.

TABLE 1   Clinical Appraisal of Problems of Hydration*

Point of Appraisal	Clinical Symptoms and Signs*	Laboratory Determination of Greatest Value
Volume	Circulatory impairment, skin changes, eye and fontanelle changes, oliguria.	Body weight, urea N in serum
Osmolality	For hypernatremia: CNS signs—disturbance of consciousness, hypertonicity of muscles, increased reflexes, marked thirst, "inapparent dehydration" with good circulation for degree of loss. For hyponatremia: Exaggeration of the signs listed under *Volume.*	Na$^+$ in serum
Hydrogen ion status	Hyperpnea in acidemia.	CO$_2$ content (HCO$_3^-$) in serum, Pco$_2$, pH
Intracellular ion deficits	Abdominal distention, muscle weakness, diminished reflexes.	K$^+$ in serum (limited use), ECG
Calcium homeostasis	Tetany, convulsions.	Ca^{++} in serum (complex interpretation), ECG

*Only the symptoms and signs of dehydration have been given in this table. A companion group of signs for the corresponding disturbances of overhydration has been omitted for simplicity. The same points of appraisal and the same laboratory examinations may be used advantageously.

The Deficit.   Deficit refers to a loss of volume or mass of water from the hydrated state. When diarrhea causes loss of water and salt in physiological proportions (about two-thirds of the time in North American experience), clinical signs first appear when about 5 per cent of the body mass (7 per cent of the body fluid) has been lost over a 1- or 2-day period. Tachycardia and dryness of the mucous membranes appear as the earliest signs. Earlier symptoms, such as thirst and a dry feeling in the mouth, are not useful in infants; moreover, thirst may be obscured by nausea. Next in order of appearance are evidences of advancing circulatory insufficiency and changes in the elasticity of the skin and subcutaneous tissue. Thus, by the time the deficit has progressed to the order of 10 per cent of the weight, the extremities show cyanosis or mottling and diminished temperature. The pulse rate may be very rapid, even for the fever which may also be present. Oliguria becomes manifest. The fontanelle, if open, will be depressed, and the eyeballs appear sunken. The skin and subcutaneous tissue of the abdomen in the infant will show loss of elasticity by sustaining folds when pinched and loss of turgor by the slow return of color after pressure. After the age of about 2 years subcutaneous tissue composition differs from that of the infant and these last signs usually cannot be elicited. When losses of water exceed 10 per cent of body weight, the circulatory failure becomes more pronounced so that, at an acute weight loss of about 15 per cent, a moribund irreversible state may occur.

From the preceding discussion, the repeated reference to weight makes it evident that this measurement delineates the deficit. Because pre-illness weights are seldom known, a clinical estimate according to the criteria discussed may be employed usefully with reasonable accuracy. When by good chance the previous weight is known, use it. A clinical axiom, applicable without significant error, states that changes in body weight within any 24-hour period may be considered to be water. However, one must remember not to extend this period of time because clinically insignificant deviations within 24 hours may be cumulative and highly significant over longer intervals.

Normal Maintenance. Though weight constitutes the direct measure of a water deficit, normal maintenance requirements of water are not a simple function of mass but rather of energy expenditure. Since the infant and the young child have a higher rate of metabolism per unit of mass than older, larger individuals,[1] their obligate water losses, hence maintenance requirements, are also greater per unit of mass. One hundred calories expended result in 100 ml of water loss through skin, lungs, urine, and stool. This relationship, in which obligate water losses directly follow energy expenditure, rougly parallels the surface area relation to mass, a fact which has led some to use surface area in calculation. In fact, neither surface area nor caloric expenditure measurements are made on clinical services. Either system requires for practical application that a table of estimates, such as Table 2, or a nomogram be used to derive from the weight a quantity of water per unit mass appropriate for age and size. The weight remains the practical measurement available.

TABLE 2   Approximate Basal Water Requirements in Relation to Age, Weight, and Surface Area

Age	Weight (kg)	Surface Area (M^2)	Minimal Basal Water Requirement		
			ml/kg or cal/kg	ml/M^2	ml/24 hrs
Newborn	2.5–4.0	0.20–0.23	50	750	125–200
1 week–6 months	3.0–8.0	0.20–0.35	65–70	1000–1100	200–520
6 months–12 months	8.0–12.0	0.35–0.45	50–60	1000–1050	500–600
12 months–24 months	10.0–15.0	0.45–0.60	45–50	1000–1050	500–750

The fact that two distinct bases, namely, the metabolic expenditure and the loss in weight, are necessary for the volume calculation remains the most fundamental contribution by pediatric clinicians to the field of hydration therapy.[1] No single reference base may be used; weight, calories, or surface area alone will not be accurate over a range of ages and sizes. The author prefers to use calories rather than surface area for maintenance calculations for two reasons: (1) for clarity of thinking in terms of physiology to stress the fundamental relationship, and (2) because the newborn and a few other states (edematous and obese patients) are exceptions to a simple surface area relationship. If these matters are understood, surface area nomogram enthusiasts may use their nomograms with results equal to those obtained by the scheme proposed here.

Using a value for caloric expenditure at basal conditions from a table requires an additional interpretation of the patient's actual state. Allowing for usual activity, temperature variation, and rate of breathing, coupled with observed urine formation, energy expenditure ordinarily may be assumed to be one and one-half times the basal rate. Persistent high fever warrants doubling the basal figure; and the extreme combination of persistent high body temperature, hyperventilation, and convulsive muscular activity might triple the basal allotment.

Abnormal Losses.   Continued abnormal losses, the third factor in assessing volume requirements, are measured or estimated by direct collection or observation, including any tube drainages as well as stool losses.

In addition to weight, though much less useful, a measure of the urea nitrogen concentration in the serum helps in assessing volume depletion. The level of this determination depends upon the duration as well as the quantity of deficit, since it reflects the effect of failure of glomerular filtration, roughly indicating the degree of severity of extracellular fluid loss. Since that compartment sustains most of the loss in volume when water and sodium salts are lost together in physiological proportion, in the absence of complicating primary renal disease the urea nitrogen level may be used for retrospective and prognostic estimates.

To illustrate the application of the foregoing, consider a 6-month-old infant weighing 5000 gm in the dehydrated state with clinical features suggesting a loss of 10 per cent of body weight. This leads to an estimate of a 500-ml (gm) deficit. (For convenience the dehydrated rather than the hydrated weight justifiably may be used by ignoring the water of oxidation which would, at the age in the example, constitute an arithmetical quantity of similar magnitude in the opposite direction.) Estimating the usual requirement figure at this age and size ($5 \times 65 \times 1\frac{1}{2}$) adds about another 500 ml per day (Table 2). Together these total 1000 ml, if the volume of the deficit is to be repaired in 1 day. Continued abnormal losses are observed and added. Details concerning rate of administration and solute content at the various time segments are best considered after the remainder of the appraisal is completed. In general, however, except as noted, a volume of water roughly equal to one-half the volume allotment for the first 24 hours (500 ml) will have been administered in 6 to 8 hours; the remaining 500 ml plus the volume of any abnormal losses will have been administered by the end of 24 hours.

Osmolality

Osmolality of body fluids is the second most important general element in evaluation. In a somewhat simplified sense, the content of sodium salts in the body determines the physiologically significant osmolality because Na^+ and Cl^-, owing to their relative exclusion from intracellular fluid, by their content determine the distribution of body water into its two main compartments: extracellular fluid (ECF) and intracellular fluid (ICF). Therefore, sodium concentration constitutes a more clinically relevant determination than the actual osmolality because those solutes which are distributed evenly in body water do not affect the relative size of the compartments.

This knowledge, together with the clinical appearance and course, has led to a classification of dehydration on the basis of sodium concentration in serum. In North America, isonatremic dehydration accounts for about 65 per cent of patients, hypernatremic dehydration for 20 to 25 per cent, and hyponatremic dehydration for about 10 per cent of those admitted to hospitals with dehydration. These incidence values vary from one region to another and also vary with the season and the prevailing feeding practices. In countries in which dry whole milk is promoted and made available as an inexpensive food for infants, the incidence of hypernatremic dehydration is higher.[2]

A high sodium concentration, defined as > 150 mEq/L of serum, implies relative cellular desiccation and relative preservation of ECF volume; conversely, a low sodium, < 132 mEq/L, denotes relatively greater ECF depletion per unit volume lost. Hypernatremic dehydration then has, for a given degree of loss in volume, less than the expected evidence of circulatory failure and subcutaneous tissue changes, frequently justifying the description "deceptively inapparent" dehydration. The cellular desiccation produced by hypernatremia leads to a preponderance of central nervous system symptoms, signs, and pathological damage. These manifestations usually occur at about the same volume loss as do the circulatory signs of classic or isonatremic dehydration.

Certain features from the history and physical findings enable one to recognize hypernatremia prior to laboratory confirmation. Younger infants have a higher incidence. Intake usually has stopped abruptly fairly early in the course of the disease. Less constant features that suggest the possibility include a high solute intake (e.g., full-strength skim milk) just before cessation of intake, persistent high fever, a hot, dry environment (e.g., heated apartment in winter), and hyperventilation. On examination, disturbance of consciousness usually is manifested by a peculiar combination of marked lethargy or somnolence, coupled with hyperirritability when the infant is stimulated by touch, noise, or light. Hypertonicity of muscles, often producing mild nuchal rigidity, may occur. More extreme manifestations of central nervous system involvement include muscle twitchings, tremors, and frank convulsions. The abdominal skin has a velvety feel and inconstantly a "doughy" consistency. Circulation usually is maintained, but, if the dehydration exceeds 10 per cent weight loss or if the hypernatremia is very severe ($Na^+ > 180$ mEq/L), shock may complicate even this variety of dehydration.[3]

Hyponatremic dehydration is most likely to appear when protracted stool losses have produced large electrolyte losses, and especially when this circumstance is accompanied by an ample water intake very low in solute (i.e., water without electrolyte). The clinical manifestations consist of an increase of circulatory failure per unit of volume lost. Thus extreme shock may appear at an earlier stage of volume deficit. The low sodium concentration in patients with kwashiorkor represents a different and more complex phenomenon requiring an approach not applicable in this discussion of a better nourished population.

The most common osmolal occurrence in dehydration, a normal concentration of sodium (isonatremia), produces the well-known picture of extracellular depletion with moderate circulatory deficit when about 10 per cent of body weight has been lost over a day or two. In isonatremic dehydration, balance studies have shown losses of Na^+ in the order of 8 to 15 mEq/kg.[4] Patients with hypernatremic dehydration have lost as little as 2 to 5 mEq/kg; hyponatremic patients may have deficits up to 20 mEq/kg.

With regard to solute loss, hence osmolality, treatment should take into account not only the magnitude of sodium loss but also the important fact that brain swelling results when dilute solutions of electrolyte are administered rapidly. Therefore, in hypernatremic dehydration, when the solute requirement is low, to avoid central nervous system insult on the one hand or edema from excessive isotonic ECF expansion on the other, the deficit replacement should be spread evenly over a period of at least 48 hours.

Except as noted in hypernatremic dehydration, the sodium salt replacement should be planned to take place during the first 24 hours of therapy. During this period, the deficit of sodium so exceeds that necessary for normal maintenance that no provision need be made for sodium "requirement." In the 5-kg infant not thought to have hypernatremia in our previous example, the sodium deficit of about 12 mEq/kg (range, 8 to 15 mEq/kg) would be 5 × 12 or 60 mEq (or a range of 40 to 75). Administering this amount of sodium to the infant would produce the necessary expansion of ECF to carry out life functions, including urine formation. The average concentration of sodium in the first day's therapy would thus be 60 mEq/L (range, 40 to 75 mEq/L). If the hypothetical patient was diagnosed as hypernatremic, the recommended average concentration would be lower, e.g., 25 to 40 mEq/L. The sodium administered to patients with hypernatremia may even have to exceed the deficit slightly in order to avoid too rapid infusion of water without electrolyte, a circumstance which produces brain swelling.

If restoration of volume and sodium replacement are achieved in patients with reasonably intact functioning renal and pulmonary systems, the remaining three points of assessment will require little or no attention other than the provision of the intracellular ions by mouth.

Hydrogen Ion Status

Patients with diarrhea usually have a primary excess of H^+ for four reasons: (1) stool water may contain a relatively large amount of HCO_3^-; (2) starvation and dehydration lead to increased production of keto acids (non-volatile acid production); (3) diminished perfusion of tissue causes increased lactic acid release; and (4) perhaps most importantly, progressive reduction of renal function leads to retention of non-volatile acids (H^+). In spite of compensatory blowing off of CO_2 reducing the Pco_2, pH may fall. The CO_2 content of the serum will be low, and, for reasons beyond the present scope of discussion, Cl^- ion concentration is usually increased in this type of acidosis.

Unless these changes are very severe (CO_2 content < 3 mEq/L) or some persistent impairment of kidney or lung exists, no specific administration of alkali ordinarily will be required. The physiological proportion of basic anions to the total in extracellular fluid is about 1:5 or 1:4. Thus, all deficit repair solutions for acidotic states and all maintenance solutions should have from one-fifth to one-quarter of the anions as base. While this may be safely increased slightly in diarrheal disease, experience shows that this extra base usually is not necessary so long as volume and osmolality needs are met and, very important, urine formation occurs. For this reason, the emergency phase of therapy will be optimal if it promotes urine formation.

Intracellular Ion Deficits

The loss of potassium from cells, first demonstrated more than 20 years ago, has proved to be an important cause of the physiological disturbance of severe diarrheal disease.[5] All infants with severe diarrheal disease will sustain potassium loss, and replacement is necessary during the phases of repletion and early recovery. Clinical signs often not seen until unmasked by initial hydration include hypotonia of muscles, abdominal distention, and weakness. The level of K^+ in serum may be high because of poor glomerular filtration, even in severe K^+ deficit. Because the myocardium is quite sensitive to small (absolute) changes in K^+ levels in serum, caution is required in administration, particularly prior to the establishment of urine output. Even afterwards, parenteral K^+ must be given carefully, and experience has shown that the safer oral route may be employed in most instances. The magnitude of the deficit may be as much as 10 mEq/kg.[4] This does not necessarily represent a corresponding volume of loss of ICF, because probably not all the K^+ is osmotically active.

Generally, 3 mEq/kg per day is a reasonably effective and safe rate of replacement. If parenteral K^+ must be given, concentrations greater than 40 mEq/L should be avoided and rates greater than 4 mEq/hour may be risky for small infants.

Correcting Mg^{++} and $PO_4^=$ deficits has not been shown to be clinically important.

Homeostasis

Calcium homeostasis occasionally goes awry during dehydration, especially with hypernatremia, with resultant hypocalcemia. However, this rarely leads to tetany.[3] For this reason, during the management of hypernatremic dehydration, the addition of 10 ml of 10 per cent calcium gluconate to every 500 ml of intravenous solution has seemed a wise precaution.

IMPLEMENTATION OF THERAPY

Having presented the principles, let us return to the example. At this point a volume of 1000 ml has been tentatively established for administration during the first 24 hours of treatment. The sodium content will be approximately 60 mEq and the potassium content will be about 15 mEq. The 75 mEq of anions should be apportioned approximately 55 mEq as chloride and 20 mEq as base, e.g., bicarbonate, lactate, or acetate. The solution should also include glucose to supply calories.

As previously stated, this therapy should be considered in three phases: emergency, repletion, and early recovery.

Phase 1 — Emergency

Immediate infusion of a volume of fluid over a 10- to 15-minute period to expand the intravascular compartment and thus restore circulation should begin therapy for every patient in circulatory distress. The following fluids have been used successfully: whole blood, single donor plasma, 5 per cent albumin, and a 10 per cent glucose solution with a sodium concentration of 75 mEq/L, bicarbonate of 20 mEq/L, and chloride of 55 mEq/L. Blood and plasma have fallen into mild disfavor because of suspected problems with hepatitis and actual problems of availability. The albumin solutions are not available everywhere but have proved particularly useful for the coincidence of shock and hypernatremia, a potentially deadly combination. The author prefers hypertonic glucose (10 per cent) to plain electrolyte solutions (e.g., Ringer's lactate) because of the more immediate expansion of the intravascular space and the empirical impression of more rapid urine formation. Solutions containing albumin are preferred for malnourished infants and those presenting with hypernatremia plus circulatory embarrassment.

The volume of these rapid infusions should be 20 ml/kg of body weight for blood, plasma, or 5 per cent albumin and 40 ml/kg for the solution of 10 per cent glucose with 75 mEq/L of sodium. The larger volume (40 ml/kg) will require 30 to 40 minutes for administration.

Phase 2 — Repletion

The remaining water volume with electrolytes may now be combined as a single solution for the rest of the 24 hours, with the rate adjusted appropriately. The glucose concentration now should be reduced to 5 per cent. In the example of the 5-kg infant, with estimated deficit of 500 ml, if the amount already administered in Phase 1 was 40 ml/kg, then 200 ml subtracted from 1000 ml leaves 800 ml to be infused. Fifteen milliequivalents of sodium have been given, leaving 45 to be given. Potassium will be added after urine formation has been assured by clinical observation; 15 mEq will be added in a concentration not to exceed 40 mEq/L. The anions for Na^+ and K^+ combined should be approximately one-quarter base (HCO_3^-, acetate$^-$, or lactate$^-$) and three-quarters chloride. The rate of administration should be adjusted to deliver the remaining one-half of the estimate for the first 24 hours, 300 ml (500 − 200 = 300), by the time 8 hours have elapsed from the onset of therapy. Even though body composition remains abnormal, the circulation and renal function will be adequately restored, enabling physiological mechanisms to operate maximally in the final recovery phase. Because ongoing losses have occurred, the patient's water volume remains somewhat less than the estimated normal.

Note that all of the plan outlined has been based on clinical observations and general principles. If laboratory values are available during this phase of therapy, suitable adjustments may be made—if, for instance, the Na$^+$ concentration is in an unexpected range or the acidosis is more severe than supposed. Only occasionally will such adjustments be truly necessary, since the model permits treatment of a fairly wide latitude of disturbances narrowed by decisions derived from clinical data.

In hospitals in which only commercial polyionic solutions are available, they may be readily modified to the compositions indicated herein. Small differences, even up to 20 per cent in concentration values, need not be adjusted. The author does not use these solutions because of the inflexibility their exclusive use imposes.

If the example had been a patient suspected to have hypernatremia, the rate of fluid administration would have been slower during repletion, which then would have been planned for a 48-hour period. In that event, the Na$^+$ concentration of the intravenous infusion would be at the lower level (25 to 40 mEq/L), and K$^+$ salts would be added at the earliest safe moment. The rate should then deliver the deficit volume plus 2 days' maintenance volume added together in equal hourly increments over 48 hours.

Phase 3—Early Recovery

After 8 hours many patients may take fluids by mouth, and their therapy may be continued with an oral electrolyte-glucose solution containing sodium and potassium salts. Those more severely ill will remain on the same infusion, now slowed in rate to deliver the rest of the calculated volume by the end of 24 hours. Observed abnormal losses will be added quantitatively to the infusion as 120 mEq/L sodium chloride for gastric drainage and 40 mEq/L sodium chloride plus 40 mEq/L of potassium acetate for intestinal loss. Several interim weighings will give valuable information about success of therapy. The example given and the use of solutions described in the preceding text may be summarized as shown in Table 3.

Ideally, the patient should show a 7 to 9 per cent gain in weight at

TABLE 3 Summary of Therapeutic Measures Used in the
Example in the Text

Phase	Time	Water (ml)	Na⁺ (mEq)	K⁺ (mEq)	Cl⁻ (mEq)	Base (mEq)	Glucose (gm)
1	0–20 min	200	15	0.0	11.0	4.0	20
2	20 min–8 hr	300	15	5.6	16.5	4.1	15
3	8–24 hr	500	30	9.4	27.5	11.9	25
TOTAL	24 hr	1000	60	15.0	55.0	20.0	60

24 hours. Too little or too much suggests an error in appraisal or technique. Except as previously noted for hypernatremic dehydration, the next 24 hours will, in most instances, be calculated as maintenance plus any continuing abnormal losses; the deficit usually will have been overcome. The same five-point analysis should be repeated, and individual variation should be managed accordingly. In most patients, recovery from the critical phases of the illness will be indicated by ability to take fluid and solute by mouth. On the second day, whether oral feeding containing calories as carbohydrate and protein may be added or whether high caloric parenteral feedings should be used depends upon the state of nutrition, the etiology and duration of the disorder, and a number of other factors. These matters have become increasingly important as the problems of hydration have yielded to understanding and techniques.

REFERENCES

1. Darrow, D. C.: The significance of body size. Am. J. Dis. Child., *98*:416, 1959.
2. Taitz, L. S., and Byers, H. D.: High calorie/osmolar feeding and hypertonic dehydration. Arch. Dis. Child., *47*:257, 1972.
3. Finberg, L.: Hypernatremic dehydration. Adv. Pediatr., *16*:325, 1969.
4. Darrow, D. C., Pratt, E. L., Flett, J., Jr., Gamble, A. H., and Wiese, H. F.: Disturbances of water and electrolytes in infantile diarrhea. Pediatrics, *3*:129, 1949.
5. Govan, C. D., and Darrow, D. C.: The use of potassium chloride in the treatment of diarrhea in infants. J. Pediatr., *28*:541, 1946.

ADDITIONAL READING

Winters, R. W., ed.: The Body Fluids in Pediatrics. Boston, Little, Brown and Co., 1973, esp. chaps. 5, 6, 7, and 18.

Chapter Twenty-One

INTRAVENOUS ALIMENTATION

ROBERT M. FILLER, M.D.,
JOHN B. DAS, M.D., PH.D.,
ARNOLD G. CORAN, M.D.

Insufficient caloric intake for a prolonged period contributes appreciably to mortality in infants and children with lesions of the gastrointestinal tract. Not uncommonly, patients with persistent intestinal obstruction, bowel fistulas, or short-bowel syndrome die solely of inanition and its complications before curative treatment or appropriate surgical procedures have been carried out.

Dudrick and co-workers[1, 2] first demonstrated that the intravenous infusion of a fat-free, amino acid, glucose solution could support normal growth and development. Filler and co-workers[3] reported the successful long-term use of this solution in 14 critically ill infants with a variety of gastrointestinal disorders. Our experience since then and reports from other institutions indicate the lifesaving potential of total parenteral nutrition (TPN) in infants and children with inadequate gastrointestinal tract function.

Success of this mode of treatment was brought about by the development of special techniques so that nutrient solutions which could not be delivered into peripheral veins because of their high glucose content could be administered safely into a central vein for prolonged periods.

In recent years, with the development of an intravenous fat solution an alternative approach to TPN in infants and children has been adopted in the United States and abroad. Because of the calories provided by the fat, the glucose content of the nutrient solution can be

---

From the Department of Surgery, Children's Hospital Medical Center, Harvard Medical School, Boston, Massachusetts, and University of Michigan Medical Center, Ann Arbor, Michigan.

286

lowered so that infusions through peripheral veins are not associated with rapid phlebothrombosis.[4, 5, 6, 7] This program obviates the need for a central venous catheter, thereby eliminating some of the attendant complications. Recently, in a number of institutions parenteral nutrition has been provided through peripheral veins even when intravenous fat has not been available. This approach is possible in the patient who can tolerate large volumes of nutrient solutions which must contain no more than 10 per cent glucose.[8] In many clinical situations, the choice of one technique over the others involves individual patient consideration.

Because of problems not ordinarily seen with routine intravenous therapy, intelligent use of these life-sustaining systems requires the careful selection of patients for therapy, constant surveillance for the early signs of complications, and persistent attention to the minute details of procedures that minimize these dangers.

INDICATIONS

Central venous TPN has been used extensively at the Children's Hospital Medical Center since 1968, and to date, more than 325 infants and children have been treated. During the two and one-half year period from January, 1972 to June, 1974, 80 infants and children at the Los Angeles County-USC Medical Center and Los Angeles Children's Hospital received intravenous feeding through peripheral veins using the fat emulsion Intralipid.* In addition, from July, 1974 to July, 1975, over 30 infants and children at the Mott Children's Hospital in the University of Michigan Medical Center were treated with peripheral hyperalimentation composed of fat-free solutions.

TPN is reserved for those infants and children whose lives are threatened because feeding by means of the gastrointestinal tract is impossible, inadequate, or hazardous. The goal of treatment depends on the patient's underlying condition. In some instances, such as in those infants with chronic non-specific diarrhea, placing the gastrointestinal tract at rest for a prolonged period is curative. In others, the restoration and maintenance of adequate nutrition permits corrective surgery.

The common conditions for which this treatment has been used include chronic intestinal obstruction due to adhesions or peritoneal sepsis, bowel fistulas, inadequate intestinal length, chronic non-remitting severe diarrhea, extensive body burns, and abdominal tumors

---

*Manufactured by Vitrum Company, Stockholm, Sweden, and kindly supplied by Cutter Laboratories, Berkeley, California, 94710.

treated by surgery, irradiation, and chemotherapy. Although TPN is used to replete the malnourished child, it may be started prophylactically in clinical situations in which prolonged starvation is expected (Table 1).

As confidence and experience with the method have grown, additional indications for its use have developed. For example, with certain modifications, we have employed TPN in very small premature infants (less than 1 kg) who, despite an apparently normal gastrointestinal tract, constantly regurgitate feedings placed in the stomach either by gavage or by gastrostomy. Dudrick and others[9] have successfully treated uremia and hyperkalemia of acute renal failure with intravenous infusions of purified amino acids and glucose, thus reducing the need for dialysis.

The decision to begin a program of total intravenous alimentation requires mature clinical judgment. Such a decision can be made readily for an infant with complicated omphalocele (Fig. 1), or for one in whom a large portion of the midgut has been resected because of volvulus. In others, the decision may be more difficult. For example, in a child with chronic diarrhea and malnutrition, one must be certain that customary therapy has failed before beginning total intravenous therapy (Fig. 2). Although anorexia, vomiting, and diarrhea commonly accompany irradiation and chemotherapy, only the occasional patient becomes so markedly debilitated that treatment is required (Fig. 3).

One must weigh the need for improved nutrition to save life and reduce morbidity against the possibility of serious complications, especially sepsis. TPN should not be employed in those children in whom nutrients can be safely delivered and absorbed from the gastrointestinal tract by careful oral feedings, gavage, or gastrostomy. On the other hand, our experience indicates that when the technique is applied with proper care, the threat of serious morbidity is sufficiently low to justify its use in an ever-increasing number of patients.

TABLE 1 Indications for Long-Term Intravenous Alimentation by Central Vein in 328 Children

Diagnosis	Number of Patients
Chronic intestinal obstruction	45
Intraperitoneal sepsis and bowel fistulas	22
Omphalocele and gastroschisis	35
Complicated esophageal abnormalities	26
Chronic diarrhea	47
Enteritis during tumor therapy	42
Prematurity (less than 1000 gm)	10
Inflammatory bowel disease	39
Miscellaneous	62

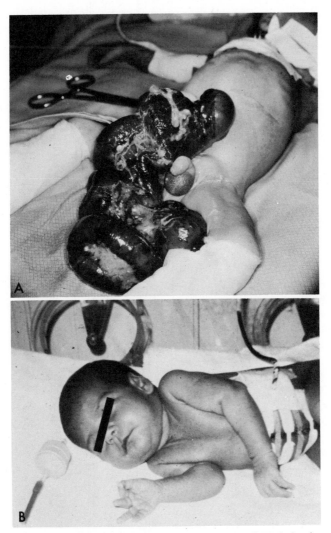

Figure 1. C.D., a 1.9-kg infant with antenatal rupture of omphalocele, repaired in six stages over 10 days. Total parenteral nutrition was started on the first day of life and was maintained for 23 days. *A*, Infant at admission, showing the obstructed, densely adherent, edematous dilated intestinal loops. *B*, Infant after completion of abdominal closure on the 23rd day of life. Good wound healing occurred and satisfactory nutrition is apparent.

Illustration continued on opposite page

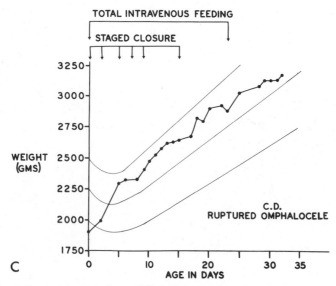

Figure 1 *Continued.* *C,* Infant's daily weights compared to expected weight curve. Sustained weight gain during the period of total intravenous alimentation paralleled expected growth pattern.

SOLUTIONS USED FOR TPN

The composition of the basic glucose-protein hydrolysate solutions currently prepared in our hospital pharmacy is noted in Table 2 (p. 293). Vitamins and trace elements are added as shown. Bottles are labeled to designate the glucose concentration in the nutrient solution. Thus PN-20 contains 20 per cent glucose, a solution designed for infusion through a central venous catheter. Solutions PN-20-I and PN-20-II are similar except for the lower vitamin, calcium, and trace metal content of the latter solution. Solutions PN-8 and PN-5 contain 8 per cent and 5 per cent glucose, respectively, and are infused into a peripheral or a central vein. Intralipid is supplied as an isotonic 10 per cent fat solution containing 1100 cal/L and usually is administered into peripheral veins. To date, supplies of Intralipid have been limited.

MANAGEMENT OF CENTRAL VENOUS FEEDING PROGRAM

For patients receiving nutrients through a central vein, the infusion of 135 ml/kg/day of PN-20-I provides an appropriate mixture of glucose, amino acids, and other nutrients to meet the normal infant's

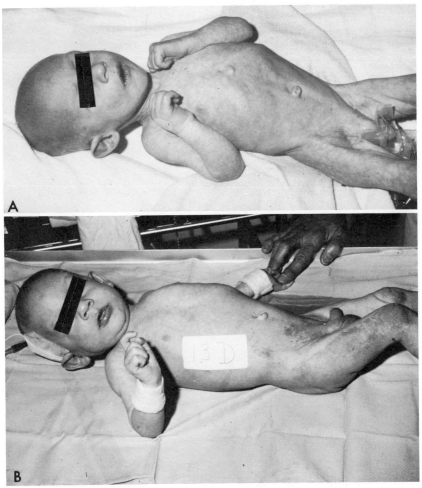

Figure 2. C.S., an 11-week-old child who developed explosive diarrhea with associated projectile vomiting 2 weeks prior to admission. No specific cause of diarrhea could be found and symptoms did not improve with routine treatment, which included intravenous fluids and drugs to decrease intestinal motility. Attempts to administer even clear fluids by mouth increased the diarrhea. Because of life-threatening unremitting starvation, all oral feedings were withheld and total nutrition was provided by vein for 21 days. Thereafter oral feedings were progressively increased and IV feedings eventually terminated 10 days later. *A*, The appearance of patient just prior to institution of total parenteral alimentation. Weight, 3.6 kg. *B*, After 13 days the patient's nutrition has improved markedly. Weight, 4.20 kg.

Illustration continued on opposite page

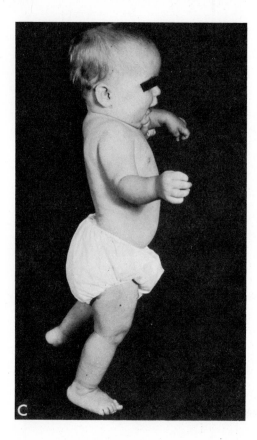

Figure 2 Continued. C, Patient at 18 months of age, tolerating a normal diet with no evidence of persistent bowel dysfunction.

need for tissue repair and growth. Even in the older child whose basic caloric requirements are less, 135 ml/kg/day may be administered safely. However, to avoid vitamin, calcium, and trace metal excesses in these older patients, PN-20-II should be given for nutritional needs in excess of 1000 ml/day.

More dilute glucose solutions (PN-8 or PN-5) are used during the first day or two of therapy. During this period, the child is adapting to the very high glucose load and the high concentration of glucose may produce an osmotic diuresis which will lead to hypertonic dehydration. As the patient's tolerance develops, as judged from diminishing glycosuria, PN-20 solutions may be used. In patients with exceptionally high extrarenal fluid losses, PN-8 is used instead of PN-20. Large volumes of this solution will supply the fluid and caloric needs of such patients without causing hyperglycemia and glycosuria. The administration of insulin is not necessary for non-diabetic children.

In most patients, additional potassium and sodium chloride are necessary. Usually the addition of 30 mEq of NaCl and 20 mEq KCl (per liter) to the standard infusate will suffice and will not overburden the normal infant kidney or cardiovascular system. The electrolyte content

TABLE 2   Solutions for Parenteral IV Alimentation

PN-20-I

Each 1000 ml contains:

Protein hydrolysate (108 cal)	30.0 gm
Dextrose (hydrous) (668 cal)	196.6 gm
Potassium	12.0 mEq
Sodium	15.0 mEq
Calcium	540 mg (27.0 mEq)
Phosphorus (P)	155.0 mg
Magnesium	92 mg (7.6 mEq)
Chloride	10.8 mEq
Folic acid	0.5 mg
Multivitamins (MVI)	5.0 ml
Vitamin K_1	0.2 mg
Vitamin B_{12}	6.6 mcg
Trace elements	
(Zn, Cu, I, F, Mn) sol	2.0 ml

Each 1000 ml contains approximately
4.1 gm nitrogen and 800 cal.

PN-20-II

Each 1000 ml contains:

Protein hydrolysate (108 cal)	30.0 gm
Dextrose (hydrous) (668 cal)	196.6 gm
Potassium	12.0 mEq
Sodium	15.0 mEq
Calcium	60 mg (3.0 mEq)
Phosphorus (P)	155.0 mg
Magnesium	92 mg (7.6 mEq)
Chloride	10.8 mEq
Folic acid	0.5 mg
Vitamin K_1	0.2 mg
Vitamin B_{12}	6.6 mcg

Each 1000 ml contains approximately
4.1 gm nitrogen and 800 cal.

PN-8

Each 1000 ml contains:

Protein hydrolysate (70 cal)	20.0 gm
Dextrose (hydrous) (272 cal)	80.0 gm
Potassium	8.0 mEq
Sodium	10.0 mEq
Calcium	270 mg (13.5 mEq)
Phosphorus (P)	103.0 mg
Magnesium	92 mg (7.6 mEq)
Chloride	7.2 mEq
Folic acid	0.5 mg
Multivitamins (MVI)	5.0 ml
Vitamin K_1	0.2 mg
Vitamin B_{12}	6.6 mcg
Trace elements	
(Zn, Cu, I, F, Mn) sol	2.0 ml

Each 1000 ml contains approximately
2.7 gm nitrogen and 350 cal.

PN-5

Each 1000 ml contains:

Protein hydrolysate (70 cal)	20.0 gm
Dextrose (hydrous) (175 cal)	50.0 gm
Potassium	8.0 mEq
Sodium	10.0 mEq
Calcium	540 mg (27.0 mEq)
Phosphorus (P)	103.0 mg
Magnesium	92 mg (7.6 mEq)
Chloride	7.2 mEq
Folic acid	0.5 mg
Multivitamins (MVI)	5.0 ml
Vitamin K_1	0.2 mg
Vitamin B_{12}	6.6 mcg
Trace elements	
(Zn, Cu, I, F, Mn) sol	2.0 ml

Each 1000 ml contains approximately
2.7 gm nitrogen and 250 cal.

M.V.I.*

Each 10 ml contains:

Ascorbic acid (C)	500 mg
Vitamin A	10,000 IU
Vitamin D	1,000 IU
Thiamine	50 mg
Riboflavin	10 mg
Pyridoxine	15 mg
Niacinamide	100 mg
Dexpanthenol	25 mg
Vitamin E	5 IU

Trace Element Solution

Each 1000 ml contains:

Zinc sulfate	800 mcg
Copper sulfate	400 mcg
Sodium fluoride	20 mcg
Sodium iodide	118 mcg
Manganese sulfate	4000 mcg

*USV Pharmaceutical Corp., Tuckahoe, New York, 10707.

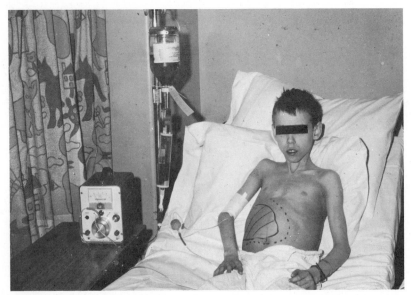

Figure 3. F.H., a 13-year-old boy with very large Wilms' tumor and pulmonary and groin metastases. Because of the massive tumor and the boy's poor general condition, x-ray therapy and chemotherapy were administered prior to surgical excision. Concurrent vomiting and diarrhea caused further deterioration in this boy's general condition. Oral feedings were withheld and nutrition was improved by parenteral alimentation during preoperative antitumor therapy. Surgery 3 weeks later was well tolerated.

of different amino acid sources varies, a factor which must be considered if an amino acid preparation other than that listed in Table 2 is used. Children with normal renal function rarely have serum electrolyte abnormalities with this program. However, more caution is necessary for those with reduced renal function and other metabolic defects.

Iron requirements are met either by weekly intramuscular injections of iron-dextran or by blood transfusion. Trace elements now are added to the basic mixture routinely (Table 2). A recent study suggests that significant essential fatty acids can be supplied by the daily application of sunflower seed oil to the child's chest and back.[10]

Hypertonic infusates (PN-20) must be delivered through a central venous catheter to avoid peripheral venous inflammation and thrombosis. For this purpose, a silicone rubber catheter is passed through the internal or external jugular vein to the superior vena cava. This procedure is best carried out in an operating room or cardiac catheterization laboratory in which adequate exposure, proper instruments, and strict aseptic conditions are available. To minimize blood stream contamination, the venous catheter is tunneled from the vein entry point to a skin exit site which is placed 2 to 4 inches away. In the infant, it is brought out on the scalp, whereas in the older child, the exit site may be the neck or upper extremity. Central venous intubation by percutaneous subclavian vein puncture also has been used. The silicone rubber venous line may be left in place until the completion of therapy unless it becomes dislodged accidentally or septic complications develop. We have had a single catheter in place for as long as 120 days.

The central venous catheter can be inserted under local or general anesthesia. The head is turned to the side and the scalp carefully shaved. A transverse incision, 1 to 2 cm long, is made over the sternocleidomastoid muscle at the junction of the middle and lower third of the neck. The external or internal jugular vein is prepared for cannulation. The external jugular vein ordinarily is preferred' and usually can be cannulated successfully even in the premature infant. However, if either external jugular vein is unavailable because of previous use or small caliber, or if entrance of the catheter from the external jugular vein into the vena cava is not possible, the internal jugular vein can be used for cannulation. A long hollow needle with an obturator in place is passed beneath the skin of the neck from the incision to the scalp (Fig. 4). If the internal jugular vein is being used, the needle also pierces the belly of the sternocleidomastoid muscle. After the obturator is removed, the silicone rubber catheter (for an infant, the internal diameter is 0.025 in and the outside diameter is 0.047 in) is passed through the needle. When the needle is withdrawn, the catheter resides in its subcutaneous tract. Prior to cannulation, the vein is ligated distally and an incision is made between this point and a proximal controlling ligature. If the internal jugular vein has been selected, ligature of the vein sometimes can be avoided by passing the cannula into the vein through an incision made in the center of a pursestring suture. The jugular vein then is cannulated and the tubing advanced to the region of the right atrium (approximately 5 cm in an infant). Occasionally, some manipulation is necessary to obtain entry into the superior vena cava from the external jugular vein. The exact location of the catheter is confirmed radiographically by taking a single x-ray with the catheter filled with radiopaque contrast material, a procedure necessary because of the small size of such catheters.

The silicone rubber catheter slides easily and is soft and compressible. Therefore, the ligature which holds it in the lumen of the vein must be tied so that it neither occludes the lumen of the tube nor allows the catheter to slip out of the vessel. To fix the tube properly, we use a circular sleeve of silicone rubber to which Dacron wings have been bonded* (Fig. 4). After venous cannulation, the sleeve of silicone rubber is opened, and the venous catheter is placed within the lumen of the sleeve at its entrance into the jugular vein. The venous catheter is glued to the sleeve with silicone cement. The Dacron wings are sutured with non-absorbable sutures to the surrounding tissues. To remove the central venous line, the sleeve and its Dacron attachments must be cut by opening the neck wound under local anesthesia.

Antibiotics are administered only when indicated by the child's primary illness, but not specifically to prevent sepsis that might occur from the presence of a central venous line.

An antibacterial ointment and sterile dressing are applied to the skin exit site, and to avoid accidental displacement a coil of catheter is

---

*Manufactured by Medical Devices, Inc., Seattle, Washington.

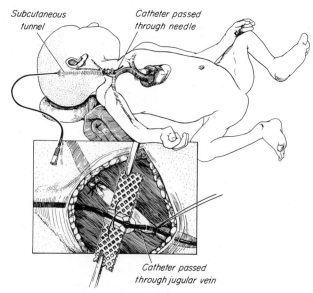

Subcutaneous tunnel

Catheter passed through needle

Catheter passed through jugular vein

Figure 4. Insertion and fixation of silicone rubber central venous catheter in an infant. The catheter is passed through a hollow needle which has created a subcutaneous tunnel from the venous cutdown site in the neck to the appropriate skin exit site behind the ear. After the vein is intubated a vein flange of silicone rubber with Dacron wings is attached to the tubing and secured in the neck wound to prevent accidental dislodgement of the catheter.[21] (Reprinted with permission from Ghadimi, H.: Total Parenteral Nutrition — Premises and Promises, New York, John Wiley & Sons, 1975.)

included in the dressing. Every 2 days the dressing is removed aseptically, the skin cleansed with an antiseptic, and a sterile dressing and antibacterial ointment reapplied. Povidone-iodine (Betadine) ointment now is used routinely because of its effectiveness against both bacteria and fungi. Before the infusion is started, a Millipore filter (0.22 μ) is placed in line to remove particulate matter, or microorganisms, or both which may have contaminated the solution. A calibrated burette is placed in the circuit to accurately monitor the volume delivered. An injection tubing ("T" connector*) may also be added to the circuit so that intravenous tubings and the bottle of infusate are changed daily. Since the high sugar content of these infusates supports the growth of yeast, the external surfaces of all intravenous tubings should be washed with Betadine solution twice a day to remove traces of nutrient solution that may have inadvertently dripped from the bottle onto the tubing. Betadine ointment also should be applied to all joints in the circuit to prevent entry of microorganisms at these points.

The infusate must be delivered at a slow uniform rate to insure

---

*Manufactured by Abbott Laboratories, South Pasadena, California, 91030.

proper utilization of the glucose and amino acids. In the small infant, this is accomplished most readily by the use of a constant infusion pump. In some centers gravity drip is used for older patients. The entire system, locally referred to as the "lifeline," is shown in Figure 5.

In many institutions, patients on TPN are treated in one intensive care area. Because of our geographic and departmental structure, and the diversity of disease states we have encountered, we have found it more efficient to treat these children on the medical or surgical divisions where they would be if they were not on TPN. To provide standardized optimal care, we employ a nurse who oversees the care of every patient on TPN. This nurse makes rounds twice a day to check the intravenous tubings, pumps, and infusates. She advises and instructs the floor nurse and house staff on proper techniques and management. She is on call for any unforeseen mechanical problems that may develop. On alternate days, she changes the dressings over the central venous catheter and is the only person who is permitted to draw blood from the central venous line to obtain samples for routine weekly analysis or for additional studies which may be required by special protocol.

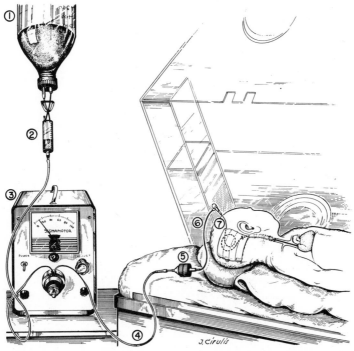

Figure 5. System for long-term intravenous alimentation ("lifeline"). (1) Amino acid-glucose infusate. (2) Calibrated burette. (3) Constant infusion pump. (4) Disposable tubing with a compressible section which adapts to pump head. (5) Millipore filter. (6) "T" connector. (7) Silicone rubber intravenous catheter.

MANAGEMENT OF PERIPHERAL VENOUS FEEDING PROGRAM

Eighty to 100 cal/kg/day usually can be supplied by administering large volumes of the dilute glucose-protein hydrolysates into peripheral veins. Using PN-8, 200 to 250 ml/kg/day are necessary. Caution is required to prevent fluid overload, and indeed some patients cannot tolerate these large volumes. Electrolytes may be added to the stock solutions as necessary. Heparin 0.5 u/ml also may be added to reduce the incidence of phlebitis. The techniques involved are the same as those used for routine intravenous therapy. The solution is infused into a small needle in a peripheral vein on the scalp or in an extremity. A Millipore filter is placed in line and the entire circuit is changed daily. An intravenous site which usually lasts from 24 to 48 hours must be changed promptly when infiltration or phlebitis occurs. Warm soaks over an infiltration site reduce the swelling quickly.

When Intralipid is used, more than 100 cal/kg/day can be given safely through a peripheral vein. Since this fat solution is not miscible with the glucose solutions, it must be infused through a separate bottle and tubing. However, only a single venous entry site is necessary if the Intralipid enters the circuit containing the glucose solution close to the venous entry site. This is accomplished by inserting a needle on the end of the tubing from the Intralipid bottle into the injectible rubber segment at the end of the tubing from the glucose bottle.

Needles as small as #28 may be used according to the size of the child. A constant infusion pump is used for both the Intralipid and the glucose circuits. Bacterial filters are not recommended because they block the passage of the fat emulsion.

At the start of therapy with Intralipid, 15 ml/kg/day are given. If the serum does not become lipemic, the dose is increased by 5 ml/kg each day until maintenance volumes are achieved (Table 3).

Iron requirements with the peripheral venous feeding program are met by intramuscular iron-dextran or by blood transfusion.

TABLE 3 Maintenance Schedule for Peripheral TPN with Intralipid

	Solution	ml/kg/day	cal/kg/day
Infants less than 1 year	Intralipid	35	39
	PN-8	150	60
		185	99
Children over 1 year	Intralipid	30	33
	PN-8	100	40
		130	73

METABOLIC OBSERVATIONS

Clinical measurements which have been found essential to evaluate the child's metabolic response include daily body weight, accurate volume of urine, and other body fluid losses. The urine sugar content is monitored at each voiding. The important blood tests and the frequency of study in the usual patient are given in Table 4. More frequent monitoring of some variables may be necessary in patients with specific metabolic abnormalities, such as those with renal or hepatic disease.

Weight changes during the period of intravenous feeding will vary with the patient's overall clinical status. Weight gains comparable to those of normal infants may be expected in those children who are not malnourished at the time intravenous feedings are instituted or in whom sepsis is not a part of the clinical picture (Fig. 1). In the patient with infection or another clinical problem which increases metabolic requirements, a flatter growth curve may be observed. A significant weight gain in the first 2 weeks of therapy usually is not seen in those infants and children who are severely depleted at the start of treatment. The weight gains observed with the three different techniques are comparable, averaging 20 to 30 gm per day in the neonate.

Despite the variations in weight curves, positive nitrogen balance has been noted in all patients studied in detail. Fecal loss of nitrogen is usually negligible, since stools are infrequent and scanty during periods of intravenous feeding. Urinary amino acid losses have been found to be negligible and not sufficient to produce osmotic diuresis except in infants weighing under 1 kg and in those children with severe renal disease.

In most patients, the large quantity of intravenous glucose is well tolerated without the addition of exogenous insulin. Blood sugar levels remain in the normal range, but urinary sugar content usually varies between 0 and 3+ by the Clinitest method. Urinary sugar levels gen-

TABLE 4 Blood Values Monitored Routinely During TPN

| | Frequency of Monitoring | |
At Start of Therapy and Weekly	At Start of Therapy and Every 2 Weeks	As Indicated
Na, K, Cl	SGOT, LDH, ALP	Copper
Urea	Bilirubin	Zinc
Glucose	Creatinine	Iron
Magnesium		Ammonia
Calcium, phosphorus		Osmolarity
Total protein		pH
Hgb, Hct, WBC		
Blood culture		
Candida precipitins		

erally are highest during the first day or two of treatment. Qualitative urine sugars consistently above 3+ may cause an osmotic diuresis and often signal the likelihood of blood stream infection, especially in the patient who has been treated for many days without glycosuria. A temporary decrease in hourly infusion rate or use of a more dilute solution usually corrects the problem if it is not due to sepsis.

Water balance is maintained even in infants weighing under 2.5 kg and in those following surgery despite the infusion of hypertonic PN-20 solutions. Urinary solute excretion on this intravenous diet is usually greater than that observed during oral feeding, but this increased load does not exceed the concentrating capability of the normal infant kidney.

COMPLICATIONS

Metabolic.   The metabolic complications that have occurred during TPN in infants and children are listed in Table 5. The potential complications are many, but most patients tolerate all these intravenous mixtures quite well. Although some of the complications are unavoidable, most can be prevented by appropriate adjustments of the infusate based on careful clinical monitoring.

Glucose intolerance and hyperglycemia have been observed (in the absence of sepsis) only in low birth weight premature infants and others with severe renal and central nervous system abnormalities. In some of these cases, widely fluctuating blood sugar levels even with the use of insulin forced us to abandon the intravenous feeding program.

Although hypoglycemia has been reported when TPN is stopped abruptly, we have not observed this complication despite the many accidental interruptions of the infusion. Nevertheless, when TPN is no

---

TABLE 5   Metabolic Complications of Intravenous Alimentation

Persistent hyperglycemia and glycosuria
Osmotic diuresis
Postinfusion hypoglycemia
Acidosis
Hyperammonemia
Amino acid toxicity
Hypomagnesemia
Hypocupremia
Essential fatty acid deficiency
Hypocalcemia, hypercalcemia, hypophosphatemia
Hepatic impairment (toxic)
Hypercholesterolemia
Hypertriglyceridemia

---

longer needed and oral intake starts, we recommend a gradual weaning from the intravenous diet to avoid this potential complication.

Metabolic acidosis has occurred as a complication of TPN. Although the composition of all TPN solutions presently available produces an acid load, pediatric patients do not become acidotic. The acidity and free water content of our mixtures are such that the acid-base regulatory mechanisms of the average infant and child provide adequate compensation. When a more concentrated preparation (5.25 per cent FreAmine* and 25 per cent glucose) was used in the past, the smaller infants developed acidosis with serum pH as low as 7.0. In susceptible individuals such as the low birth weight premature infant and those with renal or hepatic disease, frequent monitoring of blood pH is necessary to avoid acidosis even when using present mixtures.

Hyperammonemia generally has been reported in infants less than 6 months of age.[11, 12] It has been postulated that it is due to one or a combination of the following factors: (a) infusion of large quantities of ammonia that are present in protein hydrolysate solutions; (b) the administration of an intravenous diet which contains inappropriate proportions of amino acids; (c) subclinical liver disease or hepatic immaturity; and (d) arginine deficiency. We have measured blood ammonia at varying intervals after the institution of TPN in 23 infants. In 12 infants with elevated SGOT, LDH, and bilirubin, blood ammonia levels were normal. In 11 others with normal liver function tests, blood ammonia was elevated (75 mg per 100 ml) in two but normal in the others. Clinical signs of ammonia intoxication were never evident in any of these 23 patients or in any other patient whom we have treated.

Plasma and urine amino acids were measured in a small group of children, and in some abnormal serum values were detected. Histological examination of the central nervous system in children who have died while on TPN did not reveal the hypothalamic lesions which Olney, Ho, and Rhee[13] produced in mice by the administration of protein hydrolysate or acidic amino acids.

Hypomagnesemia causing seizures was seen in several patients early in our experience. In each case, the patient had prolonged diarrhea prior to the institution of TPN. Typically, seizures occurred within the first week of TPN therapy. Seizures due to hypomagnesemia largely have been eliminated since the magnesium content of the standard infusate has been increased, and additional magnesium has been administered at the start of therapy to patients with hypomagnesemia due to chronic diarrhea.

Copper deficiency has been observed recently as a result of chronic diarrhea and diets with insufficient copper such as TPN programs.[14, 15] Copper now is given routinely to all patients. The features that have been ascribed to lack of copper include anemia, neutropenia, hypopro-

---

*Manufactured by McGraw Laboratories, Glendale, California, 91201.

teinemia, osteoporosis, deep pigmentation of skin and hair, hypotonia, and psychomotor retardation. In the malnourished patient with depleted copper stores, overt signs of copper deficiency are most likely to develop when weight gain and growth occur on a high caloric, high protein diet low in copper. In the last 3 years, serum copper was measured in 76 infants and children on TPN. In 23 cases, serum copper was low and ranged from 20 to 75 mcg per 100 ml (normal 87 to 150 mcg per 100 ml). Nineteen of these 23 patients were on TPN because of chronic diarrhea and had a low serum copper content at the onset of therapy. The other four were not depleted at the start, but developed low serum copper before copper was added to the intravenous mixture routinely from 1 month to 5 months after the start of therapy. Anemia, which was noted in 15 of these copper-deficient patients, at least in part was caused by copper deficiency. Clinical evaluation for bone abnormalities was not performed. Increase in the serum copper was noted in depleted patients who were treated with small quantities of copper sulfate by mouth and in the others when oral feedings resumed.

Serum zinc was measured in conjunction with serum copper in these 76 patients. Low serum zinc was never observed (even after 6 months of TPN), even when the only source of zinc available was from transfusion. Nevertheless, zinc is now given to all patients in the trace metal solution.

Clinical signs of essential fatty acid deficiency have been apparent in only two children on the central feeding program, although in our series and others,[16] serious abnormalities in serum lipids have been noted after prolonged fat-free therapy. Each patient had been on TPN longer than 3 months when a severe generalized skin rash typical of essential fatty acid deficiency developed. Fortunately, at this stage of therapy, each infant was able to tolerate a small quantity of fat by mouth and the skin lesions soon disappeared. Essential fatty acid deficiency did not develop in any of the patients on Intralipid, nor was this syndrome seen in the infants receiving sunflower seed oil cutaneously. Most of the patients on Intralipid had normal triglyceride and cholesterol levels in their serum; however, a few who were on hyperalimentation for longer than one month ran serum triglycerides in the range of 300 to 350 mg per cent (normal 150 to 250 mg per 100 ml) and serum cholesterols of 150 to 250 mg per 100 ml (normal 100 to 150 mg per 100 ml). These mild elevations returned to normal once the Intralipid was stopped.

Hypocalcemia, hypercalcemia, hypophosphatemia, and hyperphosphatemia all have occurred in patients being fed solely by vein.[17, 18] Quantities of calcium and phosphorus in our present intravenous mixtures appear sufficient to avoid these problems in the vast majority of patients treated. Weekly monitoring of serum calcium and phosphorus suffices to detect an abnormality which might require modification in the quantities of calcium and phosphorus infused.

Signs of abnormal liver function often have been observed during TPN. Transient hepatic enlargement, with or without abnormal liver function tests, has been noted during the first week of therapy in most small infants. Variable and intermittent elevations of serum SGOT, LDH, and bilirubin have occurred throughout the course of treatment in many patients. The histological appearance of the liver either by biopsy or autopsy fails to reveal a consistent pathological alteration, although cholestasis is often prominent in our patients and in reports of others.[19] Sometimes the underlying clinical problem for which TPN is required sufficiently explains the liver abnormalities, but often such a cause is not apparent. We must remain alert to the possibility that these liver abnormalities may be due to a harmful substance in the infusate or to a dietary imbalance. The liver abnormalities seen with and without Intralipid appear to be the same and disappear once the intravenous feeding is stopped. In addition, intravenous fat pigment usually is seen in the Kuppfer cells of the liver in most patients on Intralipid for more than 1 month. This pigment deposition appears to have no effect on liver functions.

About 80 per cent of the patients on Intralipid develop a peripheral eosinophilia in the range of 5 to 10 per cent and in a few this may rise to 35 per cent. There are no clinical manifestations of this abnormality, such as skin rashes, urticaria, and so forth.

Osmotic diuresis secondary to significant glycosuria occasionally occurs when the 20 per cent glucose infusate is used. The premature infant with underdeveloped renal tubules is most susceptible to this complication. This phenomenon is not seen with peripheral hyperalimentation because of the lower tonicity of the infusates used.

No instance of fluid overload in the form of pulmonary edema, peripheral edema, or congestive heart failure was seen in any of the patients treated with the three techniques. This is especially important to note in the group with peripheral hyperalimentation without fats, in which the volume of fluid infused is quite high.

Technical. Many of the early technical problems associated with the catheter now either have been corrected or reduced in frequency. The use of polyvinyl catheters was associated with a high incidence of sterile inflammation and thrombosis; non-reactive silicone rubber catheters have minimized these hazards. Transitory arrhythmias may occur during the insertion of the catheter, especially if the tip enters the heart. The position of the catheter tip must be checked radiographically to be certain that the irritating hyperosmolar solution is delivered into the superior vena cava and not into a smaller vein with a lower blood flow, such as the hepatic. Dislocation of the catheter is less frequent since a vein flange is used to secure it.

Venous Perforation. This complication, although reported in the literature, has not occurred in our patients. Thrombosis of the vein in which the catheter resides can occur, especially in the critically ill patient with sepsis and inadequate circulation. When thrombosis occurs in the superior vena cava, it is better tolerated than in most other vessels. Although evidence of thromboembolism has been noted at autopsy in children dying with the central venous catheter in place, manifestations of this phenomenon *in vivo* are extremely rare.

Nevertheless, it should be avoided if possible. Among the important factors in its prevention are the use of jugular veins rather than femoral or umbilical veins for intubation, x-ray control of the catheter position, the avoidance of sepsis, and the use of a silicone rubber catheter.

No cases of phlebitis were seen in patients treated with Intralipid peripherally, in spite of the fact that the entire infusate is slightly hypertonic. In some unknown fashion Intralipid appears to protect the vein. When infiltration does occur, it is usually bland and the fluid is reabsorbed rapidly. Phlebitis occasionally is seen in the patients fed peripherally without fat, but it disappears when the infusion site is changed. In the 35 patients treated with peripheral hyperalimentation without fat, three cases of skin slough at the infusion site were seen, but these all healed spontaneously without the need for skin grafting.

Infection. Sepsis remains the major complication of central TPN in the pediatric patient. Long-term indwelling venous cannulas are a well-documented source of blood stream infection. Organisms may enter the blood stream along the catheter tract or with a contaminated intravenous solution. The catheter, a foreign body in the blood stream, may act as a focus for bacterial growth even if organisms enter from a distant septic site. To minimize the risk of sepsis, the following measures and precautions should be taken. Catheters should be placed under aseptic conditions in an operating room. Silicone rubber catheters rather than polyethylene or polyvinyl catheters should be used because they cause less tissue reaction and are less likely to produce a thrombus which will support the growth of microorganisms along the wall of the intubated vein. The skin exit site for the catheter should be placed in an area which can be aseptically and meticulously cleansed. Proper care of this site and all the connectors and tubings between the intravenous bottle and the patient is essential. Withdrawal of blood from the central venous catheter for chemical and bacterial testing should be done only by properly trained personnel.

Any relaxation in strict adherence to the standard technique of catheter care is followed by sharp rise in the incidence of infective complications. Some institutions[20] have reported such an extremely high incidence of fungal septicemia and death that treatment with TPN in such a hospital is unsafe.

A review of the Children's Hospital Medical Center experience indicated that 42 of 264 patients (16 per cent) had one or more septic complications. The incidence of sepsis was not related to the patient's age or diagnosis. Analysis of our septic complications reveals that the likelihood of sepsis clearly was related to the duration of therapy. For each week of therapy after the first, the risk of sepsis increases by about 5 per cent.

Fever, leukocytosis, and/or unexplained glycosuria were usually the first clues to blood stream infection. Infection was confirmed when microorgani ms were cultured from blood obtained through the central venous line. *Candida* was isolated in 18 blood cultures, a variety of gram-negative bacteria in 9 cultures, and staphylococci, streptococci, or diphtheroids in 20. In five cases more than one organism was found.

Infants with proven *Candida* blood stream infection were treated by removal of the central venous line; chemotherapy usually was withheld because of the toxicity of amphotericin. In those with bacterial sepsis, the line usually was withdrawn and appropriate antibiotics were given. In five patients with bacterial infection, the venous catheter was left in place and antibiotic therapy alone was curative. Recovery from septicemia usually was evident within 24 hours. Forty of 42 patients survived the septicemia episode, although six eventually died of their primary disease. Two deaths could be attributed directly to catheter sepsis. One infant, a newborn with gastroschisis and intestinal obstruction, developed *Candida* septicemia on the sixteenth day of TPN and the line was removed. The central venous line was inserted 5 days later, but septicemia recurred and the infant expired. The other death occurred in an 8-week-old infant with a complicated esophageal abnormality including tracheoesophageal fistula and massive chalasia. The patient developed *Candida* septicemia on the twenty-second day of TPN. The line was removed, blood cultures became negative, and a second line was inserted 10 days later. On the following day, bilateral overwhelming monilial pneumonia due to embolization of a septic thrombus in the superior vena cava resulted in the death of this infant. Therefore, despite the relatively high incidence of infection, the overwhelming majority of affected patients recover without serious sequelae.

Invasive sepsis related to hyperalimentation was not seen in any of the 80 patients treated with Intralipid or in any of the infants and children managed with peripheral intravenous feeding without fat.

CONCLUSION

When patients are properly selected for treatment and appropriate precautions are exercised, the benefits of parenteral alimentation far outweigh the risks. It has been most gratifying to be able to salvage the lives of many children who otherwise would have died of starvation in the past.

REFERENCES

1. Dudrick, S. J., Wilmore, D. W., Vars, H. M., and Rhoads, J. E.: Long-term total parenteral nutrition with growth, development, and positive nitrogen balance. Surgery, *64*:134, 1968.
2. Dudrick, S. J., Wilmore, D. W., Vars, H. M., and Rhoads, J. E.: Can intravenous feeding as the sole means of nutrition support growth in the child and restore weight loss in an adult? An affirmative answer. Ann. Surg., *169*:974, 1969.
3. Filler, R. M., Eraklis, A. J., Rubin, V. G., and Das, J. B.: Long-term parenteral nutrition in infants. N. Engl. J. Med., *281*:589, 1969.
4. Borresen, H. C., Coran, A. G., and Knutrud, O.: Metabolic results of parenteral feeding in neonatal surgery: A balanced parenteral feeding program based on a synthetic L-amino acid solution and a commercial fat emulsion. Ann. Surg., *172*:291, 1970.
5. Coran, A. G.: The intravenous use of fat for the total parenteral nutrition of the infant. Lipids, *7*:455, 1972.
6. Coran, A. G.: Total intravenous feeding of infants and children without the use of a central venous catheter. Ann Surg., *179*:445, 1974.
7. Coran, A. G.: The long-term total intravenous feeding of infants using peripheral veins. J. Pediatr. Surg., *8*:801, 1973.
8. Fox, H. A., and Krasna, I. H.: Total intravenous nutrition by peripheral vein in neonatal surgical patients. Pediatrics, *52*:14, 1973.
9. Dudrick, S. J., Steiger, E., and Long, J. M.: Renal failure in surgical patients: Treatment with intravenous essential amino acids and hypertonic glucose. Surgery, *68*:180, 1970.
10. Press, M., Hartop, P. J., and Prottey, C.: Correction of essential fatty-acid deficiency in man by the cutaneous application of sunflower seed oil. Lancet, *1*:579, 1974.
11. Johnson, J. C., Albritton, W. L., and Sunshine, P.: Hyperammonemia accompanying parenteral nutrition in newborn infants. J. Pediatr., *81*:154, 1972.
12. Ghadimi, H., Abaci, F., Kumar, S., and Rathi, M.: Biochemical aspects of intravenous alimentation. Pediatrics, *48*:955, 1971.
13. Olney, J. W., Ho, O. L., Rhee, B.: Brain-damaging potential of protein hydrolysates. N. Engl. J. Med., *289*:391, 1973.
14. Karpel, J. T., and Peden, V. H.: Copper deficiency in long-term parenteral nutrition. J. Pediatr., *80*:32, 1972.
15. Ashkenazi, A., Levin, S., Djaldetti, M., Fishel, E., and Benvenisti, B.: The syndrome of neonatal copper deficiency. Pediatrics, *52*:525, 1973.
16. Paulsrud, J. R., Pensler, L., Whitten, C. F., Stewart, S., and Holman, R. T.: Essential fatty acid deficiency in infants induced by fat-free intravenous feeding. Am. J. Clin. Nutr., *25*:897, 1972.
17. Travis, S. F., Sugarman, H. J., Ruberg, R. L., Dudrick, S. J., Papadopoulos, M. D., Miller, L. D., and Oski, F. A.: Alterations of red cell glycolytic intermediates and oxygen transport as a consequence of hypophosphatemia in patients receiving intravenous hyperalimentation. N. Engl. J. Med., *285*:763, 1971.
18. Shils, M. E.: Guidelines for total parenteral nutrition. J.A.M.A., *220*:1721, 1972.
19. Touloukian, R. J., Downing, S. E.: Cholestasis associated with long-term parenteral hyperalimentation. Arch. Surg., *106*:58, 1973.
20. Curry, C. R., and Quie, P. G.: Fungal septicemia in patients receiving parenteral hyperalimentation. N. Engl. J. Med., *285*:1221, 1971.
21. Filler, R. M.: A new method of fixation of silicone rubber catheters for long-term hyperalimentation. J. Pediatr. Surg., *8*:395, 1973.

Chapter Twenty-Two

DISSEMINATED INTRAVASCULAR COAGULATION

WILLIAM E. HATHAWAY, M.D.

Disseminated intravascular coagulation (DIC) is a disease process characterized by intravascular consumption of plasma clotting factors and platelets. In many clinical instances, this process results in widespread deposition of fibrin thrombi within the peripheral vascular system and a generalized hemorrhagic diathesis. As outlined in Figure 1 (p. 314), several events can initiate or trigger the process of DIC. Activation of the coagulation mechanism through Hageman factor (XII) or by tissue thromboplastin leads to the formation of fibrin. During coagulation certain factors are consumed. These factors, depleted during active DIC, are antihemophilic factor (VIII), proaccelerin (V), platelets, prothrombin (II), and fibrinogen. In addition, clotting factors may be activated or complexed with other factors during the coagulation sequence. Depending upon the clotting factor activity assay used, the activated factors actually may appear increased during the process, i.e., factors XI, VIII, and V. The complexing of factor VII with tissue thromboplastin may lead to lowered levels of factor VII during DIC. As fibrin is deposited in the small vessels and capillaries, the fibrinolytic system is activated, and the newly formed fibrinolysin splits the fibrin into fragments. Limited action of thrombin may produce fibrin monomer which can complex with native fibrinogen or fibrin split products. These fibrin split products (FSP) and fibrin complexes are cleared from the circulation by action of the reticuloendothelial system (RES). While circulating, the FSP have several functions. They act as an

From the Department of Pediatrics, University of Colorado Medical Center, Denver, Colorado.

anticoagulant on the initial as well as later stages of coagulation; they decrease platelet function; and they may exhibit vasoactive properties. Naturally occurring anticoagulants or protease inhibitors also are involved by binding and inactivating the activated clotting factors (thrombin, activated factor XI and factor X). The most important protease inhibitor is an alpha-2-globulin called antithrombin III. This inhibitor may be consumed during DIC.

The end results of this process include: (1) thrombi and emboli which produce *tissue ischemia and necrosis* in various organs (principally lungs, kidneys, gastrointestinal tract, adrenal glands, brain, liver, pancreas, and skin); (2) depletion of clotting factors, plus the antihemostatic effect of FSP, which lead to widespread *hemorrhage;* (3) a *microangiopathic hemolytic anemia* due to red cell fragmentation by strands of fibrin in the peripheral vasculature; and (4) finally *shock* and death. At the onset, it should be emphasized that DIC can occur with varying degrees of severity. This fact, and the variability of physiological compensation mechanisms (fibrinolysis, clotting factor synthesis), lead to different clinical expressions of the disorder which may not always include diffuse thrombi or hemorrhagic diathesis. DIC may occur acutely and be an important contributing factor to the demise of a severely ill patient (severe asphyxia or septic shock). Chronic or subacute DIC also occurs in many disorders in which the process may be confined largely to the microvasculature either diffusely or localized to one organ or tissue (giant hemangioma, malignancy, necrotizing enterocolitis).

Table 1 lists the many diseases in which DIC has been documented or suspected as an etiological or complicating mechanism.

RECOGNITION OF DISSEMINATED INTRAVASCULAR COAGULATION

Clinical Aspects

The preceding paragraphs suggest that any severely ill child may develop the complication of disseminated intravascular coagulation. Indeed, the multiple and frequently non-specific features may well explain why the condition may be diagnosed either too often or not often enough. Suspicious clinical signs are: (1) evidence of multiple organ involvement by thrombi and emboli, i.e., respiratory distress; hematuria and progressive renal shutdown; deterioration of consciousness, coma, and convulsions; gastrointestinal distention, ileus, vomiting, and diarrhea; and thrombotic lesions of the skin; (2) a bleeding tendency which initially may be only skin purpura or oozing from puncture sites, but which may progress to widespread hemorrhage; (3)

TABLE 1   Diseases in Which Disseminated Intravascular Coagulation has Been Documented or Suspected

Infection:	
Bacterial sepsis[1]	Meningococcus, *E. coli, A. aerogenes,* Clostridia, *Pasteurella pestis, Pseudomonas aeruginosa,* β-hemolytic streptococcus, *H. Influenzae, Staphylococcus aureus*
Viral infections[2]	Varicella, vaccinia, variola, rubella, rubeola, arboviruses, herpes,[3] cytomegalovirus, influenza A,[4] psittacosis[5]
Other	Malaria, rickettsia (Rocky Mountain spotted fever)
Surgical conditions:	Burns (thermal, electrical)[6]
	Trauma
	Hemorrhagic shock
	Renal transplants[7]
	Liver transplants[8]
	Fat embolism
Neonatal conditions:	Asphyxia neonatorum
	Idiopathic respiratory distress syndrome[9,10]
	Infant born to mother with toxemia, abruptio placentae, or diabetes mellitus
	Twin with dead fetus[11]
	Necrotizing enterocolitis[12]
	Chorioangioma of placenta[23]
Malignancies:	Disseminated cancer: neuroblastoma, carcinoma[13]
	Leukemia: acute promyelocytic,[14] acute lymphatic, or stem cell
Metabolic disorders:	Cirrhosis,[15] hepatitis,[15] diabetic coma[16]
	Hyperthermia: heat stroke,[17] anesthesia[18]
Miscellaneous conditions:	Snake bite
	Purpura fulminans
	Giant hemangioma[19]
	Hemolytic transfusion reactions
	Thrombotic thrombocytopenic purpura
	Cyanotic congenital heart disease
	Acute anaphylactic reaction[20]
	Hemolytic-uremic syndrome[21,22]
	Disseminated lupus erythematosus[24]
	Cardiac arrest[25]
Pharmacological agents:	Crude opium[26]
	Stibophen[27]
	Dilantin[28]

pallor or slight jaundice due to an acute hemolytic anemia; (4) shock. Corrigan[29] and McKay[30] have emphasized the association of hypotension leading to peripheral vascular collapse in patients with DIC. Obviously, accurate diagnosis requires not only clinical suspicion but laboratory confirmation.

Laboratory Tests

The laboratory signs of DIC usually produce evidence of the following: (1) consumption of factors utilized when blood clots (fibrinogen, V, VIII, II, and platelets); (2) secondary fibrinolysis leading to fibrinogen-fibrin split products; and (3) microangiopathic hemolytic anemia. Table 2 outlines the coagulation tests which can be abnormal in DIC. Both the author's and published experience[31, 32, 33] with the use of clotting tests to detect DIC indicate that the simple screening tests most frequently are abnormal. The platelet count, prothrombin time, partial thromboplastin time (PTT), fibrinogen level, and some indicator of intravascular fibrinolysis, such as the thrombin time or fibrin-fibrinogen split product test, are the most useful laboratory determinations. Specific factor assays may be useful in the differential diagnosis of complex coagulopathies (see further on), but usually are not necessary in the laboratory confirmation of DIC. As discussed earlier, specific factor assays of clotting activity may vary greatly depending upon the severity and stage of the DIC process. For example, factor VIII appears elevated early in the disorder and frequently does not fall to abnormal levels even in severe DIC. These findings may be due in part to the one-stage (PTT) method commonly used for the factor VIII determination.[34] In our experience, factor V levels usually are depressed in acute DIC. The determination of the degradation products of fibrinogen-fibrin (FSP) is helpful to indicate that excessive fibrin deposition and lysis have occurred intravascularly. The most sensitive tests for FSP are those based on hemagglutination inhibition of fibrinogen-coated, tanned red cells.[35] Fibrinogen-antibody-coated latex particles are used in a sensitive and widely available slide test for FSP (Thrombo-Wellcotest). Other immunological methods for FSP measurement are too cumbersome or slow to be of significant clinical benefit. Rapid and simple tests for FSP or complexes of fibrin monomers and fibrinogen have been described as helpful in diagnosis of DIC; of these tests the protamine precipitation test appears to be the most useful.[36, 37] Reviews of the limitations and usefulness of tests for FSP[38, 39] indicate that these tests are helpful in the diagnosis of DIC but may also be positive in

TABLE 2   Coagulation Tests Which May Be Abnormal in Intravascular Coagulation

Test	Pathophysiological Abnormality Detected
Bleeding time (tourniquet test)	Thrombocytopenia and platelet hypofunction due to fibrin split products (FSP)
Platelet count	Platelet consumption
Partial thromboplastin time	Factors VIII, V, II, fibrinogen consumption; anti-coagulant effect of FSP
Prothrombin time	Factors VII, II, V, fibrinogen consumption
Thrombin time	Fibrinogen consumption; presence of FSP
Fibrinogen, II, V, VIII, VII assays	Factor consumption
Euglobulin lysis time	Presence of fibrinolysins
Immunoassay for FSP (protamine precipitation test)	Presence of degradation products of fibrin and complexes of fibrin monomer with fibrinogen or FSP

other conditions associated with inflammation. The proof of the diagnosis of intravascular coagulation is the demonstration of thrombin generation in the circulation. The development of a radioimmunoassay for detection of fibrinopeptides A and B[40] and a method for measurement of ^{14}C glycine-ethyl ester incorporation into circulating fibrin[41] may prove useful tools for detection of DIC.

Fragmented, burred, microspherocytic, and helmet-shaped erythrocytes frequently are seen in the peripheral blood in DIC.[42] These cells are the basis for the hemolytic anemia (microangiopathic anemia) noted earlier. Therefore, careful examination of a freshly made blood smear should be done in all suspected cases of DIC.

The laboratory diagnosis of disseminated intravascular coagulation during the neonatal period may be difficult. The physiological alterations of the coagulation system in the newborn cause a few seconds prolongation of the clotting tests that are most helpful in the older child, i.e., the prothrombin time, partial thromboplastin time, and thrombin time (see Table 3). A microfibrinogen test[43] and the platelet count may be helpful in diagnosis since both preterm and term infants have values for these tests like those of older children. If care is taken in collection of newborn infant blood (into tubes containing fibrinolytic inhibitors), increased amounts of FSP should be considered of pathological significance and as reflecting increased fibrinolysis. Discussions of the bleeding and thrombotic disorders in the newborn have been presented recently.[44, 45] (See also Chapter 15 in this book.)

When the process of DIC is interrupted, a rebound increase of the consumable factors occasionally is seen. When hepatic function is normal, this rebound can be helpful in confirmation of the diagnosis. An

TABLE 3 **Coagulation Tests in the Newborn***

Test	Normal Adult	Normal Newborns (Full Term and Premature)
Kaolin partial thromboplastin time	38–50 sec	41–80 sec
Prothrombin time	12–14 sec	12–20 sec
Thrombin time	8–10 sec	10–17 sec
Platelet count	200,000–450,000/cu mm	200,000–400,000/cu mm
Factor assays:		
I (fibrinogen)	190–420 mg/100 ml	157–369 mg/100 ml
II (prothrombin)	70–120%	24–66%
V (proaccelerin)	70–150%	60–140%
VIII (antihemophilic factor)	60–150%	64–147%
Euglobulin fibrinolysin time	90–300 min	21–145 min†

*Values are from the author's laboratory.
†Cord blood.

exception is the persistent thrombocytopenia frequently seen after an episode of DIC.[31]

With so many possible laboratory approaches, the author would advise concentrating on the following tests for laboratory confirmation of DIC: red cell smear, platelet count, partial thromboplastin time, prothrombin time, thrombin time or test for FSP, and fibrinogen.

Differential Diagnosis

Several conditions causing critical illness in a child may be confused with DIC on clinical grounds. Patients with massive hepatitis, severe cirrhosis, or acute hepatic necrosis as seen in Reye's syndrome may develop a severe bleeding diathesis with depression of fibrinogen, factors V and II, and platelets. Factor VIII levels remain normal or elevated in liver disease but may be decreased in severe DIC. Rarely, primary fibrinolysis may occur in children in association with liver disease. Release of activators from the damaged liver causes pathologically increased fibrinolysis, thus resulting in decreased fibrinogen and increased FSP. Direct action of the proteolytic enzyme may cause decreased levels of factors V and VIII as well. Platelets usually remain normal. The process may not be as severe as acute DIC, but the differential diagnosis is obviously a difficult one; often serial measurements, or cautious therapeutic trials, or both may be necessary to establish the diagnosis. Whether DIC occurs in liver disease has been questioned.[15]

Severe uremia often is seen with a bleeding diathesis which is associated with decreased platelets, prolonged prothrombin and thrombin times, and increased levels of FSP. However, fibrinogen and factors V and VIII levels usually remain normal or even increased.

Infections, especially meningococcemia, Rocky Mountain spotted fever, and certain viral diseases, can present with thrombocytopenia, and even prolongation of the prothrombin time,[46] without other evidence of DIC. In septicemia the platelet count may fall precipitously without evidence for DIC.[47] Demonstration of a prolonged thrombin time and decreased fibrinogen level would be necessary in order to confirm the diagnosis of DIC in such patients.

Patients with cyanotic congenital heart disease and polycythemia may have marked derangement of the coagulation mechanism without definite consumption coagulopathy. These abnormalities include prolonged bleeding times, thrombocytopenia, increased prothrombin and euglobulin lysis times. The thrombocytopenia has been associated with decreased platelet survival,[48] the precise mechanism of which is as yet unclear. An occasional patient with cyanotic heart disease can develop DIC as a complication during the natural course of the disorder.[49]

Fibrin split products and thrombocytopenia may be present in several conditions without other evidence of diffuse intravascular coagulation. These syndromes, which have been associated with platelet consumption without significant fibrinogen consumption,[50] include renal disease,[51] hemolytic-uremic syndrome,[52] thrombotic thrombocytopenic purpura,[50] and necrotizing enterocolitis.[12] Acute DIC may occur in any of these disorders, but the usual manifestation is increased platelet destruction with evidence for chronic or low-grade DIC (increased FSP, low antithrombin III).

Since therapy with heparin may aggravate the bleeding in many of the aforementioned conditions, i.e., liver disease or renal disease, presence of a consumption coagulopathy must be proved before therapy is started. This may require extensive studies, including factor assays.

In these seriously ill children positive answers to the following questions should be obtained before therapy is instituted:

1. Does the patient have a triggering event present such as infection, tissue damage, or endothelial damage?

2. Is hypotension or multiple system involvement present?

3. Is there laboratory evidence of a consumption coagulopathy?

TREATMENT

In the past several years many articles have appeared in the medical literature which discuss treatment of DIC in various clinical situations. Essentially all of these discussions are based on practical experience without carefully controlled prospective studies. Heparin therapy does not appear to decrease the mortality due to severe septic shock in children.[53] The use of heparin in meningococcemia has been reviewed,[54] with the conclusion that in selected cases heparin is an effective adjunct to total therapy. Reversal of the primary disease usually ameliorates DIC, frequently without need for specific therapy with heparin.[55] Hemorrhagic shock and DIC are best managed without the use of heparin.[56] Heparin therapy does not affect the death rate in acute renal failure with DIC.[57] Exchange transfusion with citrated whole blood is effective therapy for DIC.[58] In the absence of controlled studies, these reports and personal experiences have led the author to adopt the following empirical approach to the management of DIC.

The triggering events, clinical and laboratory manifestations, and end results (Figure 1) should be kept in mind when therapy is considered. In assessing the need for treatment in DIC, one should determine the triggering event and note the severity of the clinical and laboratory manifestations. The following guide then can be used to determine the specific therapeutic modalities.

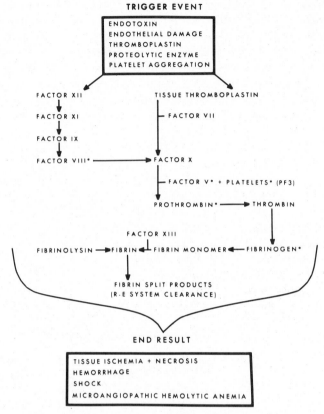

Figure 1.   Scheme of disseminated intravascular coagulation.

1. Triggering event controlled or relieved; manifestations minimal (slight bleeding, blood pressure normal, slight to moderately severe laboratory abnormalities); *no therapy.* Example: neonatal asphyxia after resuscitation, posthemorrhagic or septic shock state.

2. Triggering event controlled or relieved; manifestations severe (frank bleeding, mild hypotension, markedly abnormal laboratory tests); *treatment by platelet and coagulation factor replacement or exchange transfusion in the newborn or infant.* Example: after severe asphyxia, abruptio placenta, or hemorrhagic shock.

3. Triggering event controlled or relieved; clinical manifestations include evidence for definite thrombosis (renal cortical necrosis, large vessel thrombi, gangrene); *therapeutic trial of heparin.* Example: purpura fulminans, renal vein thrombosis.

4. Persistent triggering event; mild to absent clinical manifestations, mild to moderate laboratory findings; *no therapy.* Example: viral infection, sepsis without shock.

5. Persistent triggering event; clinical manifestations include frank bleeding or organ damage by microthrombosis: *heparinization and replacement of platelets and clotting factors.* Example: early, severe meningococcemia; neonatal sepsis with shock; necrotizing enterocolitis.

6. If the triggering events are being relieved but secondary events (persistent shock or hypoxia) persist and clinical manifestations are severe, *replacement therapy or exchange transfusion may be indicated; heparin usually is not indicated.* Example: sepsis with "intractable" shock; severe idiopathic respiratory distress syndrome.

The therapeutic modalities which may be used are as follows:

Prompt Removal of Triggering Event. Maintenance of blood pressure, institution of antimicrobial therapy,[7] correction of hypoxia and acidosis, and restoration of peripheral perfusion often are all that is needed to effectively interrupt the DIC process.

Heparinization. When indicated, heparin may be given in intravenous "push" doses of 100 units/kg body weight every 4 hours. Dosage may be adjusted according to clinical response or effect on laboratory tests. Duration of therapy is based on removal of triggering event and cessation of clinical manifestations; this may be only 24 hours in many instances. When longer term heparinization is necessary, monitoring of heparin effect may be done by adjusting the dosage (adjust dose or time interval, 4 to 6 hours) according to the partial thromboplastin time or thrombin time measured just before the next dose. These tests should show definite but slight heparin effect at that time. Heparin should be used with great caution, if at all, in clinical situations in which impaired coagulation factor synthesis is seen (i.e., severe liver disease) or when the platelet count is 20,000/cu mm or less. Severe thrombocytopenia becomes less of a contraindication if adequate platelet replacement is assured. Heparinization may be neutralized by giving 0.75 to 1 mg protamine sulfate for each 100 units of heparin estimated to be circulating in the patient.

Replacement Therapy. Replacement of consumed clotting factors and platelets is often necessary in severe DIC associated with bleeding. A hemostatic level of plasma factors can be achieved by 10 ml/kg of fresh or fresh-frozen plasma. Platelets can be raised to a hemostatic level by administering 1 unit platelet concentrate per 6 to 8 kg body weight (should give 80,000 per cu mm rise). In the newborn, 10ml/kg of platelet concentrate will give hemostatic levels of both platelets and clotting factors.

Exchange Transfusion. In the neonate and small child, exchange transfusion is an efficient way to replace depleted clotting factors and to remove fibrin degradation products without volume overload. This procedure usually is reserved for the severely ill infant with marked depletion of clotting factors and clinical bleeding. In this situation, acid-citrate-dextrose or citrate-phosphate-dextrose blood is used rather than heparinized blood in order to minimize the risk of serious hemorrhage.

Other Pharmacological Agents. In instances of disseminated microthrombosis of the microvasculature in which platelet consumption is the major abnormality, consideration of antiplatelet agents (aspirin, dipyridamole) is indicated. The effectiveness of such drugs in preventing platelet consumption in the hemolytic uremic syndrome has been reported.[59] Amicar (E-aminocaproic acid) and other antifibrinolytic agents are contraindicated in DIC.

SUMMARY

The complication of disseminated intravascular coagulation should be suspected in a critically ill child when evidence of the following signs and symptoms is present: (1) the potential of a triggering event, such as endotoxin, tissue thromboplastin (damaged tissue), endothelial damage, or proteolysis; (2) multiple system involvement producing coma, renal shutdown, respiratory disease, and shock; (3) a bleeding diathesis; and (4) a hemolytic anemia associated with fragmented and burred red cells. Laboratory confirmation should include evidence for depletion of coagulation factors consumed during clotting, i.e., platelets, fibrinogen, and factors II, V, and VIII. Treatment consists of removal of the triggering event, replacement of depleted factors and platelets, and supportive care. In specific instances exchange transfusion or heparinization may be indicated.

REFERENCES

1. Yoshikawa, T., Tanaka, K. R., and Guze, L. B.: Infection and disseminated intravascular coagulation. Medicine, *50*:237, 1971.
2. McKay, D. C., and Margaretten, W.: Disseminated intravascular coagulation in virus diseases. Arch. Intern. Med., *120*:129, 1967.
3. Miller, D. R., Hanshaw, J. P., O'Leary, D. S., and Hnilick, J. V.: Fatal disseminated herpes simplex virus infection and hemorrhage in the neonate. J. Pediatr., *76*:409, 1970.
4. Davison, A. M., Thomson, D., Robson, J. S.: Intravascular coagulation complicating influenza A virus infection. Br. Med. J., *1*:654, 1973.
5. Hamilton, D. V.: Psittacosis and disseminated intravascular coagulation. Br. Med. J., *4*:370, 1975.
6. McManus, W. F., Eurenius, K., and Pruitt, B. A.: Disseminated intravascular coagulation in burned patients. J. Trauma, *13*:416, 1973.
7. Starzl, T. E., Lerner, R. A., Dixon, R. J., Groth, C. G., Brettschneider, L., and Terasaki, P.: Schwartzmann reaction after human renal transplantation. N. Engl. J. Med., *278*:642, 1968.
8. Groth, C. G., Pechet, L., and Starzl, T. E.: Coagulation during and after orthotopic transplantation of the human liver. Arch. Surg., *98*:31, 1969.

9. Hathaway, W. E., Mull, M. M., and Pechet, C. S.: Disseminated intravascular coagulation in the newborn. Pediatrics, *43*:233, 1969.
10. Altstatt, L. B., Dennis, L. H., Sundell, H., Malan, A., Harrison, V., Hedvall, G., Eichelberger, J., Fogel, B., and Stahlman, M.: Disseminated intravascular coagulation and hyaline membrane disease. Biol. Neonate, *19*:227, 1971.
11. Moore, C. M., McAdams, A. J., and Sutherland, J.: Intrauterine disseminated intravascular coagulation: A syndrome of multiple pregnancy with a dead twin fetus. J. Pediatr., *74*:523, 1969.
12. Hutter, J. J., Hathaway, W. E., and Wayne, E. R.: Hematologic abnormalities in severe neonatal necrotizing enterocolitis. J. Pediatr., *88*:1026, 1976.
13. Peck, S., and Reiquam, C. W.: Disseminated intravascular coagulation in cancer patients: supportive evidence. Cancer, *31*:1114, 1973.
14. Gralnick, H. R., and Sultan, C.: Acute promyelocytic leukaemia: Haemorrhagic manifestation and morphologic criteria. Br. J. Haematol., *29*:373, 1975.
15. Bloom, A. L.: Intravascular coagulation and the liver. Br. J. Haematol., *30*:1, 1975.
16. Nicholson, G., and Tomkin, G. H.: Disseminated intravascular coagulation in diabetic coma. Br. Med. J., *4*:450, 1974.
17. Weber, M. B., and Blakely, J. A.: The haemorrhagic diathesis of heatstroke. Lancet, *1*:1190, 1969.
18. Purkis, I. E., Horrelt, O., De Young, C. G., Gleming, R. A. P., and Langley, G. R.: Hyperpyrexia during anesthesia in a second member of a family, with associated coagulation defect due to increased intravascular coagulation. Can. Anaesth. Soc. J., *14*:183, 1967.
19. Thatcher, L. G., Clatanoff, D. V., and Stiehm, E. R.: Splenic hemangioma with thrombocytopenia and afibrinogenemia. J. Pediatr., *73*:345, 1968.
20. Blombäck, M., Johnsson, S. A., and Sjöberg, H. E.: Coagulation factors and defibrination syndrome in anaphylaxis. Acta Physiol. Scand., *69*:313, 1967.
21. Piel, C. F., and Phibbs, R. H.: The hemolytic-uremic syndrome. Pediatr. Clin. North Am., *13*:295, 1966.
22. Sanchez Avalos, J., Vitacco, M., Molinas, F., Penalver, J., and Gianantonio, C.: Coagulation studies in the hemolytic-uremic syndrome. J. Pediatr., *76*:538, 1970.
23. Jones, C. E., Rivers, R. P., and Taghizadeh, A.: Disseminated intravascular coagulation and fetal hydrops in a newborn infant in association with a chorangioma of placenta. Pediatrics, *50*:901, 1972.
24. Beall, C. L., and Pierce, L. E.: Intravascular coagulation in acute lupus erythematosus. J.A.M.A., *234*:518, 1975.
25. Mehta, B., Briggs, D. K., Sommers, S. C., and Karpatkin, M.: Disseminated intravascular coagulation following cardiac arrest: A study of 15 patients. Am. J. Med. Sci., *264*:353, 1972.
26. Bernheim, J. L., Cate, J. W. ten, and Heide R. M., van der: Disseminated intravascular coagulation, uremia and liver damage after intravenous crude opium. Acta. Med. Scand., *191*:63, 1972.
27. Weiss, H. J., Berger, R. E., Tice, A. D., and Phillips, L. L.: Fatal disseminated intravascular coagulation and hemolytic anemia following stibophen therapy: A study of basic mechanisms. Am. J. Med. Sci., *264*:375, 1972.
28. Targan, S. R., Chassin, M. R. G., and Guze, L. B.: Dilantin-induced disseminated intravascular coagulation with purpura fulminans. Ann. Int. Med., *83*:227, 1975.
29. Corrigan, J. J., Jr., Ray, W. L., and May, N.: Changes in the blood coagulation system associated with septicemia. N. Engl. J. Med., *279*:851, 1968.
30. McKay, D. G.: Progress in disseminated intravascular coagulation. Part I. Calif. Med., *111*:186, 1969.
31. Colman, R. W., Robboy, S. J., and Minna, J. D.: Disseminated intravascular coagulation (DIC): An approach. Am. J. Med., *52*:679, 1972.
32. Whaun, J. M., and Oski, F. A.: Experience with disseminated intravascular coagulation in a children's hospital. Can. Med. Assoc. J., *107*:963, 1972.
33. Regan, D. H., and Lackner, H.: Defibrination syndrome: changing concepts and recognition of the low grade form. Am. J. Med. Sci., *266*:84, 1973.
34. Niemetz, J., and Nossel, H. L.: Activated coagulation factors: in vivo and in vitro studies. Br. J. Haematol., *16*:337, 1969.
35. Mersky, C., Lalezari, P., and Johnson, A. J.: A rapid, simple, sensitive method for

measuring fibrinolytic split products in human serum. Proc. Soc. Exp. Biol. Med., *131*:871, 1969.

36. Seaman, A. J.: The recognition of intravascular clotting. The plasma protamine paracoagulation test. Arch. Int. Med., *125*:1016, 1970.

37. Kidder, W. R., Logan, L. J., Rapaport, S. I., and Patch, M. J.: The plasma protamine paracoagulation test: clinical and laboratory evaluation. Am. J. Clin. Pathol., *58*:675, 1972.

38. Thomas, D. P., Niewiarowski, S., Myers, A. R., Bloch, K. J., and Colman, R. W.: Four methods for detecting fibrinogen degradation products. N. Engl. J. Med., *283*:663, 1970.

39. Marder, V. J., Matchett, M. O., and Sherry, S.: Detection of serum fibrinogen and fibrin degradation products. Am. J. Med., *51*:71, 1971.

40. Nossel, H. L., Younger, L. R., Wilner, G. D., et al.: Radioimmunoassay of human fibrinopeptide A. Proc. Natl. Acad. Sci. U.S.A., *68*:2350, 1971.

41. Kisker, C. T., and Rush, R.: Detection of intravascular coagulation. J. Clin. Invest., *50*:2235, 1971.

42. Baker, L. R. I., Rubenberg, M. L., Dacie, J. V., and Brain, M. C.: Fibrinogen catabolism in microangiopathic haemolytic anaemia. Br. J. Haematol., *14*:617, 1968.

43. Searcy, R. L., Simms, N. M., and Low, E. M. Y.: A simple method for rapid detection of hypofibrinogenemia. Am. J. Med. Technol., *33*:326, 1967.

44. Chessels, J. M., and Hardisty, R. M.: Bleeding problems in the newborn infant. Progr. Hemost. Thromb., *2*:333, 1974.

45. Hathaway, W. E.: The bleeding newborn. Semin. Hematol., *12*:175, 1975.

46. McGehee, W. G., Rapaport, S. I., and Hjort, P. R.: Intravascular coagulation in fulminant meningococcemia. Ann. Intern. Med., *67*:250, 1967.

47. Reidler, G. F., Straub, P. W., and Frick, P. G.: Thrombocytopenia in septicemia. Helv. Med. Acta, *36*:23, 1971.

48. Waldman, J. D., Czapek, E. E., Paul, M. H., Schwartz, A. D., Levin, D. L., and Schindler, S.: Shortened platelet survival in cyanotic heart disease. J. Pediatr., *87*:77, 1975.

49. Dennis, H. L., Stewart, J. L., and Conrad, M. E.: A consumption coagulation in congenital cyanotic heart disease and its treatment with heparin. J. Pediatr., *71*:407, 1967.

50. Harker, L., and Slichter, S. J.: Platelet and fibrinogen consumption in man. N. Engl. J. Med., *287*:999, 1972.

51. George, C. R. P., Slichter, S. P., Quadracci, L. J., Striker, G. E., and Harker, L. A.: A kinetic evaluation of hemostasis in renal disease. N. Engl. J. Med., *291*:1111, 1974.

52. Katz, J., Krawitz, S., Sacks, P. V., Levin, S. E., Thomson, P., Levin, J., and Metz, J.: Platelet, erythrocyte, and fibrinogen kinetics in the hemolytic-uremic syndrome of infancy. J. Pediatr., *83*:739, 1973.

53. Corrigan, J. J., and Jordan, C. M.: Heparin therapy in septicemia with disseminated intravascular coagulation. N. Engl. J. Med., *283*:778, 1970.

54. Hathaway, W. E.: Heparin therapy in acute meningococcemia. J. Pediatr., *82*:900, 1973.

55. Marcus, A. J.: Heparin therapy for disseminated intravascular coagulation. Am. J. Med. Sci., *264*:365, 1972.

56. Hardaway, R. M., III: Disseminated intravascular coagulation (DIC). J.A.M.A., *227*:657, 1964.

57. Ribes, E. A., Daménech, J. C., Nicolás, J. M. M., and Gaspar, M. L.: Risk of acute renal failure associated with disseminated intravascular coagulation. Br. Med. J., *3*:745, 1975.

58. Gross, S., and Melhorn, D. K.: Exchange transfusion with citrated whole blood for disseminated intravascular coagulation. J. Pediatr., *78*:415, 1971.

59. Arensen, E. B., and August, C. S.: Preliminary report: Treatment of the hemolytic-uremic syndrome with aspirin and dipyridamole. J. Pediatr., *86*:957, 1975.

Chapter Twenty-Three

SICKLE CELL DISEASE CRISES AND THEIR MANAGEMENT

HOWARD A. PEARSON, M.D.,
LOUIS K. DIAMOND, M.D.

The population shifts which have characterized American demography during the past few generations have made it imperative that practicing physicians throughout the country learn to recognize the protean manifestations of the most common hematological abnormality of the black race — sickling of the red cells. Because the clinical consequences and sequelae of the sickling phenomenon frequently present life-threatening emergencies, successful management requires prompt diagnosis, ready application of rational therapy, and alertness in an often rapidly changing clinical situation.

This brief review will be confined to the recognition and treatment of the acute crises seen in infants and children with sickle cell diseases. The term Hgb S disease as we employ it refers to major sickle hemoglobin syndromes in which quantitatively more than 50 per cent of the total hemoglobin is hemoglobin S and spontaneous *in vivo* sickling occurs under physiological conditions. Specifically Hgb SC, S-β thalassemia and Hgb SS diseases are considered "major" Hgb S diseases. Homozygous Hgb SS disease is the most severe of these and will be the major focus of this discussion.

Although the child with Hgb SS disease always has anemia, its severity varies in degree in different patients and even in the same individual from time to time. A well-compensated hemolytic anemia may be aggravated by infections, dietary deficiencies — especially of folic

From the Departments of Pediatrics, Yale University, New Haven, Connecticut, and University of California, San Francisco Medical Center, San Francisco, California.

319

acid—dehydration, and occasionally by certain drugs. In these clinical situations damage to the circulatory red cells or their precursors in the bone marrow may occur.

Hgb SS disease is associated with an accelerated hemolytic process, so that symptoms and signs of anemia (pallor, weakness, fatigability, growth failure, and leg ulcerations) are usually prominent. In addition to these features of any chronic anemia, unique clinical aspects of sickle cell disease result from occlusion of blood vessels and subsequent tissue infarction, caused by the distorted sickled red cells found in large numbers in the circulation of these patients. The clinical and hematological manifestations of Hgb SS disease thus reflect two processes: (1) severe hemolysis and the compensatory mechanisms evoked by hemolytic anemia; and (2) widespread vaso-occlusive phenomena involving many tissues and organs.

There are four types of episodic events which are usually called "crises" and which can threaten the comfort or life of the pediatric patient with Hgb SS disease. These are: (1) vaso-occlusive crises; (2) acute splenic sequestration crises and chronic splenic dysfunction (functional asplenia) with increased susceptibility to certain bacterial infections; (3) aplastic crises; and (4) hyperhemolytic crises.

In order to put the laboratory findings during the episodic crises into perspective, the average values found in patients with Hgb SS disease during intercritical periods are listed in Table 1. These values, rather than those of normal children, must be considered in the evaluation of these patients.

VASO-OCCLUSIVE CRISES

These painful episodes are by far the most common type of crises seen in children with Hgb SS disease. The manifestations may vary markedly, depending upon the tissues or organs involved and the extent of the ischemic damage. The basic cause of such a crisis is obstruction of blood flow by tangled masses of sickled cells and an immeasur-

TABLE 1   Selected Laboratory Values in Hgb SS Disease

| | | Values in Sickle Cell Disease | |
	Normal Values	Average	Range
Hemoglobin (gm/dl)	12	7.5	5.5–9.5
Hematocrit (%)	36	22	17–29
Reticulocytes (%)	1.5	12	5–30
Nucleated RBC/100 WBC	0	3	1–20
White blood cell count (per mm^3)	7500	20,000	12,000–35,000
Bilirubin (mg/dl)	<1.0	2.5	1.5–4.0

able degree of vasospasm. There are usually few or no changes in the hematological parameters during these episodes. The events which trigger vaso-occlusion are largely undefined, but a number of distinctive syndromes can be recognized.

"Hand-Foot Syndrome"

A common initial manifestation of sickle cell disease during infancy is dactylitis resulting from symmetrical involvement of metacarpals and metatarsals and manifested as painful swelling of the dorsa of the hands and feet. Low-grade fever may accompany this — occasionally there may be high fever — but without characteristic hematological changes. X-ray films show no abnormalities initially, but later areas of osteolysis, periostitis, and bone reabsorption may appear. The diffuse symmetrical pattern of involvement of multiple bones and the finding of sterile blood cultures differentiate the "hand-foot syndrome" from osteomyelitis, which is so often suggested by the roentgenographic appearance. There is no specific therapy. Repeated attacks may occur over many months but after the second or third year of life the syndrome does not usually recur. There are no permanent orthopedic sequelae.

Involvement of the Joints and Extremities

Symptomatic, painful crises involving the joints and extremities usually begin during the second or third year of life. Pains in the extremities may be due to areas of infarction of the long bones or the bone marrow or involvement of the periosteum or of periarticular tissues of the larger joints. There is swelling and limitation of motion but no redness. Joint pain may mimic acute rheumatic fever or rheumatoid arthritis. X-ray studies may show areas of bone infarction and periostitis but also may be negative, especially at the onset, and even for the following week or so. There are, in general, no hematological changes during these crises and significant fever usually is not observed.

Abdominal Involvement

These episodes are due to areas of infarction in abdominal structures such as the liver, spleen, and abdominal lymph nodes, with stretching of their capsules. Occasionally the pain may be incapacitatingly severe and episodic in character. Signs of peritoneal irritation are sometimes present but peristalsis usually persists. This finding may differentiate the abdominal crisis from an inflammatory process, such as appendicitis or peritonitis, which requires surgical intervention. Painful abdominal crises often are associated with low-grade fever but when very severe may be accompanied by hyperpyrexia and prostration.

The duration of the painful crises averages from 3 to 4 days. There may be early termination, but protracted episodes also can occur. This variability makes evaluation of any specific drug therapy or new method of treatment very difficult.

Hepatic Involvement

Some degree of hyperbilirubinemia is usual in Hgb SS disease; however, an episode of severe obstructive jaundice also may occur, and may even end in death. The basis of this is extensive intrahepatic sickling with subsequent hepatocellular necrosis and swelling. The level of serum bilirubin may increase to 25 mg/dl or more, mostly of the conjugated variety. These findings may suggest biliary obstruction by a stone in the common duct, a diagnostic dilemma compounded by the finding of pigmentary cholelithiasis in many of these patients. As treatment for severe obstructive jaundice we recommend multiple transfusions of packed red cells. Emergency gallbladder surgery is *not* performed unless the obstruction is chronic. The necessity for surgery in the patient with asymptomatic gallstones is controversial. We have not advocated cholecystectomy routinely.

Central Nervous System Crises

Children with sickle cell disease may develop monoplegia or hemiplegia with other neurological findings suggestive of upper motor neuron damage. The sequelae of these "strokes" are variable. Some patients recover rapidly and completely, even after apparent widespread involvement, indicating that there is a significant element of vasospasm and edema. Others are left with permanent neurological deficits, showing that actual infarction may occur. Angiographic studies are not indicated in the early stages of these attacks. We have noted *in vitro* that the high tonicity of contrast media produces immediate sickling of the red cells suspended in them. This could aggravate the vaso-occlusive component. The treatment of central nervous system episodes includes prompt and vigorous hydration, administration of oxygen, and multiple transfusions of packed red cells. Recent reports state that repeated transfusions for 1 year result in marked improvement of vascular abnormalities in patients with Hgb SS disease who have suffered strokes. Such a program clearly seems warranted.[1]

Pulmonary Crises

Children with Hgb SS disease often have severe and protracted episodes of pulmonary disease. Although the precipitating event may be bacterial infection due to the pneumococcus or even mycoplasma organisms, infarction may be a significant component. It may be very difficult to separate infection from infarction; in fact, both processes may be operative. After appropriate cultures are taken, antibiotic therapy, including penicillin, is given. Multiple transfusions of packed red cells also are indicated if the pulmonary involvement is extensive or protracted and is causing significant pulmonary insufficiency. In our experience this shortens the clinical course.

TREATMENT

There is no specific drug therapy for vaso-occlusive crises. Many medications of possible value have been proposed at various times. These include anticoagulants, low molecular weight dextran, alkalis, phenothiazines, and many others as well. Most recently, urea and cyanate have been extolled. Suitably controlled studies have not proved the efficacy of most of these.

Management of the vaso-occlusive crises must include therapy directed at reversal of the following conditions that are known to enhance sickling:

Dehydration.   Hypertonicity enhances the sickling process *in vitro.* The expanded plasma volume may show a sharp constriction during painful crises or infection. In addition, these patients are hyposthenuric and may become dehydrated very easily; therefore, optimal hydration should be ensured. Oral fluids can be encouraged in the milder episodes, but if the pain is severe, and particularly when fever, vomiting, or other processes which contribute to dehydration are present, parenteral hydration is indicated. The use of a half and half mixture of normal saline in 5 per cent dextrose, infused at a rate of 2000 to 2500 ml/m^2/day, is advised.

Acidosis.   This also aggravates sickling, and pain can be produced by the infusion of acidifying compounds such as ammonium sulfate. Accordingly, alkali therapy is administered to rectify potential or actual acidosis. Although data to prove the effectiveness of such therapy are contradictory, in mild vaso-occlusive crises oral sodium bicarbonate is given in a dose of 3 to 4 gm/m²/day in four divided doses, or polycitrate (Shohl's solution) in a dose of 3 tablespoons four times a day. If intravenous therapy is used, sodium bicarbonate is added to the hydrating solution and the urine pH is maintained at 6.5 to 7.0.

Hypoxia.   Since reduced oxygenation increases sickling, an atmosphere of well-humidified oxygen may be used so long as the child is experiencing severe pain; the modest increase in oxygenation attained with an oxygen tent is, however, of uncertain value.

Infection.   Many clinicians believe that infection may be a precipitating cause of vaso-occlusive crises. The patient should be examined carefully. If evidence of bacterial infection is found, antibiotic therapy is indicated after appropriate cultures are taken.

Besides attention to these four contributing factors, the possible use of transfusion must be considered. Since the ordinary vaso-occlusive crisis is not associated with hematological changes, blood is not routinely administered for anemia. The beneficial effects of a single blood transfusion of 10 to 15 ml/kg may be counterbalanced by the increased blood viscosity caused by an increase in hematocrit. But in severe or prolonged vaso-occlusive crises, more vigorous, multiple transfusion therapy to "dilute" the patient's sickle cells may be considered.

If the number of sickle cells in the circulation can be reduced effectively, many of the clinical manifestations of the disease will cease. The most effective way to accomplish this reduction is by transfusion of normal red blood cells from proved non–sickle cell donors. When at least 60 per cent of the patient's circulating red blood cells are replaced by normal red cells, vaso-occlusive symptomatology usually will stop. Transfusions of fresh packed red blood cells, 10 to 15 ml/kg, are infused every 12 hours until the hemoglobin is increased to 12 to 13 gm/dl. At this point, simple dilution will have decreased the circulating complement of the patient's red blood cells and his erythropoiesis will be suppressed. Because of their 15 to 20 day survival, the patient's own red blood cells, which contain hemoglobin S, disappear rapidly. With small packed cell transfusions given as indicated, the proportion of circulating cells containing hemoglobin S will fall to very low levels, thus effectively producing an exchange transfusion in a few days. Packed cell transfusions every 2 to 3 weeks will ensure that the circulating blood will contain predominantly normal red blood cells. A quantitative sickle cell preparation using sodium metabisulfite is a rapid and accurate method for assessing the completeness of replacement transfusion. Red cells of the patient and donor can be differentiated quantitatively on the basis of sickling morphology. Although this "hypertransfusion regimen" is symptomatically effective, there are inherent risks of isoimmunization, hepatitis, and hemosiderosis. This type of program usually is used, therefore, only for specific indications, such as prolonged or very severe vaso-occlusive crises, especially those involving the central nervous system, preparation for anesthesia and surgery, management of pregnancy in sickle cell anemia, and as supportive therapy during complicating medical conditions. In critical situations exchange transfusions with fresh packed red cells may be the most effective way to rapidly reduce the proportion of cells containing Hgb S.

Sedation and Analgesia

Considerable relief of pain and discomfort may be obtained with the judicious use of sedatives and analgesics. Aspirin in large doses should be avoided so as not to aggravate a tendency to metabolic acidosis. Acetaminophen (Tylenol) in a dose of 120 to 240 mg every 4 to 6 hours may provide some relief in mild painful crises and may act as an antipyretic. When pain is more severe, codeine sulfate (30 to 60 mg) may be necessary. Use of meperidine hydrochloride or morphine sulfate may lead to addiction, so these are not employed unless pain is extreme.

Compounds such as prochlorperazine and chlorpromazine are useful adjuncts for treatment of painful crises. Because of their sedative and tranquilizing action, 0.5 mg/kg of chlorpromazine every 6 to 8 hours or prochlorperazine in a dose of 2 to 5 mg every 8 hours may reduce the need for narcotics.

Urea and Cyanate Therapy

The history of the sickle cell diseases is studded with enthusiastic preliminary reports of effective therapies, but when these are subjected to tests in larger controlled studies, usually no significant benefit can be shown. The problems of evaluation are compounded by the diversity and extreme variability of the sickle cell "crises." Ultimately, any beneficial therapy of sickle cell disease must be reflected in a decrease in *in vivo* sickling. Unless such unequivocal proof can be demonstrated, a degree of healthy skepticism must be maintained, especially if the proposed treatment involves real or potential hazards. Two forms of therapy proposed recently, namely the use of urea and cyanate, merit special attention.

Considerable publicity — much of it in the press — has extolled the possible benefit of intravenous urea in invert sugar for the painful crises of sickle cell diseases. The supposed reason for this therapy was that high concentrations of urea disrupt the molecular bonds which participate in the sickling process. The use of urea increases the patient's BUN to from 150 to 200 mg/dl and produces a profound diuresis which must be treated vigorously if dehydration is to be avoided. Despite preliminary and uncontrolled clinical reports indicating the efficacy of urea therapy,[2] the "therapeutic" level of urea attained in patients was shown to have no effect on *in vitro* sickling.[3] Controlled studies on both intravenous and oral urea have not demonstrated any significant benefit.[4, 5] The use of urea is not indicated in the management of sickle cell disease.

More recently, the possible value of cyanate — an invariable contaminant of commercial urea preparations — has been investigated vigorously in patients with Hgb SS disease. This compound interacts with the sickle hemoglobin molecule by a process called carbamylation. Probably by changing the affinity between hemoglobin and oxygen, cyanate directly inhibits the sickling process. Oral cyanate treatment decreases the rate of destruction of sickle red cells and leads to an increase in hemoglobin levels.[6] However, a recently reported controlled study demonstrated that cyanate treatment did not significantly reduce the number or severity of vaso-occlusive episodes. In addition, considerable drug toxicity was observed including peripheral neuropathy, interference with nutrition, and in two patients the development of cataracts.[7] The use of cyanate is not indicated in sickle cell disease.

SPLENIC SEQUESTRATION CRISES, ACUTE AND CHRONIC

Acute Crises

Infants and young children with Hgb SS disease whose spleens have not yet undergone multiple infarctions and subsequent fibrosis and children with other major Hgb S syndromes whose spleens remain enlarged into adult life may suddenly pool vast amounts of blood in the spleen. During these sequestration crises the spleen becomes enormous, even reaching to the pelvis. The hemoglobin level may drop so precipitously that hypovolemic shock and death may occur. This is the most immediately dangerous crisis in the life of the young child with this disease; it must be recognized and treated promptly. Infants between 8 months and 5 years of age are particularly susceptible and may succumb within hours of the first signs of this disturbance. The sudden development of weakness, pallor of the lips and mucous membranes, breathlessness, rapid pulse, and faintness should never be ignored.[8]

An illustrative case history follows:

A 5-year-old black girl known to have Hgb SS disease was admitted to the hospital with a markedly enlarged spleen. She had been taken to her private physician on the preceding day with a slight fever. He noted an enlarged spleen, pale conjunctivae, a rapid pulse, and a hemoglobin of 4.0 gm/dl. On the following day, her hemoglobin level had dropped to 3.4 gm/dl. On admission, she was alert but breathing rapidly. The abdomen was distended; a hard mass was felt on the left side extending across the midline and down to the iliac crest. The liver was about 2 cm below the right costal margin. X-rays revealed a large heart and the abdominal mass which was said to be the spleen. At this time, her hemoglobin level was 2.1 gm/dl, reticulocytes 50 per cent, platelet count 53,000/mm^3. Her vital signs included a blood pressure of 110/70, a respiratory rate of 36, and a pulse of 140 at rest. The patient was transfused over a 5 to 6-hour period with 100 ml of sedimented red blood cells. Another transfusion of the same amount was given on the second hospital day; both transfusions were well tolerated. Her hemoglobin level was then found to be 8 gm/dl; that calculated from the estimated blood volume and the mass of transfused cells would have predicted a rise to only 5 to 6 gm/dl. Following transfusion, there was a marked reduction in splenic size; over the next 3 days her hemoglobin level increased further to 9.6 gm/dl. A bone marrow examination showed marked erythroid hyperplasia.

The patient was discharged from the hospital on the fifth day. One week later, she appeared in excellent health with a hemoglobin of *11 gm/dl*, and a palpable spleen estimated to be less than one-third the size noted on admission. On the next visit, one week later, the spleen size was unchanged, her hemoglobin was 10 gm/dl, and she appeared well. The following week, she again appeared to be well, but examination revealed pale conjunctivae, with her spleen again enlarged down to the left iliac crest, and a hemoglobin of 3.8 gm/dl. There was also a fall in platelet count from 209,000/mm^3 to 82,000/mm^3. The reticulocyte level was 16 per cent.

The patient was readmitted and transfused with 100 ml sedimented cells on two successive days. On the third hospital day, hemoglobin was 10.2 gm/dl and the spleen had decreased to 3 to 4 cm below the left costal margin. The patient was then discharged and was followed weekly for 3 months, at which time she was readmitted for transfusions and elective removal of what had been called a "yo-yo" spleen.

It is somewhat paradoxical that the spleen, which is markedly inactive in reticuloendothelial functions ("functional asplenia"), can still act as an enormous reservoir and trap for blood cells.

Treatment of the sequestration crisis is directed toward the prompt correction of hypovolemia with plasma expanders and, particularly, with whole blood transfusion. If the shock can be reversed, much of the blood sequestered in the spleen appears to be remobilized and dramatic regression of splenomegaly may occur in a short time. Because of the rapidity with which a sequestration crisis can occur and even recur and because of its potential fatality in a matter of hours, we recommend splenectomy if a child has had one or two of these crises of a severe degree.

Chronic Splenic Dysfunction (Functional Asplenia)

Increased susceptibility to pneumococcal infection of the pharynx, lungs, meninges, and even of the blood stream has long been a puzzling occurrence in infants and children with sickle cell disease. It has been estimated that the young child with sickle cell anemia is 600 times more likely to develop pneumococcal meningitis than normal children,[9] while as many as 25 per cent of Hgb SS children may die in the first 5 years of life—most from severe infection.[6, 11] To perhaps a lesser extent, they show diminished resistance to infections with *Salmonella*, often localized as osteomyelitis, and also to *H. influenzae* bacilli and meningococci. Taken in conjunction with observations of nucleated red cells, Howell-Jolly bodies, and bizarre-shaped erythrocytes in peripheral blood smears, the specific immunological deficiency involving the pneumococcus strongly resembles the changes seen in young children lacking spleens, either congenitally or postsurgery, despite the presence of considerable splenomegaly! This apparent paradox has been clarified at least in part by demonstrating with radioactive tagging techniques that "functional asplenia" exists in these patients, possibly as the result of temporary vaso-occlusive episodes or of puddling in the splenic circulation.[12, 13] Such an occurrence could cause shunting of the blood so as to bypass the splenic sinusoids, in which defective and particle-containing red cells ordinarily are sequestered or are culled and, more important, in which bacteria are removed and processed preparatory to antibody action. In essence, therefore, such patients have the handicaps and face the hazards of the asplenic infant or young child.

An illustrative case report is described here.*

A black female was born to a 25-year-old healthy mother. Labor, delivery, and newborn course were uncomplicated. There was no family history of sickle cell anemia. Physical examination was normal except for pallor of the conjunctivae and mucous membranes; the spleen was not palpable. Hemoglobin level was 8.6 gm/dl, hematocrit 25 per cent, and reticulocytes 5.9 per cent. Sickle cell preparation was positive. Anisocytosis, poikilocytosis, moderate polychromasia, and a few target cells were noted on blood smear but no sickled forms or Howell-Jolly bodies were present. Hemoglobin electrophoresis revealed a 52 per cent Hgb F. By 15 weeks of age, moderate splenomegaly and hepatomegaly were present. Hgb was 6.6 gm/dl and hematocrit was 20 per cent. Sickled red cells, but no Howell-Jolly bodies, were seen on peripheral blood smear. Hgb S was 60 per cent, Hgb F was 40 per cent, and A_2 was 1.2 per cent. ^{99m}Tc sulfur colloid scan at age 6 months revealed outlines of both liver and spleen.

At age 8 months the patient was seen because of fever and symptoms of an upper respiratory infection, and bilateral otitis media was detected. A nasopharyngeal culture grew a heavy growth of pneumococcus. The spleen was palpable 3 cm below the left costal margin. Hemoglobin was 6.5 gm/dl and hematocrit 22 per cent. Howell-Jolly bodies were noted on the blood smear. Hgb F level was 20 per cent, Hgb S 80 per cent. Spleen scan was repeated. No splenic uptake of the radio-colloid could be identified despite clinical splenomegaly. She was treated with oral penicillin and rapidly improved.

At 16 months of age she developed fever, cough, and nasal discharge and

---

*Case provided by Dr. J. C. Parke, Charlotte, North Carolina.

was treated with intramuscular procaine penicillin for an upper respiratory infection. Five days later she was brought to the hospital because of persistent fever, cough, and irritability. Upon admission she was febrile, comatose, and moderately dehydrated. The cerebrospinal fluid was grossly cloudy and contained 1000 neutrophils/mm³. Gram-positive diplococci were seen on smear and a culture of the CSF grew diplococcus pneumonia. Hgb was 5.7 gm/dl and platelets were plentiful. Howell-Jolly bodies and sickled forms were present on the peripheral blood smear.

The child deteriorated despite intravenous penicillin and fresh whole blood transfusions. Left-sided focal seizures began and continued until cardiorespiratory arrest occurred 17 hours after admission.

Diffuse purulent meningitis due to pneumococcus was found at postmortem examination. Vascular congestion and pulmonary edema were noted in the dependent portions of both lungs, but no growth of bacteria was obtained on culture of the lung. The spleen weighed 30 gm (normal, 26 gm). Blood vessels were patent, the follicular architecture was retained, and there was slight accentuation of the fibrous trabeculae. On microscopical examination the splenic sinusoids were congested with sickled red blood cells but no fibrosis was identified.

It has also been shown that transfusion with normal blood to a level of 50 per cent or more of hemoglobin A restores the splenic circulation to its normal pathways and corrects the functional asplenia, at least for a few weeks or months.[14] At any rate, because of this susceptibility to overwhelming bacterial infection, ampicillin therapy is indicated in the treatment of sickle cell disease in an infant who develops unexplained significant fever. Persistent functional asplenia usually is not seen in major Hgb S syndromes other than Hgb S disease, although it may occur transiently in Hgb SC or S-β thalassemia.

APLASTIC CRISES

In patients with Hgb SS disease the red cell survival is only between 15 and 20 days compared with 120 days in normal individuals. Despite this extreme hemolysis, the patient with Hgb SS disease usually maintains a hemoglobin of 5.5 to 9.5 gm per dl by increasing red cell production five- to eightfold. If this maximal compensatory response is compromised, profound anemia can be explained without invoking "hyperhemolysis" as the cause. Diminished red cell production superimposed on the usual rapid destruction is the basis of the "aplastic crisis." A number of infections, usually viral in type, may in some way damage the erythroid bone marrow and result almost in a cessation of red cell production which may persist for 10 to 14 days.[15] Aplastic crises may occur in several members of a family—further evidence of their infectious origin. Although nutritional deficiencies of folic acid have been invoked in the genesis of some of these crises, other studies did not confirm a relationship.[16] During these "aplastic" episodes, reticulocytes disappear from the blood and a markedly reduced number of erythroid precursors are present in the bone marrow.

The hematological findings during aplastic crises differ, depending on the stage at which the patient is studied. Early, the degree of anemia is progressively more extreme and the numbers of reticulocytes in the blood and nucleated red cells in the bone marrow are sharply decreased. However, platelet and white blood cell counts usually are not affected, and jaundice may even decrease. At the nadir of the aplastic crisis, the hemoglobin level may fall as low as 1 gm/dl and death may result from severe anemia and congestive heart failure.

Erythroid aplasia usually terminates spontaneously after 7 to 10 days and recovery is accompanied by a surge of reticulocytes and nucleated red cells in the blood. Reticulocyte count may then climb as high as 50 to 60 per cent. Shortly thereafter the hemoglobin returns to precrisis levels. If the patient is first studied early in the recovery stage from an aplastic crisis, a mistaken diagnosis of "hemolytic" crisis may be entertained because of the still present severe anemia and the marked reticulocytosis.

The treatment for an aplastic crisis is transfusion of relatively fresh packed red cells, given slowly in a dose of not more than 2 to 3 ml/kg of body weight every 8 hours until the hemoglobin level is increased by about 5 gm/dl. For the small child, a whole unit of packed cells (250 to 300 ml) can be divided and used sequentially, thereby reducing the risk of transfusion hepatitis associated with multiple donors. When profound anemia is present, fresh blood, preferably collected with CPD anticoagulant, should be used to assure normal levels of 2,3-diphosphoglyceride so that oxygen transport of the transfused red cells is normal.[17] Oxygen may be administered if the patient is dyspneic, but digitalis is not recommended nor usually needed. If signs of congestive heart failure are present, venous pressure may be monitored by a central venous catheter during transfusion, and blood can be withdrawn from the patient as the donor blood is given, resulting in a partial exchange transfusion.

Parents of children with major Hgb S diseases should be made aware of the manifestations of the aplastic crisis. They should seek medical attention promptly if the child becomes pale or weak, especially following an infection.

HYPERHEMOLYTIC CRISES

The frequency of so-called hyperhemolytic crises is somewhat controversial, owing to the difficulty in proving a more rapid rate of hemolysis superimposed upon an already severe process.[18] Nevertheless, in association with certain drugs or acute infections, hyperhemolysis may ensue.[5] During these episodes the patient begins to feel weak, look more pale, and show more scleral icterus. There may be abdominal pain and an increase in splenomegaly. The hematocrit may fall from its usual 21 to 25 per cent to 15 per cent or less in a few days. The reticulocytes may rise to 35 per cent or more. The urine may darken with excess urobilinogen. After several days to a few weeks, the excessive hemolysis tends to subside gradually, especially if treatment is prompt.

Treatment consists of a search for sites of infection, culture of the nose and throat, sputum, blood, urine, and stools; if pathogenic organisms are found or their presence suggested (e.g., pneumonic consolidation by x-ray), antibiotics should be given. Drugs that may produce hemolysis should be discontinued. At the same time, dehydration and acidosis must be corrected promptly and completely. Adequate and careful blood transfusion of packed or sedimented red cells should be given to reverse or prevent incipient heart failure from anemic hypoxia. Persistence of a hyperhemolytic state suggests residual infection, which must be identified and treated vigorously.

SICKLE CELL TRAIT

The heterozygous state for Hgb S is not classified as a "disease." Only 35 to 45 per cent of the hemoglobin in the sickle trait person is of the Hgb S variety and there is no evidence of intravascular sickling or hematological abnormalities. Under situations of severe and nonphysiological hypoxia *in vivo* sickling may occur, usually manifested as splenic infarction. Although a wide variety of conditions have been reported to occur in individuals with sickle trait, a cause and effect relationship has been defined for only a few. The individual with sickle trait may develop renal abnormalities, especially painless renal hematuria, almost always from the left kidney. Postoperative deaths and deaths associated with severe exertion have been reported in individuals with sickle cell trait, but the exact cause of death and whether there is a significant increase of risk in such individuals have never been established.

At the present time there is no consensus that the individual with sickle trait needs to take special precautions other than avoiding extremes of altitude or situations that might result in hypoxia. Clearly, hypoxia and shock should be avoided during anesthesia and surgery. No restrictions in physical activity are necessary. It is reassuring to note that the proportion of professional football players (including the Denver Broncos, whose home playing field is at 6000 ft elevation) with sickle trait is the same as the proportion of those with the traits in the national population. [9]

SUMMARY

This brief review, being limited in scope to the recognition and management of the life-threatening and painful crises in infants and children with sickle cell diseases, has not even touched on the intriguing mystery of the molecular basis for the sickling phenomenon—how one amino acid substitution (gene-controlled) in the beta chain sequence of 146 amino acids can cause such serious disruption in form and function, or how this mutation occurred in the first place and why it has persisted in contrast to the rapid disappearance of many other deleterious mutants. The accumulated knowledge about this mutant gene, its biochemical effects, and its geographic distribution is enormous. From a fundamental scientific standpoint, sickle cell disease is one of the best understood of human afflictions.

However, from a practical point of view, treatment of the patient is often only symptomatic and palliative. Nevertheless, prompt and effective therapy of the myriad manifestations of sickle cell disease can effectively reduce morbidity and mortality. The pediatrician with black children in his or her practice should be familiar with the cardinal diagnostic and clinical aspects of the major sickle cell diseases and their crises.

REFERENCES

1. Russell, M. O., Goldberg, H. I., Reis, L., Friedman, S. H., Slater, R., Reivich, M., and Schwartz, E.: Transfusion therapy for cerebrovascular abnormalities in sickle cell disease. J. Pediatr., 88:382, 1976.
2. Nalbandian, R. M.: Urea for sickle-cell crises (Letter). N. Engl. J. Med., 284:1381, 1971.
3. Segal, G. B., Feig, S. A., Mentzer, W. C., McCaffrey, R. P., Wells, R., Bunn, H. F., Shohet, S. R., and Nathan, D. C.: Effects of urea and cyanate on sickling in vitro. N. Engl. J. Med., 287:59, 1972.
4. Kraus, A. P.: Clinical trials of therapy for sickle cell vaso-occlusive crises. Blood, 42:979, 1973.
5. Lubin, N. H., and Oski, F. A.: Oral urea therapy in children with sickle cell anemia. J. Pediatr., 82:311, 1973.
6. Gillette, P. M., Peterson, C. M., Lu, Y. S., and Cerami, A.: Sodium cyanate as a potential treatment for sickle-cell disease. N. Engl. J. Med., 290:654, 1974.
7. Harkness, D. R.: Preliminary results of a double-blind clinical trial of oral sodium cyanate (NaNCO) in patients with sickle cell anemia. Blood, 46:1001, 1975.
8. Jenkins, M. E., Scott, R. B., and Baird, R. L.: Studies in sickle cell anemia. XVI. Sudden death during sickle cell crises in young children. J. Pediatr., 56:30, 1960.
9. Barrett-Connor, E.: Bacterial infection and sickle cell anemia. Medicine, 50:97, 1971.
10. Diggs, L. W.: Anatomic lesions in sickle cell diseases. In Abramson, H., Bertles, J. F., and Wethers, D. L., eds.: Sickle Cell Disease—Diagnosis, Management, Education, and Research. St. Louis, C. V. Mosby, 1973.
11. Powars, D. R.: Natural history of sickle cell disease—the first ten years. Semin. Hematol., 12:267, 1975.
12. Pearson, H. A., Spencer, R. P., and Cornelius, E. A.: Functional asplenia in sickle cell anemia. N. Engl. J. Med., 281:293, 1969.

13. Diamond, L. K., Price, D. C., and Young, E.: Functional asplenia, a newly recognized splenic disorder. Clin. Res., *18*:209, 1970.
14. Pearson, H. A., Cornelius, E. A., Schwartz, A. D., Zelson, J. H., Wolfson, S. L., and Spencer, R. P.: Transfusion-reversible functional asplenia in young children with sickle-cell anemia. N. Engl. J. Med., *283*:334, 1970.
15. MacIver, J. E., and Parker-Williams, E. J.: The aplastic crisis in sickle cell anaemia. Lancet, *1*:1086, 1961.
16. Pearson, H. A., and Cobb, W. T.: Folic acid studies in sickle cell anemia. J. Lab. Clin. Med., *64*:913, 1964.
17. Oski, F. A., and Delevoria-Papadopoulos, M.: The red cell, 2,3-diphosphoglycerate and tissue oxygen release. J. Pediatr., *77*:941, 1970.
18. Diggs, L. W.: Sickle cell crisis. Am. J. Clin. Pathol., *44*:1, 1965.
19. Murphy, J. R.: Sickle cell hemoglobin (Hg AS) in black football players. J.A.M.A., *225*:921, 1973.

Chapter Twenty-Four

ANAPHYLAXIS

C. WARREN BIERMAN, M.D.

Anaphylaxis* is an acute reaction, which may range from mild self-limited symptoms to a grave medical emergency. It is caused by a variety of agents, usually occurs unexpectedly, frequently is iatrogenic, and can be fatal if not treated promptly and appropriately. The mechanism of anaphylaxis involves sequentially: (1) the interaction of antigen and antibody or of a substance acting directly on the mast cell or other target tissue, (2) the release of such pharmacologically active mediators as histamine, slow reactive substance of anaphylaxis, or activated kinins, and (3) the response of the individual to these substances. Every physician's and dentist's office, pediatric outpatient clinic, hospital emergency room, allergy clinic, and radiology department should be equipped to treat this potential disaster.[1]

This chapter was reviewed by the Committee on Drugs of the American Academy of Pediatrics. It was originally published as a commentary by the Committee[2] as a guide to physicians in the management of this medical emergency.

CLINICAL PICTURE

Anaphylaxis usually is characterized by the following sequence of signs and symptoms: generalized flush, urticaria, paroxysmal coughing,

---

From the Department of Pediatrics, University of Washington School of Medicine, Seattle, Washington.

*In this chapter, anaphylactic reactions (which result from specific allergy, i.e., prior sensitization) and anaphylactoid reactions (which do not require prior sensitization and can occur on the first administration of a substance) are combined, since the clinical picture and management are identical.

severe anxiety, dyspnea, wheezing, orthopnea, vomiting, cyanosis, and shock.[3] The sooner symptoms develop after the initiating stimulus, the more intense the reaction. Symptoms beginning within 15 minutes after administration of the inciting agent require the most expeditious management.[4]

The primary cause of death in the child is laryngeal edema. In the adult, cardiac arrhythmias may be superimposed on acute upper airway edema.[5]

MAJOR CAUSES OF ANAPHYLAXIS

Table 1 lists the most common agents associated with anaphylaxis in children. The severity and acuteness of onset depend upon both the type of agent and the route of administration. Generally, agents administered parenterally are more apt to result in severe life-threatening or fatal anaphylactic reactions than those ingested orally or administered topically to mucous membranes. Medications administered orally, such as aspirin or penicillin, however, have been associated with fatal reactions; therefore, the oral route cannot be utilized with impunity.

Before administration of substances such as are listed in Table 1, the physician should inquire carefully for a history of reactions. If the patient thinks he or she is allergic to a drug, it would be preferable to select an alternate drug. If there is a possibility of sensitivity to foreign proteins, such as horse serum or egg-based vaccines, or to penicillin, skin testing for immediate hypersensitivity to the agent should be performed prior to its therapeutic administration. Since even skin testing may induce anaphylaxis, such testing should be done carefully with emergency equipment on hand. Vaccines containing foreign proteins should be diluted 1:100 with saline for skin testing and penicillin should be diluted to 1000 units per ml.[6] The intracutaneous injection of 0.01 ml of the material into the forearm should be preceded by a preliminary scratch test. A wheal 5 mm greater than the saline control should be considered evidence of allergy and an indication for an alternate preparation. Skin testing is of little value in predicting anaphylactic sensitivity to human gamma globulin, local anesthetics, aspirin, or to most diagnostic agents listed in Table 1.[7]

MANAGEMENT OF ANAPHYLAXIS

Recognizing the early signs of anaphylaxis will save valuable minutes.[8] By initiating treatment early, the life-threatening stages of anaphylactic shock may be avoided or minimized. The physician should always have basic emergency equipment available to treat this condi-

TABLE 1   Major Causes of Anaphylaxis[3]

1. *Antibiotics*
   Penicillin and its semisynthetic derivatives
   Cephalosporins: cephaloxin (Keflex), cephaloglycin (Kafocin), cephaloridine
      (Loridine), cephalothin (Keflin)
   Chloramphenicol
   Colymycin
   Kanamycin
   Polymyxin B
   Streptomycin
   Tetracyclines
   Troleandomycin (Cyclamycin, TAO)
   Vancomycin (Vancocin)
   Amphotericin B (Fungizone)

2. *Biologicals*
   Foreign serums (antitoxins, antilymphocyte globulins — ALG)
   Chymotrypsin
   Gamma globulin
   Asparaginase
   Polypeptide hormones (ACTH, TSH, insulin)
   Influenza vaccine
   Tetanus toxoid
   Measles and other egg-based vaccines

3. *Injectable Medications*
   Iron-dextran (Inferon)
   Dextran
   Methylergonovine maleate (Methergine)
   Nitrofurantoin

4. *Local Anesthetics*

5. *Aspirin* (acetylsalicylic acid)

6. *Diagnostic Agents*
   Iodinated contrast media
   Sulfobromophthalein (BSP)

7. *Hymenoptera Stings* (bee, yellow-jacket, wasp, and hornet)

8. *Allergic Extracts* (skin-testing and treatment solutions)

9. *Foods* (especially eggs, nuts, cottonseed, and shellfish)

10. *Intravenous Narcotics* (heroin)

---

tion. The quantity of equipment and medication to be kept on hand for immediate therapy of anaphylaxis will depend upon the location of the practice and the secondary support available to the physician. For example, the physician who is located miles from the nearest hospital, or the allergist who is more likely to encounter anaphylaxis, needs more equipment than the physician attending patients within a medical center who can summon an emergency team within minutes.

Principles of Therapy

In anaphylaxis there is a massive release into the cardiovascular system of allergic mediator substances, including histamine, slow reactive substance of anaphylaxis (SRS-A) and kinins as well as activated complement fractions such as anaphylatoxin.[9] These substances cause generalized vasodilation and urticaria, increase vascular permeability, induce bronchospasm, and produce glottid and subglottid edema. This results in upper and lower airway obstruction, a fall in blood pressure, and usually in vomiting, which may present an additional hazard of aspiration pneumonia.

Therapy designed to counter these factors thus may be divided into three stages:

Stage 1 — Immediate Therapy: To be initiated with any patient presenting the early signs of anaphylaxis.

Stage 2 — Supportive Therapy: For patients who have not responded to the immediate therapy.

Stage 3 — Therapy of Complication: For those few patients who have developed the most severe complications of anaphylaxis — occlusion of the upper airway, cardiac arrhythmias, or severe derangement of acid-base balance.

The physician should monitor the patient for the following manifestations:

1. *Upper Airway Obstruction.* One of the most dramatic aspects of acute anaphylaxis in the pediatric age group frequently is overlooked, though pharyngeal and uvular edema develop acutely in children and are readily visible. The pharynx should be observed frequently. At the first sign of upper airway obstruction an oral or endotracheal airway should be inserted.

2. *Lower Airway Obstruction.* Dyspnea, frequently without wheezing, accompanies anaphylaxis in children. Bronchospasm may be so severe that wheezing is not heard because of a markedly diminished tidal volume.

3. *Hypotension.* Frequent blood pressure determinations should be taken. Every effort should be made to keep pressure stable using plasma volume expanders and vasopressor medications if necessary.

4. *Aspiration of Gastric Contents.* Vomiting usually accompanies anaphylaxis in children. Aspiration of gastric contents should be anticipated.

Stage 1 — Immediate Therapy. *All* patients with early signs of anaphylaxis should receive the following therapy at once. Its prompt initiation may prevent subsequent complications which would require further therapy. Table 2 lists primary equipment and medications which should be present in an emergency kit.

1. *Tourniquet.* If subcutaneous or intramuscular injection has been

TABLE 2   Primary Equipment and Medications for Anaphylaxis

To be kept by all physicians in an emergency kit:
  A. Tourniquet
  B. 1-ml and 5-ml disposable syringes
  C. Oxygen tank and mask
  D. Epinephrine solution (aqueous) 1:1000
  E. Diphenhydramine (Benadryl), injectable 50 mg/ml

given into an extremity, a tourniquet should be applied immediately proximal to the site to obstruct venous return from the injection.

2. *Epinephrine.* 0.1 to 0.3 ml of 1:1000 aqueous epinephrine should be injected subcutaneously. An equal amount may be injected around the site of injection or sting to decrease absorption of antigen. If the patient is in shock, the physician may administer 1 or 2 ml 1:10,000 aqueous epinephrine, intravenously.

3. *Oxygen.* Since hypoxemia associated with hypotension or upper airway edema contributes to myocardial irritability and ventricular fibrillation as major causes of death, oxygen should be administered by mask early in the course of anaphylaxis.

4. *Antihistamines.* Diphenhydramine (Benadryl) may be administered intravenously (2 mg/kg) or orally (5 mg/kg/24 hours) for the therapy of urticaria. Such therapy should be considered of *secondary importance* and should not delay more therapeutic steps.

Stage 2—Supportive Therapy. If the patient fails to respond to initial therapy or is in shock when first seen, the following therapy should be given immediately after steps 1, 2, and 3 of initial therapy. Table 3 lists the necessary supporting equipment and medication,

TABLE 3   Supporting Equipment and Medication for Anaphylaxis

These should be available within minutes;
though not necessarily in the primary emergency unit:
  A. Intravenous infusion sets
  B. Intravenous needles
  C. Laryngoscope with interchangeable pediatric and adult blades
  D. Oral airway—infant to adult
  E. Apparatus to establish airway patency:[12]
      1. #12 needles for temporary airway
      2. Endotracheal tubes (#'s 18, 22, 26, and 30 French)
      3. Cricothyrotomy tube or tracheotomy setup
  F. Suction apparatus
  G. Bag resuscitator for assisted ventilation[13, 14] (Resusci-Folding bag, P.M.R., or Ambu bag)
  H. Sterile surgical cutdown set
  I. Aminophylline solution (injectable), 25 mg/ml
  J. Hydrocortisone/hemisuccinate (Solu-Cortef) or equivalent
  K. 5% glucose in isotonic saline (two 500-ml bottles)
  L. Metaraminol bitartrate (Aramine), 1% for injection

which need not be in the emergency kit but should be readily available to the physician.

1. *Intravenous fluids.* If the patient does not respond promptly to the initial therapy, intravenous fluids should be initiated immediately to support blood pressure to treat hypovolemia. In anaphylaxis, shock, resulting primarily from vasodilation and loss of plasma volume, should be treated by rapid infusion of saline or other plasma volume expanders. (See also pp. 11–15, this book.)

2. *Aminophylline solution.* Seven mg/kg diluted in 2 equal volumes of saline, given intravenously over a 5- to 10-minute period followed by 9 mg/kg/24 hours[10] aids in reversing bronchospasm and may inhibit further mediator release from mast cells.[11]

3. *Adrenocorticosteroids* have little effect during the initial crucial few minutes of anaphylaxis treatment and should be used only to supplement the major therapeutic steps. Hydrocortisone 7 mg/kg immediately, followed by 7 mg/kg/24 hours, administered intravenously may aid during the later recovery phase.

4. *Metaraminol bitartrate (Aramine).* If the blood pressure fails to respond to saline, Aramine 0.5 mg to 5 mg (0.4 mg/kg) may be added to the intravenous fluids, but cardiac side effects should be closely monitored.

Stage 3 — Therapy of Complications. Late complications of anaphylaxis include occlusion of the airway, cardiac arrhythmias, hypoxic seizures, and metabolic acidosis. For therapy of these conditions a hospital intensive care unit and blood gas laboratory are essential.[15] Table 4 lists equipment and supplies which are necessary in the therapy of these late complications.

Detailed description of this tertiary therapy is not included here, since therapy varies greatly with the patient's clinical course, and needs to be individualized by the physician or the consultants. Basically an airway must be established, blood gas derangements corrected, aberrant cardiac rhythms corrected, seizures treated, and tissue hypoxemia corrected.

TABLE 4   Optional Equipment and Supplies for Anaphylaxis

These items are desirable but may be available only in a well-equipped emergency room or intensive care unit:

   A. EKG monitor
   B. Defibrillator
   C. Calcium gluconate 10% (parenteral)
   D. Digoxin (Lanoxin) 0.25 mg/ml
   E. Diazepam (Valium), injectable, 5 mg/ml
   F. Lidocaine (Xylocaine) 2% with 1:1000 epinephrine for injection
   G. Lidocaine (Xylocaine) 2% for injection
   H. Sodium bicarbonate 3.75 gm in 500 ml

COMMENT

Since most anaphylaxis results from iatrogenic causes, it may be prevented or minimized by (1) obtaining an adequate history of drug reactions prior to drug administration, (2) minimizing the use of foreign biological products, and (3) testing for hypersensitivity prior to administering agents such as penicillin to a patient with a history of penicillin allergy if an alternate antibiotic cannot be employed. No physician can afford to administer a drug which can induce an anaphylactic reaction without appropriate emergency equipment on hand. Finally, when an agent capable of inducing anaphylaxis, such as an allergy vaccine or penicillin, has been administered, the patient should be required to remain in the immediate vicinity of the physician's office or the emergency room for at least 20 minutes so that appropriate therapy can be initiated at the first sign of a constitutional allergic reaction. Anaphylaxis occurs unexpectedly and suddenly and may occur in spite of extensive precautions. Appropriate and prompt therapy increases the chances of a favorable outcome.

REFERENCES

1. Van Arsdel, P. P., Jr.: Anaphylaxis and serum sickness. *In* Conn, H. L., ed.: Current Therapy. Philadelphia, W. B. Saunders Co., 1965, p. 415.
2. American Academy of Pediatrics, Committee on Drugs: Anaphylaxis. Pediatrics, *51*:136, 1973.
3. Austen, K. F.: Current concepts: Systemic anaphylaxis in the human being. N. Engl. J. Med., *291*:661, 1974.
4. James, L. P. J., and Austen, K. F.: Fatal systemic anaphylaxis in man. N. Engl. J. Med., *270*:597, 1961.
5. Siegel, S. C., and Heimlich, E. M.: Anaphylaxis. Pediatr. Clin. North Am., *9*:29, 1962.
6. Bierman, C. W., and Van Arsdel, P. P., Jr.: Penicillin allergy in children. J. Allergy, *43*:267, 1969.
7. Zweiman, B., Mishkin, M. M., and Hildreth, E. D.: An approach to the performance of contrast studies in contrast material-reactive persons. Ann. Int. Med., *83*:159, 1975.
8. Frick, O. L.: Anaphylaxis. *In* Gellis, S. S., and Kagan, B. M., eds.: Current Pediatric Therapy 4. Philadelphia, W. B. Saunders Co., 1970, p. 934.
9. Kelly, J. F., and Patterson, R.: Anaphylaxis. J.A.M.A., *227*:1431, 1974.
10. Pierson, W. E., Bierman, C. W., Stamm, S. J., and Van Arsdel, P. P., Jr.: Double blind trial of aminophylline in status asthmaticus. Pediatrics, *48*:642, 1971.
11. Orange, R. P., Austen, W. G., and Austen, K. F.: Immunologic release of histamine and slow reactive substance of anaphylaxis from human lung. J. Exp. Med., *134*:136 (Suppl.), 1971.
12. Safar, P.: Recognition and management of airway obstruction. J.A.M.A., *208*:1008, 1969.
13. Manually operated emergency ventilation devices. Med. Letter, *11*:53, 1969.
14. Manually operated emergency ventilation devices. Med. Letter, *13*:76, 1971.
15. Hanashiro, P. K., and Weil, M. H.: Anaphylactic shock in man. Arch. Int. Med., *119*:129, 1967.

Chapter Twenty-Five

PSYCHIATRIC EMERGENCIES

MYRON L. BELFER, M.D.

INTRODUCTION

Psychiatric emergencies in children require of the pediatrician: *first,* recognition that an emergency is, indeed, present; *second,* diagnostic acumen, sharpened by instruction and experience; *third,* a willingness to persist until intervention is effective or referral adequate; and *fourth* (and always), the caution that avoids making a bad situation worse by involvement beyond one's own depth.

These qualifications should be within the powers of pediatricians. For their application to specific situations, this brief article first will describe the general approach to a disturbed child. It will then present the more common psychiatric emergencies encountered in children, not each of them perhaps "critical" but all serious, and capable of resulting in more significant psychopathology if not treated appropriately. In any of them, therefore, if the chosen intervention does not bring prompt resolution, psychiatric consultation, or even hospitalization, is recommended.

The History: General

The history must be both comprehensive and focused. It should explore the emotional state of the family fully enough to make sure the emergency in the child is not merely one part of more global family distress.[1] In that case, such emergencies may well have been recurrent,

---

From the Department of Psychiatry, Children's Hospital Medical Center, and Harvard Medical School, Boston, Mass.

and prior attempts at intervention ineffective. The physician must be alert to possible elements of "secondary gain" either for the child or for the family. At the time of crisis, it is often easy to see the child's and the family's weaknesses but to overlook current or potential strengths. A child doing well in school, with good peer group relationships and without significant prior psychopathology, has strengths on which one can capitalize in management. If, on the other hand, a psychiatric emergency has nevertheless occurred in such a child, the immediate stress must have been significant and warrants prompt and definitive intervention. Finally, when the history shows the previously enumerated strengths to be lacking, one should consider again whether the urgent situation is but one of many signals that extensive intervention is required. Here the physician must deal for the moment with the so-called "emergency" but then also seek means of resolving what may be deep-seated or family conflict.

The History: Details of Procedure

Once the appropriate emergency care has taken place (in the case of a life-threatening situation), the physician should seek in his* interview to understand the exact circumstances of the present crisis and to accumulate the information which will permit a definitive intervention. A place removed from distractions will be helpful. Whether in the setting of the child's home, a private office, clinic, or hospital admitting room, the atmosphere must be one in which the child and the parents (or responsible others) can relate to the doctor. While introducing himself to all parties concerned, the physician must judge as best he can whether circumstances are best served by sitting down first with parents and child, or parents alone, or child alone, for a brief assessment of the probable interaction and the tone of the dialogue.[2] There can be no rule as to which is preferable, because the child's age and emotional state (and that of the parents) will influence the decision. Whichever choice is made, it is important that the pediatrician present himself as a responsible and competent person who will help to sort out the current and presumably confused situation. It is unwise to ally oneself prematurely with either child or parents, or to ask obviously pointed questions while seeking the views of each participant on what has happened.

If a social worker is available to see the parents, she† may be introduced to them and they may be encouraged to speak together while the physician talks with the child. If not, the pediatrician may simply tell the parents he wishes that opportunity. While the interview with

---

*The masculine pronouns, rather than choices of either, are used hereafter, but purely for convenience.

†Necessary exception to the rule above.

the child may not lead to an alliance, the early establishment of a personal acquaintance should later help in the child's acceptance of an intervention. The occasion will also allow an evaluation of the child's current mental state (to be discussed later). If the child seems out of touch with reality, is grossly inappropriate in words or actions, or is profoundly withdrawn, the pediatrician should be prepared to make an immediate referral for psychiatric consultation and consider possible hospitalization. If the objective signs are unclear, a sense of unease in the pediatrician should alert him to the advisability of referral to a psychiatric resource at this point.[3]

If the child is able to relate satisfactorily, he should be encouraged to tell his story. The critical questions are the following: (1) Was the episode impulsive? (2) Has it occurred before? (3) Did it "solve" a particular problem? (4) What alternatives did the child consider? (5) Has anyone else in the family or neighborhood carried out a similar act? (6) Is the child guilty over the act? (7) Does he intend to repeat it? (8) Does he plan to hurt himself or others? (9) What might he gain from it? Other important data relate to how the child sees his environment: Does he have friends? Does he now feel supported? Does he have positive future plans? If the act was not under the child's control, or if he denies control, does he feel the danger has passed, or that he can avoid circumstances that led to his being a "victim"? Many children will be able to report involvement with a significant adult: a local minister, a teacher, or school counselor. Such individuals, if identified, can provide further information as to the safety of the child's current life situation.

The interview with parent(s) or caretaker(s) should elicit *their* understanding of what has happened, and their view of the child's responsibility. Do they see him as at fault or as victimized? Are the parents angry with the child or sympathetic with his distress? Are they in agreement with each other and with the child? Are there, or have there been, ongoing conflicts relating to the child, which the child may be "acting out"? How have the parents responded to past episodes? Have there been changes in the home environment, disruptions, or losses? Are the parents willing to take responsibility for the child? If so (or indeed if not), what alternatives do they see for the child's management? What action do they desire? The all too common equation of psychiatric disturbance with the conviction that the child is "bad," which may emerge in this phase, should be firmly dispelled.

Evaluation

Once the information is gathered, the data must be evaluated. Calls to schools, agencies, and significant others need to be made at this time. Since the pediatrician is expected to be a source of strength, his plans should be well thought out before they are shared with the child and the parents, though there will be a need for airing any ambivalences and determining the feasibility of the plans. In most cases, the physician, social worker, or nurse should not only assist in the planning but provide for some follow-up to determine if the plan has been carried out.

APPLICATION TO SPECIFIC PSYCHIATRIC DISTURBANCES

Given the foregoing general procedures, the following section describes the specific issues of diagnosis and management in six common emergencies.

Anxiety Reaction. The acute anxiety reaction can be a nonspecific response to a variety of stresses. The most commonly seen manifestations are "nervousness," hyperventilation, crying, obsessive thoughts, rapid activity, and a feeling of losing control. Since such a reaction may be seen in response to school examinations, trauma, novel experiences, or the anticipation of a stressful event, specific elements of the history should include past episodes, the response to various kinds of intervention, and the nature of possible current precipitants. The anxiety can be expected to diminish with a reduction of or removal from the acute stress. Parental conflicts may tend to exacerbate the child's anxiety; therefore, knowledge of the parents' feelings at the time of crisis is necessary. Children with long-standing conflicts of the neurotic type manifesting anxiety require a more intensive psychotherapeutic approach.

A diligent, firm and reassuring manner in eliciting a history can go a long way to diminish the reaction. The pediatrician will have to judge whether recommendations for alleviating the stress or removing the child from the stress are appropriate. If the anxiety does not respond to reassurance and if it has led to psychological disorganization, the use of a minor tranquilizer (such as diazepam 1.0 to 2.5 mg tid) should be considered. In children under age 13, a medication such as diphenhydramine, Benadryl (5 mg/kg/24 hr by mouth) or promethazine hydrochloride (25 mg by mouth as a single dose) may be tried. Parents should be advised to provide a relatively calm, supportive environment for the child, with an opportunity for him to ventilate his feelings. Failure of remission of the anxiety indicates either persistent stress or the onset of significant psychopathology and warrants referral to a psychiatric resource.

Depressive Reaction. An acute depressive reaction may be marked by tearfulness, abrupt loss of appetite, sleep disturbance, or withdrawal. The history usually reveals a recent, readily identifiable, real or perceived loss of a valued person, pet, or object. The depressive reaction is not necessarily pathological, but can be seen as a rational response to loss. If the depression is not openly expressed, it can be harbored as a more chronic conflict. Therefore, both the child and the parents should be encouraged to talk about the loss, to try to understand it, and to put it in perspective. If withdrawal and loss of appetite are significant, or if they are linked with a desire to die, then the intervention should parallel that discussed under suicidal behavior in a later section. Otherwise, encouraging ventilation and providing reassurance that the response is natural and time-limited will be of help. A review of available supports and alternative modes of response is indicated. The child should be helped to reenter activities and the continuation of school encouraged. The parents should be alerted to progressive withdrawal, onset of any kind of bizarre behavior, or verbalization of the wish to die. If these become apparent, then further psychiatric intervention is warranted. Psychotropic medication, such as the tricyclic antidepressants, is usually not indicated for acutely depressed children, but may be used with caution in severely depressed, nonsuicidal adolescents.

The following case is illustrative of a typical depressive reaction:

Ann, a 13-year-old girl, experienced the sudden death of her father 1 month prior to being seen by her local pediatrician for insomnia. She claimed to have grieved over her father's loss, but at the same time said that she felt she had more sadness inside her. She claimed to keep it inside her now since her father had always said that she must carry on. Since shortly after his death, Ann had experienced insomnia as well as waking several times during the night. She often thought that she heard him call her and that she saw him in her room at such times. This did not frighten her and she had some perspective on this as an intense wish fulfillment rather than reality. She specifically denied any other vegetative symptoms of depression or deterioration in her school performance.

Ann appeared as a somber girl who was reticent though not evasive. She related in a somewhat constricted manner, reflecting more on her unresolved grief than interpersonal anxiety. She acknowledged sadness and fear of further losses. Neither suicidal ideation nor evidence of a thought disorder were present.

Ann was seen as being in the throes of an unresolved grief reaction with good maternal support, sustained contact with peers, but an inability to speak about her sadness. It was clear that the insomnia was related to her sadness as opposed to evidence of some possible neurological disturbance as suspected by her mother. The pediatrician was able to speak reassuringly with Ann, and spoke at some length with Ann's mother regarding the need to be available to hear of Ann's sadness, and to acknowledge her own. Both were encouraged to return to the more active lives that they had been a part of prior to the death of Ann's father. The pediatrician made himself available to the family for follow-up or possible referral if there was persistence in the symptoms, which did not occur.

Alcohol and Drug Abuse. Alcohol and drug abuse as psychiatric emergencies require first the appropriate medical management of the illness. The history will indicate if the episode of abuse is an isolated one or if it is part of a more chronic pattern of abuse. If it is the former, then it is necessary to ascertain the precipitants and to proceed to alleviate current stresses. Alcohol or drugs may be used to diminish the psychological pain or depression accompanying a personal loss, to compensate for feelings of poor self-esteem, or to avoid a painful social or environmental stress. Following the immediate crisis, it is prudent to refer children to the specialized programs available to treat these problems. When the precipitant is clear and the psychological conflict is evident, referral to a mental health program rather than a drug or alcohol program is indicated.

Acute Psychotic Reaction.   Here not only a careful history but also an evaluation of the child's mental status is essential for the diagnosis. Physical examination and laboratory and other tests may be needed to rule out an organic cause of the psychosis (such as, among others, a brain tumor, the inhalation of a toxic substance, or trauma). Have the symptoms waxed and waned paralleling exposure to a toxic substance, recurrent bleeds, or fluctuations in intracranial pressure? Has there been a history of psychological stress, depression, preoccupation with success, concerns with sexual identity, or social isolation? Is there a family history of mental illness?

The mental status examination should reveal some or all of the following: a loss of touch with reality, private thought processes that do not make sense, bizarreness, inappropriate affect, or possibly hallucinations or delusions. Paranoia, manic behavior, and gesturing are among many other symptoms and signs that may be evident. Of specific importance in determining an organic etiology along with the physical examination is the impairment of orientation to time, place, and person; impairment of recent and remote memory; decreased attention span with secondary confusion; impaired speech; shallowness and lability of affect; impaired judgment and impaired ability to manipulate acquired knowledge such as in calculation. A precise psychiatric diagnosis need not be made, but the presence of a thought disorder must be documented.

The management of an acute psychotic reaction is very much dependent on determining and dealing with its cause, on the degree of family support, the possibility of danger to the patient or others from his actions, and the past history of psychosis. In the acute phase, a phenothiazine may be used for the control of aggressive or destructive behavior. Many psychotic children can be maintained in the home and even in their school setting with proper familial support and medication, but diagnosis of psychosis makes consultation with a psychiatrist mandatory.[4]

Suicidal Behavior.   It is not necessary to hesitate over the distinction between a suicidal gesture and a suicide attempt in the context of the emergency room.[5] The management should be much the same in the acute situation. For the pediatrician, the issue of the child's possible secondary gain is outweighed by the possible dire consequences of not responding adequately to the suicidal intent of a child in acute distress and the child's feeling that options are closed off.[6]

A suicide *gesture* involves the patient's verbalization of suicidal ideation that embodies a plan, an intent to carry it out, efforts to move into closer contact with, or to remove from, important people in the child's life, and often some minor, but psychologically significant act such as an ingestion, laceration, or "accident." In most children the suicide *attempt* is evidence of a more clear-cut break with reality and a more profound withdrawal from the world. It is reported that impulsive suicide attempts in some adolescents may be seen without prodromal signs or a break with reality.[5, 7] The expression of the "wish to die" without collateral indications of disturbance may be seen in psychologically healthy children at various developmental stages and lacks the significance of the suicidal attempt or gesture.

The acute suicidal gesture or attempt provides the opportunity for a significant therapeutic intervention, but requires the data obtainable from more lengthy evaluations. At a time of crisis for the child and the family such as this, effective intervention can result in positive psychological growth for both.[8, 9, 10] The opportunity for the therapeutic use of the shift in psychological defenses at the time of crisis diminishes with time.

The pediatrician who sees a child presenting with an overt or suspected self-destructive act should have as his first goals the protection of the child and, if necessary, the appropriate medical or surgical treatment of the child. Proper attention to the child's physical condition should increase rapport with both child and family and aid in an understanding of the context in which the gesture or attempt has occurred. In the history, acute family disruption, the loss of a significant person or object, or the threat of abandonment should be sought as critical factors. It is particularly important, in addition, to determine if there has been a familial history of suicide or major difficulties in the expression of anger, both of which increase the suicidal risk in these patients.

It is important to secure the family's cooperation in reestablishing some meaningful communication with the patient. The mental status of the patient must be determined, especially whether or not the child is psychotic (see section on acute psychotic reaction), and the degree to which depression is present (see section on acute depressive reaction). One should avoid undue reassurance to the parents that the episode was transient and not likely to progress to further symptomatology, because in most instances the data will not be at hand at this time to support any conclusion. Rather, recognition and acknowledgement of the child's and family's distress are needed.

The majority of young suicidal patients can be treated as outpatients, provided that the patient is no longer considered acutely suicidal, severely depressed, or psychotic, and that a reasonably supportive environment can be provided.[5] A history of prior suicide attempts, or other serious psychopathology may militate against outpatient care because of their indication that the present episode may represent only one step in an ongoing, downhill course requiring hospitalization. It should be clear that if the child is psychotic and the family support minimal or ambivalent, then psychiatric hospitalization must be considered.

In the outpatient management of the suicidal child, the use of psychotropic medication, including antidepressants, without close follow-up supervision tends to give the patient and the family a false sense of security or the impression that the problem has been solved or that the answer lies outside the patient and the family. This may thwart definitive intervention. Medication prescribed in the context of the acute attempt may be misused by the patient for a subsequent suicide attempt. In some cases, an attempt at manipulating the environment to alleviate the precipitating stress can be effective.

The following case is illustrative of a rather common type of suicidal gesture:

Barbara, a 12-year-old girl, was noted by her parents to have withdrawn from peer relationships, to be sulking, and to be doing poorly in school. Late one afternoon, she came running to her mother with multiple slash marks on her arms. She said she wanted to die, but couldn't kill herself—that there was nothing for her. When seen in the emergency room, the slash marks proved to be quite superficial. A history revealed that this young girl had become preoccupied with the idea that she was not developing breasts, nor had she had the onset of her menses as had her peers. Her mother had reassured her that it would not be long before she developed, and that she was quite normal. The patient had not found this explanation satisfactory and felt a sense of lowered self-esteem and ostracism. These thoughts, which went uncommunicated, culminated in the slashings. The girl was not psychotic, but depressed with an ongoing sense of futility and poor self-esteem. The pediatrician established some rapport with the mother and it was apparent that the two of them could focus on a better understanding of adolescent concerns, especially in terms of the mother's concern with her daughter's pubertal changes, a time that had been difficult for the mother. The pediatrician who had examined Barbara spoke with her about trying to "sort out" her thoughts, especially those pertaining to her physical development. A brief series of visits discussing adolescent development and communication with parents resulted in a reduction of Barbara's depression and a resolution of her suicidal ideation.

Sexual Assault.   Sexual assault is a traumatic situation with potentially long-lasting sequelae. In well-studied cases, the alleged rape (one example of sexual assault) could be viewed as a symptom of a preexisting disturbance of a child's psychosexual development, or home life, or both.[6] Frequently the complaint of rape or other sexual assault is a symptom of other disturbance in self-image or relationship with others, a sign of other psychological conflict, or a request for attention from parents or others. In the management of the alleged sexual assault, it is of critical importance to put the trauma in perspective for the child and the family, to understand the dynamics of the social situation, and to offer helpful intervention.

The parents of the sexually assaulted child usually arrive in the emergency room or pediatrician's office exhibiting much anxiety, anger, and sometimes guilt. Most often, there is a demand to have the child examined and the perpetrator apprehended.

It is important to get a precise history from the parents. Care must be taken not to be accusatory because of the frequent involvement of parents in the attack, wittingly or unwittingly. The absence of the expression of guilt, whether justified or not, should alert the physician to the possible presence of either serious psychopathology in the parent or of a major disturbance in the parent-child relationship. Although parents and child may be interviewed together, the patient must be given an opportunity for a separate interview. It is necessary to assess the emotional state of the child prior to the alleged event. It is particularly important to attempt to gain some understanding of the child's interpersonal relationships and modes of relating to children and adults.

During the interview with the child, the child's affect should be observed for appropriateness and concern. The presence of seductive or provocative elements should be noted; in many instances, the alleged assault may not have actually occurred and if it did, it may partially have been at the instigation of the child. Sometimes the allegation of an assault is a coverup for some preexisting concern or guilt about sexual intercourse, masturbation, venereal disease, sex play, or pregnancy. If there has been undue delay in making the complaint and there is no evidence of injury, with indications of a preoccupation with fantasies, or the presence of neurotic symptoms, one should consider the possibility of a false accusation, perhaps with associated emotional disturbance. Psychotic and retarded children may invent or misinterpret sexual advances, but such children are also very vulnerable to sexual abuse and their allegations must be taken seriously. If the parent is the alleged assaulter, it is important not to take an accusatory role. At this time, either the child's or parent's role should not become a particular issue for discussion, as the pediatrician's task is to help ascertain facts and recommend and carry out the appropriate treatment.

The child should be approached with respect for privacy and sensitivities, and not disrobed or examined unless the indications for this have been clearly documented by the history. The history will indicate the type of physical examination required. Care should be taken during the examination because it can be viewed by the patient as a repetition of the assault. Depending on the age of the child, the nature of the examination should be explained to the patient in terms chosen to answer the concerns of the child. A nurse must be in attendance with girls; the presence of the mother or father depends on the child's wishes and the emotional state of the parent. The results should be shared with the child and parent in a factual manner.

Early follow-up is needed in all cases. The physician's prime responsibility is to the patient and family, but he should be aware of the local laws and practices. Information should not be shared with any outside party without the express permission of the child, or the family, or both. Finally, the physician's responsibility may be as much to defuse the situation as to prevent its aftereffects.

School Avoidance.   The primary and most immediate goal in acute school avoidance is to return the child to school as quickly as possible.[12] The history is the most important diagnostic tool. School avoidance should not be considered as truancy, but as an expression of anxiety (which in the extreme is a phobia), often with a positive family history of school avoidance, and some psychopathology in the parent-child relationship.[6] The major importance of family issues in the onset of school avoidance cannot be emphasized enough because this childhood behavior is so often unconsciously induced by a parent. There is a need to know about possible family stresses, parental ill health, psychiatric disorder, and so forth.

Sometimes the avoidance of school is a symptom of separation anxiety; sometimes a response to a change in the environment such as the birth of a sibling; and sometimes a physical disability, psychosis, more general phobic concerns, or perceptual or intellectual handicaps. A child complaining of a physical ailment should receive a thorough physical examination, but this should not be repeated frequently to avoid secondary elaboration of the physical complaint.

The pediatrician should convey to the child and the parents the necessity and expectation that the child will return to school.[12] The less anxious parent, a family friend, a social worker, or other person may accompany the child initially. The pediatrician may instruct the child to call him prior to going to school or upon the child's return, so that he can reinforce the child's progress in returning to school. Supportive interviews with the child and supportive casework with the family will help to continue the progress. The school should be encouraged to receive the child openly and participate in the management of the child's return to school. When there is massive initial anxiety, imipramine, a tricyclic antidepressant, has been found to be a useful adjunct to therapy.[13] The specific effect of this medication for this use is not known and the dosage must be individualized. The persistence of school avoidance after the above interventions indicates more serious psychopathology in the child or the parents, and warrants psychiatric referral.

General Conclusion.   Psychiatric emergencies in children can be a considerable challenge to the pediatrician, as they are to the child psychiatrist, and while all pediatricians should not attempt to manage all psychiatric emergencies of all children, many can successfully handle many such problems.

REFERENCES

1. Solky, C. G., and Hoekelman, R. A.: The pediatric emergency department. Clin. Pediatr., *10*:524, 1971.
2. Morrison, G. C.: Therapeutic intervention in a child psychiatry emergency service. J. Am. Acad. Child Psychiatry, *8*:542, 1969.
3. Schowalter, J. E., and Solnit, A. J.: Child psychiatry consultations in a general hospital emergency room. J. Am. Acad. Child Psychiatry, *5*:534, 1966.
4. Renshaw, D. C.: Psychiatric emergencies of childhood and adolescence. Ill. Med. J., 143:353, 1973.
5. Mattsson, A., Hawkins, J. W., and Seese, L. R.: Suicidal behavior as a child psychiatric emergency. Arch. Gen. Psychiatry, *20*:100, 1969.
6. Lewis, M., and Lewis, D. O.: Pediatric management of psychologic crises. Curr. Probl. Pediatr., *3*:3, 1973.
7. Jacobziner, H.: Attempted suicides in adolescence. J.A.M.A., *191*:7, 1965.
8. Morrison, G. C., and Collier, J. G.: Family treatment approaches to suicidal children and adolescents. J. Am. Acad. Child Psychiatry, *8*:140, 1969.
9. Burks, H. L., and Hoekstra, M.: Psychiatric emergencies in children. Am. J. Orthopsychiatry, *34*:134, 1964.
10. Lewis, M., and Solnit, A. J.: The adolescent in a suicidal crisis. *In* Solnit, A. J., and Provence, S. A., eds.: Modern Perspectives in Child Development. New York, International Universities Press, 1963.
11. Lipton, G. L., and Roth, E. I.: Rape: A complex management problem in the pediatric emergency room. J. Pediatr., *75*:854, 1969.
12. Waldfogel, S., Tessman, E., and Hahn, P.: A program for early intervention in school phobia. Am. J. Orthopsychiatry, *29*:324, 1959.
13. Gittelman-Klein, R., and Klein, D. F.: School phobia: Diagnostic considerations in the light of imipramine effects. J. Neurol. Ment. Dis., *156*:199, 1973.

INDEX

Numbers in *italics* refer to illustrations;
numbers followed by a (t) indicate tables.

353